HEALTHY AND SUSTAINABLE FOOD SYSTEMS

This comprehensive text provides the latest research on key concepts, principles and practices for promoting healthy and sustainable food systems.

There are increasing concerns about the impact of food systems on environmental sustainability and, in turn, the impact of environmental change on the capacity of food systems to protect food and nutrition security into the future. The contributors to this book are leading researchers in the causes of and solutions to these challenges. As international experts in their fields, they provide in-depth analyses of the issues and evidence-informed recommendations for future policies and practices. Starting with an overview of ideas about health, sustainability and equity in relation to food systems, *Healthy and Sustainable Food Systems* examines what constitutes a food system, with chapters on production, manufacturing, distribution and retail, among others. The text explores health and sustainable diets, looking at issues such as overconsumption and waste. The book ends with discussions about the politics, policy, personal behaviours and advocacy behind creating healthy and sustainable food systems.

With a food systems approach to health and sustainability identified as a priority area for public health, this text introduces core knowledge for students, academics, practitioners and policy-makers from a range of disciplines, including food and nutrition sciences, dietetics, public health, public policy, medicine, health science and environmental science.

Mark Lawrence is Professor of Public Health Nutrition at the Institute for Physical Activity and Nutrition, Deakin University, Burwood, Australia.

Sharon Friel is Professor of Health Equity and Director of the School of Regulation and Global Governance (RegNet), Australian National University, Canberra, Australia.

HEALTHY AND SUSTAINABLE FOOD SYSTEMS

Edited by Mark Lawrence and Sharon Friel

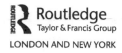

Routledge
Taylor & Francis Group

LONDON AND NEW YORK

First published 2020
by Routledge
2 Park Square, Milton Park, Abingdon, Oxon OX14 4RN

and by Routledge
52 Vanderbilt Avenue, New York, NY 10017

Routledge is an imprint of the Taylor & Francis Group, an informa business

British Library Cataloguing-in-Publication Data
A catalogue record for this book is available from the British Library

Library of Congress Cataloging-in-Publication Data
A catalog record has been requested for this book

ISBN: 978-0-8153-9326-9 (hbk)
ISBN: 978-0-8153-9327-6 (pbk)
ISBN: 978-1-351-18903-3 (ebk)

Typeset in Bembo
by Taylor & Francis Books

Mark Lawrence dedicates this book to Robert, Sarah, Anita, Andrea and June, whose futures will depend on the existence of healthy and sustainable food systems.

Sharon Friel dedicates this book to David Hughes.

CONTENTS

FIGURES

TABLES

BOXES

ACKNOWLEDGEMENTS

Our sincerest thanks to all the contributors to this book. We have been incredibly fortunate to have had the generous support of so many of the world's leading experts in disciplinary and content areas central to understanding healthy and sustainable food systems. Acknowledgement also for the invaluable editorial assistance of Kate Sievert, whose roles ranged from helping with formatting and referencing activities to tracking down supplementary materials, securing permissions and sourcing contributor biographies. Special appreciation to Sarah Lawrence for the cover design. Finally, we thank Grace McInnes and Ruth Anderson at Routledge for their guidance during the book's preparation and production, and before them Carolina Antunes and James Gemmill, also at Routledge, who supported the original book proposal and first stage of preparation.

CONTRIBUTORS

Sharon Friel is Professor of Health Equity and Director of the School of Regulation and Global Governance (RegNet), Australian National University (ANU), Canberra, Australia. She is also Director of the Menzies Centre for Health Governance ANU. She is a Fellow of the Academy of Social Sciences Australia. She is Co-Director of the National Health and Medical Research Council Centre for Research Excellence in the Social Determinants of Health Equity and has led many research projects focused on public policy and healthy eating including health and sustainable diets. She was a Commissioner on the Lancet Commission on Obesity. Between 2005 and 2008, she was the Head of the Scientific Secretariat (University College London) of the World Health Organization Commission on Social Determinants of Health. Her interests are in the political economy of health governance for healthy equity, with a focus on trade and investment, food systems, and climate change.

Mark Lawrence is Professor of Public Health Nutrition at the Institute for Physical Activity and Nutrition, Deakin University, Burwood, Victoria, Australia. He has 35 years' experience working as a practitioner and academic in food and nutrition policy at local, state, national and international levels. Mark is the Director of Deakin University's Food and Nutrition Policy Group and leads an Australian Research Council-funded project investigating the science and politics of evidence use in food and nutrition policy and regulation. He is an external advisor on healthy and sustainable diets to the World Health Organization and the Food and Agriculture Organization, a member of the International Union of Nutritional Sciences' Task Force on Sustainable Diets, Chair of the Advisory Board for Cochrane Nutrition, a Board member at Food Standards Australia New Zealand, a member of the National Health and Medical Research Council's (NHMRC's) Synthesis and Translation of Research Evidence Committee, and a former member of the NHMRC's Dietary Guidelines Working Committee.

Phillip Baker is a Research Fellow at Deakin University, and a member of the Institute for Physical Activity and Nutrition. He holds a PhD from the National Centre for Epidemiology and Population Health, Australian National University. His research focuses on understanding the inter-linkages between food systems change, the nutrition transition, public health and sustainability, and on informing governance and policy actions to prevent under-nutrition, obesity, and non-communicable diseases in Australia and internationally. Dr Baker is a member of the Independent Expert Group of the Global Nutrition Report. He was recently a fellow of the Lancet Commission on Obesity.

Liza Barbour works in the Department of Nutrition, Dietetics and Food at Monash University, Australia, where she lectures on food sustainability systems and public health nutrition. Liza's current PhD research is exploring the role of local governments in facilitating the consumption of a healthy and sustainable diet. Liza is Co-convenor of Australia's Right to Food Coalition and coordinates a community of practice for Australia's charitable food sector, which aims to increase workforce capacity to address the determinants of food insecurity. Liza has practical experience as an Accredited Practicing Dietitian in remote Western Australia, Alice Springs, the Kingdom of Tonga, metropolitan Melbourne and SecondBite, a food rescue organisation.

Nathalie Beghin is a human rights activist. She has been Head of Policy at Instituto de Estudos Socioeconômicos (INESC), Brazil, since 2012. She is an economist (Université Libre de Bruxelles, Belgium) and holds a PhD in Social Policies (Universidade de Brasilia, Brazil). She has worked as a researcher for almost 15 years with the Institute for Applied Economic Research (IPEA), linked to the Brazilian Ministry of Planning, focusing on social policies: food and nutrition security, poverty, social participation, gender and race equity. She joined Oxfam International in Brazil, first as Advocacy Advisor and then as Head of the Campaign and Advocacy Office in Brasilia. She co-created and was president for several years of a non-government organisation focused on the right to food, Ação Brasileira pela Nutrição e Direitos Humanos (ABRANDH).

Andrea Begley is an Advanced Accredited Practising Dietitian who has a focus on public health nutrition. She completed a Doctorate of Public Health, investigating cooking skills and their conceptualisation in health. She was awarded a Fellowship of the Public Health Association of Australia in 2012 in recognition of her significant contribution to the field of public health through her role as national co-convenor of the food and nutrition special interest group. Andrea currently is a senior academic in the School of Public Health at Curtin University, Perth, Australia, and has teaching and research responsibilities in dietetics and public health. Andrea's research is currently directed at evaluating effective food literacy programmes and examining ways to address food insecurity.

Jessica Bogard is an Accredited Practicing Dietitian and Nutrition Systems Scientist at the Commonwealth Scientific and Industrial Research Organisation (CSIRO) in Australia. As a dietitian and public health nutritionist, she is interested in understanding how agriculture and food systems can be leveraged to improve nutrition, particularly among vulnerable population groups, including women and young children. Prior to joining CSIRO, she worked for WorldFish, one of the Consultative Group on International Agricultural Research (CGIAR) centres in South Asia, South East Asia and the Pacific region. Her work focused on developing approaches to integrate nutrition considerations into food security research related to fisheries and aquaculture. She obtained her doctorate degree in Public Health Nutrition from the University of Queensland in 2017.

Barbara Burlingame is a scientist and Professor of Nutrition and Food Systems at Massey University, New Zealand. Her other roles include Chair of the Sustainable Diets Task Force of the International Union of Nutritional Sciences, specialty chief editor of *Frontiers in Nutrition*, scientific adviser/board member of several foundations/academies, and independent consultant for regional and global projects and programmes. Professor Burlingame is former chief of nutrition at the Food and Agriculture Organization where she worked for 16 years, and she is the author of hundreds of scientific papers and technical publications.

Martin Caraher is Professor of Food and Health Policy at the Centre for Food Policy at City University, London. He originally trained as an environmental health officer in Dublin. He spent some time working in the Irish and the English health services managing health promotion and public health services respectively. He has worked for and acted as a consultant to the UK Department of Health, the World Bank and the World Health Organization. He was a trustee of the Caroline Walker Trust. He was a member of the original London Food Board which developed the food strategy for London. He was a member of the Olympic Food Group representing public health interests on behalf of public health in the region. He also sat on the South East Food and Public Health Group which developed a food strategy for the South-east region and from which the London food strategy emerged.

Alessandro Demaio trained as a medical doctor in Australia. While practising, he completed an MPH, including diabetes fieldwork in Cambodia. In 2010, Alessandro relocated to Denmark to complete a PhD with the University of Copenhagen, focusing on non-communicable diseases in Mongolia. Alessandro held a postdoctoral fellowship at Harvard Medical School from 2013 to 2015, where he co-founded the millennial, global social movement NCDFREE. From 2015 to 2018, Alessandro was Medical Officer with the Department of Nutrition for Health and Development at the World Health Organization in Geneva, and co-host of the television series Ask the Doctor on ABC and Netflix. In 2019, he became CEO of VicHealth and currently holds fellowships at both the Johns Hopkins Bloomberg School of Public Health and the University of Melbourne.

Olivier De Schutter is a Belgian legal scholar specialising in economic and social rights. He served as the United Nations Special Rapporteur on the right to food from 2008 to 2014. He is a Professor of International Human Rights Law, European Union Law and Legal Theory at UC Louvain in Belgium and at Sciences Po in Paris. He is the first chair of the Belgian Advisory Council on Policy Coherence for Development and he co-chairs the International Panel of Experts on Sustainable Food Systems (IPES-Food), a group of experts from various disciplines and regions who work together towards developing proposals for food systems reform.

Jessica Fanzo is the Bloomberg Distinguished Associate Professor of Global Food and Agriculture Policy and Ethics at the Berman Institute of Bioethics, the Bloomberg School of Public Health, and the Nitze School of Advanced International Studies at the Johns Hopkins University, USA. She also serves as the Director of the Global Food Policy and Ethics Program at Johns Hopkins. From 2017 to 2019, Jessica served as the Co-Chair of the Global Nutrition Report and the UN High Level Panel of Experts on Food Systems and Nutrition. Before coming to Hopkins, she held positions at Columbia University, the Earth Institute,

Food and Agriculture Organization of the United Nations, the World Food Programme, Bioversity International, and the Millennium Development Goal Centre at the World Agroforestry Center in Kenya.

Sarah Gerritsen is a Research Fellow at the University of Auckland's School of Population Health, working in the field of public health nutrition and child health. Her PhD (2017) was on the potential for early childhood education services to assist with obesity prevention, and her post-doctoral research focuses on the effects of food insecurity on under-five-year-olds and ways to increase children's fruit and vegetable intake. Sarah previously worked at the Ministry of Health as a Senior Advisor in Population Health Research, and was the Research Manager for a cross-party think tank at the Royal Society of Arts in London, The Commission on 2020 Public Services.

Michalis Hadjikakou is a Research Fellow in Sustainability Assessment in the School of Life and Environmental Science at Deakin University, Burwood, Victoria, Australia. Michalis has a background in water resources management and sustainability assessment and modelling. He has a strong interest in food systems and sustainable diets, with expertise in environmental footprinting approaches. He is currently involved in a major national-scale project that aims to chart sustainable Food and Land Use Futures for Australia, and is also engaged in research at the global level examining the environmental impacts of current and future food system trajectories.

Corinna Hawkes is Professor of Food Policy and Director, Centre for Food Policy, City, University of London UK. Between 2015 and 2018, she served as the co-chair of the Global Nutrition Report. Her work focuses on supporting the design and delivery of policies and actions that effectively and equitably improve the quality of diets locally, nationally and internationally. In 2018, she was appointed Vice Chair of the Mayor of London's Child Obesity Taskforce and between 2016 and 2018 was Co-Chair of the World Economic Forum Global Future Council on Food Systems. She has previously held positions at the World Health Organization, the International Food Policy Research Institute, the University of São Paulo School of Public Health, and World Cancer Research Fund International, where she established the NOURISHING framework on policies to promote healthy diets.

Mario Herrero is Chief Research Scientist of Agriculture and Food at the Commonwealth Scientific and Industrial Research Organisation (CSIRO) in Australia. His research focuses on increasing the sustainability of food systems for the benefit of humans and ecosystems. He works in the areas of sustainable intensification of agriculture, climate mitigation and adaptation, livestock systems, and healthy and sustainable diets. Professor Herrero is a regular contributor to important global initiatives at the heart of the sustainability of global food systems, such as the Intergovernmental Panel on Climate Change, the Lancet Commission on Obesity and the EAT-Lancet Commission on Healthy Diets from Sustainable Food Systems. Professor Herrero is a Corresponding Fellow of the Royal Society of Edinburgh, an Associate Fellow of Chatham House, the Royal Institute of International Affairs, and an Honorary Professor of Agriculture and Food Innovation at the University of Queensland, Australia.

Annet Hoek is a Senior Research Fellow and consultant in the area of consumer research, food, health, and sustainability. She is passionate to improve consumer experience and food consumption by connecting insights from science, practice and consumers. Over the past 18 years Annet has worked with academia, industry and not-for-profit organisations, mostly bringing in the consumer perspective. She enjoys working in an interdisciplinary mode and is backed by qualifications in Industrial Design, Biology, Human Nutrition and a PhD in Sensory & Consumer Research. Besides healthy and sustainable foods, she has a keen interest in new health technologies and advancing food experiences and consumption of vulnerable groups.

Mark Howden is the Director of the Climate Change Institute at the Australian National University, Canberra, Australia. Mark has worked on climate variability, climate change, innovation and adoption issues for over 27 years in partnership with farmers, farmer groups, catchment groups, industry bodies, agribusiness, urban utilities and various policy agencies via both research and science-policy roles. His work has focused on how climate impacts on, and innovative adaptation options for: agriculture and food security, the natural resource base, ecosystems and biodiversity, energy, water and urban systems. He has been a major contributor to the Intergovernmental Panel on Climate Change (IPCC) Second, Third, Fourth and Fifth Assessment reports and various IPCC Special Reports, sharing the 2007 Nobel Peace Prize with other IPCC participants and Al Gore.

John Ingram leads food systems research in the University of Oxford's Environmental Change Institute, with particular emphasis on the multiple two-way interactions between food security and environment. Until 2011 he was the Executive Officer for the international research project, "Global Environmental Change and Food Systems" (GECAFS). In this role he promoted, coordinated and integrated international research related to the interactions between global environmental change and food security, as researched through analysis of food systems. On the close of GECAFS, he was appointed NERC Food Security Leader, which involves identifying and promoting NERC's contribution to the food security agenda. He also represents NERC on the UK Global Food Security Programme. John worked, until recently, on the "Climate Change, Agriculture and Food Security" (CCAFS) programme, developing regional socio-economic scenarios in East Africa, West Africa and the Indo-Gangetic Plains.

Vivica Kraak is an Assistant Professor of Food and Nutrition Policy in the Department of Human Nutrition, Foods, and Exercise at Virginia Tech in Blacksburg, Virginia, USA. She has extensive professional experience in the design, implementation and evaluation of food environment initiatives to prevent obesity and diet-related non-communicable diseases. She earned a PhD in population health from Deakin University at Burwood, Victoria, Australia, an MS degree in nutritional sciences from Case Western Reserve University, Cleveland, Ohio, and a BS degree in nutritional sciences from Cornell University, Ithaca, New York. Vivica has worked as a Research Fellow at Deakin University; as the Nutrition and Physical Activity Advisor for Save the Children in the United States; and staffed expert consensus committees at the US National Academy of Medicine in Washington, DC. Her research focuses on evaluating government and corporate accountability for healthy, resilient and sustainable food systems.

Tim Lang has been Professor of Food Policy at City University London's Centre for Food Policy since 2002. He founded the Centre in 1994. After a PhD in social psychology at Leeds University, he became a hill farmer in the 1970s in the Forest of Bowland, Lancashire, which shifted his attention to food policy, where it has been ever since. His abiding interest is how policy addresses the mixed challenge of being food for the environment, health, social justice, and citizens. He has been a special advisor to four House of Commons Select Committee inquiries, and a consultant on food security to the Royal Institute of International Affairs (Chatham House 2007–09). He was a Commissioner on the UK Government's Sustainable Development Commission (2006–11), reviewing progress on food sustainability. He has been Vice-President of the Chartered Institute of Environmental Health (since 1999) and President of Garden Organic (since 2008). He helped create City's role in the five University IFSTAL partnership (www.ifstal.ac.uk), which shares food systems thinking for post-graduates in a wide range of disciplines.

Jennie Macdiarmid is a Professor in Sustainable Nutrition and Health at The Rowett Institute, University of Aberdeen, UK. The focus of her research is food and nutrition security, in particular, sustainable diets. Her work on sustainable diets includes the impact of dietary patterns on climate change and land use as well as understanding how to shift different populations towards eating healthy and sustainable diets that are acceptable and affordable. She leads an interdisciplinary research group in Aberdeen and is the nutrition lead on a number of international projects on food systems and nutrition security in developed and developing countries.

Daniel Mason-D'Croz is a development economist working in the field of global integrated assessments, modelling the global food system to explore issues of climate change, trade, and food security. Currently, he is a Senior Research Scientist with the Commonwealth Scientific and Industrial Research Organisation (CSIRO) working on issues of food and nutrition security. Prior to joining CSIRO, he was a part of the International Food Policy Research Institute's IMPACT modelling team, where he worked on developing and using IMPACT for ex-ante analysis of the global food system. He is also a returned US Peace Corps volunteer, having served more than three years in Eastern Bolivia working on community development and education projects. He graduated from Johns Hopkins School of Advanced International Studies in 2010, with a Master's degree in International Development and International Economics.

Julia McCartan is an Accredited Practising Dietitian with experience in public health nutrition, food systems research and health promotion project management. Julia has overseen the implementation of food security and food systems projects in Victoria, Central Australia and the Kingdom of Tonga. In her current role at Monash University, Julia lectures in food sustainability systems, social justice and public health, and led data collection for a longitudinal study to monitor food cost in Victorian communities. Julia has research interests in systems-based and community coalition approaches to improve local food environments and fostering the Indigenous cultural capabilities of health professional students. Her current PhD research explores Aboriginal food discourse in South-Eastern Australia.

Sandra Murray is a Lecturer in Food, Nutrition and Public health in the School of Health Science, University of Tasmania and has over 20 years' experience as an Accredited Practicing Dietitian. She has strong research interest in food security, local food systems and sustainability and is committed to promoting the benefits of eating local food and supporting local farmers. Over the past five years she has worked on a number of food security projects investigating the cost, affordability and availability of food across Tasmania as well as a review of local food systems in Tasmania. Sandra is a member of the University of Tasmania Sustainability Committee and helped establish the Tasmanian regional centre of expertise in Education for Sustainable Development.

Gabrielle O'Kane is an Advanced Accredited Practising Dietitian and Adjunct Associate Professor with the Health Research Institute at the University of Canberra, Australia. She commenced her dietetic career in a large, metropolitan, teaching hospital in Sydney, before moving to rural NSW, where she practised in a variety of settings. After four years in private practice, Gabrielle was invited to join Charles Sturt University to contribute to the development of the first Australian rural Nutrition and Dietetic programme. Gabrielle's PhD thesis, "A moveable feast: Towards a better understanding of pathways to food citizenship" was inspired by her many years living and working in rural communities.

Christina Pollard is a 'pracademic' working in the area of public health nutrition as a practitioner and researcher for over 30 years. Christina has developed numerous public health nutrition interventions for government at national, state and local levels. She believes that nutrition-based regulatory and policy measures are essential to protect and promote public health and to protect those who are the most vulnerable to poor health due to their socio-economic circumstances. Both internal and external advocacy are key elements of her daily work. Dr Pollard has undertaken advocacy in partnership with a variety of organisations including: the World Cancer Research Fund International; the Public Health Association of Australia; the Dietitian's Association of Australia; the Red Cross; Foodbank; and, the Australian National Academy of Science.

Claire Pulker is a public health nutritionist and marketer, with 25 years' experience in Australia and the UK. She has worked predominantly in the food sector, including retailing, manufacturing, and food service, as well as for government. She was company nutritionist for two UK supermarket chains, and worked as a senior policy officer for the Western Australian Department of Health. She was responsible for launching a restaurant chain that aimed to offer healthy and sustainable food, providing nutrition information and carbon footprints on the menu. She has developed food and nutrition policy for supermarket chains and food manufacturers to guide responsible marketing of food. Drawing on her experience, Claire's PhD research investigated supermarkets' own brand foods and the implications for public health.

Elisabetta Recine is a nutritionist with a PhD in Public Health. Professor at the University of Brasília, Brazil, Department of Nutrition, Faculty of Health Sciences, she has academic and government experience in food and nutrition security policies. She coordinates the Observatory of Food and Nutrition Security Policies and is member of the Brazilian National Food and Nutrition Security Council (CONSEA), the advisory board of the Presidency of the Republic and of the Project Team for the Nutrition and Food Systems Report of the High

Level Panel of Experts/Committee on World Food Security. Her professional life has been guided by the perspective of relating the different dimensions of the food system and consumption, people's health, equity and social protection, aiming at the progressive realisation of right to adequate food.

Gyorgy Scrinis is Senior Lecturer in Food Politics and Policy in the School of Agriculture and Food at the University of Melbourne, Australia. His research covers a range of food system issues, including the philosophy of nutrition science, ultra-processed foods, corporate concentration and power, animal welfare regulations, food labelling, nutrition policy, genetically modified foods and nanotechnology. His current research focuses on how global food manufacturing corporations are re-engineering and marketing their ultra-processed products, particularly by employing the nutritional strategies of reformulation, micronutrient fortification, and functionalization. He is the author of *Nutritionism: The Science and Politics of Dietary Advice* (Columbia University Press, 2013), which presents a critique of nutritionism – or nutritional reductionism – in nutrition science research, dietary guidelines, and food marketing.

Boyd Swinburn is Professor of Population Nutrition and Global Health at the University of Auckland, New Zealand. He trained as an endocrinologist and has conducted research in metabolic, clinical and public health aspects of obesity. His major research interests are on community and policy actions to prevent obesity and reduce, what he has coined, 'obesogenic' food environments. He is Co-Chair of the World Obesity Federation's Policy & Prevention Section and Co-Chair of the Lancet Commission on Obesity. He is an Honorary Professor at Deakin University's Global Obesity Centre (GLOBE) where he established the WHO Collaborating Centre for Obesity Prevention in 2003.

Lada Timotijevic is a Principal Research Fellow at the University of Surrey, UK. Her expertise is in policy and consumer studies in the domain of food and health. She has a particular interest in processes of public and stakeholder engagement with a view to developing sustainable, ethical policies and responsible research and innovation. She publishes widely and collaborates on a number of national and international research projects.

Cristina Tirado–von der Pahlen works at the interface between science and policy related to climate, health, food and sustainability with the university, the UN, governments and NGOs worldwide. She is Director of International Climate Initiatives at the Center for Urban Resilience at Loyola Marymount University LA, Secretary of the Mediterranean Cities Climate Change Consortium MC4 and affiliated with the UCLA Institute of Environment and Sustainability. She is a lead author of the Intergovernmental Panel for Climate Change (IPCC) AR6 Health chapter, author of the Cross-Chapter Papers on Desertification and the Mediterranean and, contributing author of the Food Security and the African Region chapters. She is the President and co-founder of the Sustainability Health and Education (SHE) Foundation, and she is establishing a Climate-Resilient School and Health Center for Maasai Communities in collaboration with the Kenyan Red Cross Society.

Tony Worsley is Professor and Chair of Behavioural Nutrition at the School of Exercise and Nutrition Sciences, Deakin University, Australia. His broad interests include nutrition promotion and food communication as well the study of consumer's food and nutrition behaviours. His current research includes: examination of the food knowledge required by food consumers, fruit and vegetable promotion policies, the influence of household food purchasing and consumption on obesity risk, consumers' use of food label information, population cooking skills and the ways to increase skill levels, the food habits of baby boomers, consumers' food and health concerns, the influence of personal and cultural values and social ideologies on food behaviours.

FOREWORD: FROM REFORM TO REVOLUTION IN FOOD SYSTEMS

The systems approach adopted in this book presents us with a paradox; or perhaps, with a dilemma. On the one hand, the interconnectedness of all the factors that shape the food environment – biophysical and economic, cultural and political, technological and physiological – may lead to a sense of powerlessness. If all these factors interact with one another, and have co-evolved in time, reinforcing each other, change can only occur in food systems if all these factors are realigned with one another. We know that a shift is necessary from industrialised, input-intensive food production, leading to diets relying heavily on ultra-processed and energy-dense foods, to sustainable production and healthier consumption. But that shift, according to this view, would only be possible if everything changed at the same time – and, if not all at once, at least in a coordinated fashion, across the whole food chain, from farm to fork. In this reading, the interconnectedness of the elements of the food system is a source of inertia. Technically, one should speak of "resilience", but without the positive connotation attached to the term: a series of lock-ins exist, that can only be unlocked *together*, in a process that is more revolutionary than reformist (Naseem et al., 2010).

As Hirschman noted, this is typical of the rhetorics of reaction. Once the interdependencies between elements of a system are acknowledged, it is tempting to conclude that no change is possible unless and until the whole system changes course, and this may result in dismissing any attempt to change that does not go through a full revolution (Hirschman, 1991). On the other hand, however, this very interconnectedness may be seen as providing not one, but multiple levers for change. For instance, if industrial food production relies on cheap oil, on uncritical consumers, and on the dominant market position of large retailers, its position is in fact a fragile one, since it is threatened by peak oil, by changing expectations of eaters, as well as by the emergence of so-called "alternative food systems" that threaten the hegemony of large retail stores and the associated logistical chains.

Interconnectedness within a system, in that sense, results both in resistance to change *and* in the possibility of change occurring from different leverage points. Which of these two narratives provide the most accurate description of the challenge we face, depends largely on where the tipping point is located. Minor challenges to the dominant food system may be absorbed easily. Some more fresh produce from local farmers on the shelves of supermarkets, a gradual increase in the supply of certified organic food, some alliances between big retailers and charities for the collection of food items nearing their sell-by date in order to provide food aid to families in need, and so forth. These, however, are temporary, short-term fixes, not structural solutions; small solutions in response to minor crises, not a response to the larger crisis of food systems; reforms, not revolutions. In contrast, other challenges may be more fundamental, and oblige the system to reinvent itself. For instance, agro-ecological practices, beyond the set of agronomic techniques that favour diversity above uniformity and encourage low-input types of food production, also require that the whole food chain be rethought. This rethinking includes the processing and marketing segments, in order to ensure that farmers switching to agro-ecology are supported by improved market opportunities. Similarly, the question for food sovereignty goes beyond any specific demand (for healthier foods, or for less destructive food production techniques, for instance). Taken seriously, this demand cannot be "absorbed" within the system as it is, but requires a move from one system to another.

Once we adopt a systems perspective to the challenges facing food, we therefore face a distinction between two approaches, that may be called reformist and revolutionary respectively. Reformism may be captured, co-opted within the system; but it may produce revolutionary impacts if it cannot be so easily domesticated, and if, instead, it forces the system to reimagine itself more fundamentally.

Behind this distinction between two approaches, there lies a conflict between the economic and the ecological logics that shape the solutions we prioritise. This conflict is at the heart of many of the tensions in the food systems today. If the farmer follows a purely economic logic, agronomic choices will be made on the basis of the price signals of the market, and he or she shall grow, year after year, the crop for which demand is highest. Though there are some self-correcting mechanisms (paradoxically, the "hog cycle" referred to further below, which results from all farmers following the same price signals, while worsening price volatility, may also lead the regular rotations between cultures), the important fact about this logic is that it is entirely detached from agronomic considerations for soil health, the preservation of agrobiodiversity, or the maintenance of havens for pollinators. All that matters is price, and choices are made based purely on the basis of a cost-benefit analysis. In contrast, a farmer following an ecological logic will prioritise the agronomic choices that maintain the natural fertility of the soil (and, incidentally, its ability to function as a carbon sink, a hugely important positive externality). This farmer will plant trees, combine different plants with one another, use leguminous plants to fertilise the soil, and regularly rotate crops, even where this may result in a reduced profitability.

Such is the competition between the ecological and the economic logics. Agricultural production that maintains soil health and resilience in the face of a changing climate should prioritise diversity, through mixed cultures and frequent rotations of cultures, biological control of pests (rather than reliance on pesticides), and minimise the use of external (non-organic) inputs (IPES-Food, 2016). But the market's commands do the opposite. The negative externalities resulting from unsustainable forms of agricultural production and from a heavy reliance on fossil energy are not counted in the costs of production, and farmers are pressured to become providers of cheap raw materials to the food manufacturing industry, since that is how profits are made for shareholders – by "adding value". The result is industrialised farming on large areas of land to allow for mechanisation of production.

The future of food systems will largely depend on how the competition between these logics is addressed. The temporary, short-term fixes to the crises that the food systems regularly face remain within the mainstream, economic logic of the system, in which food is treated as a commodity, and in which consumers and producers alike are guided primarily by the price signals markets send. In contrast, the ecological logic will prevail only once more fundamental changes are made to the food system. Changes such as providing marketing opportunities to farmers switching to agro-ecology, and linking these farmers to eaters who are conscious about the impacts of their purchasing choices (whether such impacts are environmental, or whether they relate to health or to equity in food chains). The challenge therefore, as I see it, is to move beyond a reformist approach, and to reach the tipping point at which the reform becomes revolutionary – leading the system to reinvent itself.

A growing number of scholars now espouse the view that small, incremental changes may not suffice, and that we need to take bold action to redirect food systems towards sustainability. In part, this is because food markets are increasingly removed from the idealised view of "perfect" markets, in which prices reflect the match between supply and demand, and thus can be trusted to guide production choices. Concentration of power has significantly increased at various segments of food chains, both as a result of the industrialisation of agricultural production and food processing and as a result of globalisation. In the mid-twentieth century, the problem of concentration concerned primarily the big commodity traders – ADM, Bunge, Cargill, or Louis Dreyfus – dominating the networks of international trade, particularly for the major cereals. Today, concentration has increased significantly not just in the middle segment, but also at the two ends of the chain. On the side of the input providers, the US$130 billion worth merger between the US agro-chemical giants Dow and DuPont Pioneer (now Corteva), combined with Bayer's buyout of Monsanto for US$67 billion and ChemChina's acquisition of Syngenta for US$43 billion (and the planned merger with Sinochem) will result in 70 per cent of the total agrochemical industry being in the hands of only three mega companies (IPES-Food, 2017). On the side of retailers, global retailers, using their superior logistical abilities and bargaining power in upstream markets, now increasingly supply not only rich consumers – ten supermarkets supply half the food in the European Union, according to recent estimates (Oxfam, 2018) – but also the urban middle class in emerging economies (Reardon & Berdegué, 2002; Reardon et al., 2003; Reardon et al., 2010).

Moreover, concentration in one segment of the chain leads to concentration in the other segments. Large retailers tend to prefer to source from large wholesalers and large processing firms: this allows them to reduce transaction costs and have access to a diversity of product types in a "one-stop shop"; the invoicing system is formalised, allowing the retailers to discharge their accounting obligations for value-added tax accounting and product liability; and the packaging and branding of products are superior to that which smaller processors or wholesalers would be able to achieve. This leads to what some authors have called a "mutually reinforcing dual consolidation": the more that large retailers dominate consumers' markets, the more large commodity buyers tend to dominate the upstream markets.

Imperfect markets are not a new phenomenon, of course: the Cambridge economist Joan Robinson conceptualised such imperfections already in the 1930s. But the positive feedback loops (or self-reinforcing mechanisms) that now exist between the ability of the largest and more powerful players of the food systems to control the logistics and the networks, and their ability to strengthen their dominant position (as buyers) by extracting favourable conditions from their suppliers or (as sellers) from their clients, are now threatening to throw the system off balance (IPES-Food, 2017). Indeed, this process leads to a race towards the bottom: it results in lower wages for farm workers, and in a lower remuneration for independent agricultural producers that supply the raw materials. Large buyers can obtain from the sellers a number of concessions that reflect their dominant buying power. Concessions such as discounts from the market price that correspond to the savings made by the seller due to increased production, or the passing on to the seller certain costs associated with functions normally carried out by the buyer, such as grading of the livestock or stocking of shelves. This not only makes it more attractive for the retailers to source from these dominant buyers, since they may benefit from this superior buyer power that such larger suppliers have. It also further strengthens the position of the dominant buyers, who can acquire a competitive advantage over less dominant buyers in the downstream markets, leading to the acquisition by the larger agribusiness firms of dominance on both the buying and selling markets.

The end consumer may benefit from these trends, both because of the economies of scale achieved by the dominant players and because the abuse of buyer power may lead to lower prices at the end of the chain. But small food producers systematically lose. These farmers buy their inputs at retail prices, and they sell their produce at wholesale prices. Moreover, as a narrow set of large firms increasingly act as gate-keepers to the high-value markets of rich countries, small-scale farmers find it increasingly difficult to join these supply chains, and the gap is growing between large and small producers in a context in which both categories of producers compete for access to resources, to credit, and to political influence. Larger producers have easier access to capital and thus to non-land farm assets such as storage, greenhouses, or irrigation systems. They can more easily comply with the volumes and standards requirements that the agrifood companies – the commodity buyers, the processors, and the retailers, depending on which sources directly from the producer of raw materials – seek to impose. Small farmers can only compensate for these disadvantages by their lower labour costs, or because they are a less risky sourcing option to the buyers, since the larger farmers have more market options and thus can be less reliable. The disturbing consequence is that small farmers pay a high entry fee into global supply chains. These structural obstacles they face mean they can only compete by undertaking a form of self-exploitation, for instance, agreeing to low wages for those (often family members) working on the farm, and to be locked into a situation of high dependency towards the buyer. This is one major reason why undernutrition persists in many parts of the developing world, often as a result of extreme deprivation in rural areas. Only a small segment of the farming population still manages to thrive in an increasingly competitive environment, in which farmers can survive only by achieving economies of scale. They must get big or they must get out: many stay small and barely survive.

The idealised picture of well-functioning agricultural and food markets driven by price signals is unrealistic also in another way: most food producers don't respond easily. Either price increases lead them to make production choices that, six or eight months later, lead to oversupply in the markets, leading to price slumps that result in a loss of income for them, since all farmers respond to the same price signals – resulting in the "hog cycle" referred to above, well known to agricultural economists. Or alternatively, farmers are unable to adapt. When the prices of coffee or cocoa go down on international markets, for instance, the small producers of coffee or cocoa beans do not reduce production: they increase it in order to compensate for the resulting losses, and because they have to meet a number of expenses –

for education, healthcare or housing – that cannot be reduced; switching to something else is simply not an option, since they depend on soils, weather conditions, access to knowledge and seeds, and markets, that are fixed. While the "hog cycle" is more a characteristic of commodities markets dominated by large and relatively highly capitalised producers, the second problem (called the "commodity problem") is more usual for tropical crops and for relatively smaller farms. What both cases have in common is that prices cannot efficiently direct production. To believe they could do entirely ignores both the agronomic and the economic logics that are typical of agricultural production.

There is broad agreement that change is required. There is growing agreement too that such change must be radical if it is to create the kind of alternative we need. But is such change politically feasible? I believe it is, for three reasons.

First, the crises facing food systems are such that new alliances can be formed, between groups that have not been working together in the past, but that today may discover that they have a common interest in reshaping food systems. In that sense, the very size of the crisis, and its multidimensional nature, may be seen as an opportunity. Environmental NGOs can support the work of consumers' rights organisations, anti-poverty groups can team with small-scale farmers' organisations, North-South development cooperation NGOs can join forces with public health professionals, and small food entrepreneurs can partner with municipalities, in order to contribute to food systems reform. These different categories of actors pursue different aims – protecting the environment, protecting consumers' rights and improving nutritional outcomes, supporting development in the Global South, supporting peasant agriculture, or promoting local economic development. They have different histories, and they are connected to different constituencies. But they all now are realising that the current food systems, inherited from the twentieth century, are simply no longer fit for purpose: they demand something else.

Second, social innovations abound in food systems, that provide often spectacular proof that a different path can be pursued. Such innovations include short food chains and community-supported agriculture; new ways of reducing waste; various types of urban agriculture; an inventive use of public procurement schemes; or new forms of sharing food within local communities. Cities and regions are emerging as major actors in these innovations, and new alliances are being formed between public entities, local entrepreneurs, and civil society groups. The fact that such innovations exist, that they are growing exponentially, and that they are "proof of concept" that alternatives can work, should make us optimistic about the possibilities of change. The question is not whether we have examples that can provide a source of inspiration, since we do; the question is whether, by scaling up such examples, and replicating them (or "scaling out" in different locations), we can win the race against time that has now been launched against the accelerated degradation of the ecosystems and the growth of malnutrition in its various forms.

Third, the changes that are good for health and nutrition are also the changes that can reduce the ecological footprint of food, and that can support local economic development. By empowering small-scale farmers and improving their opportunities, we can at the same time reduce rural poverty and encourage the type of farming that can most effectively restore the health of the soil and maintain and enhance agrobiodiversity. Such farming is relatively labour-intensive; it is practised on relatively small farms; it relies on the use of agro-ecological techniques such as mixed cropping schemes. This type of farming is good both for the planet and for the people. The corresponding changes in diets (essentially plant-based and with a minimal use of ultra-processed foods) should keep people more healthy, at the same time allowing eaters to actively contribute to ecological outcomes, including climate change mitigation and biodiversity preservation.

For these transformative possibilities to materialise, however, any effort at food systems reform should address the question of power in food systems – asking where power resides, how the problem is framed and by whom, and which veto points exist in the system. There exists a long and respectable tradition of political economy approaches to agricultural development. Over a span of about thirty years, for instance, Robert Bates and colleagues documented the perverse role of governments in African agriculture, basically robbing farmers from the product of their work and exploiting them shamelessly in order to feed growing cities, or to export commodities on global markets in order to have access to hard currencies (Bates, 1981; 2005; Bates, Biais, & Azam, 2009). In the same vein, Michael Lipton famously denounced the "urban bias": the tendency of governments to favour the urban populations, on which their political stability depends, at the expense of the livelihoods of the rural dwellers, who, because they are often poorly educated and spread over large territories, often find it difficult to be organised (Lipton, 1977). Contrasting the situation in Africa with that of South Asia, Birner and Resnick discussed in minute detail the essential role governments played in the successes of the "first" Green Revolution, in the 1960s and 1970s (Birner & Resnick, 2010).

Power, however, does not reside only with governments; it is pervasive within food systems, and it is perhaps private power that now deserves the greatest attention, because it lacks any accountability. The challenge of the political economy to food systems is to address private government: the unchecked power of incumbents in mainstream food systems, who oppose all change, and have managed to translate their economic dominance into political influence. This is why the question of governance of food systems should be at the heart of all attempts to change.

I welcome this book as a major contribution to this debate on how food systems reform can be encouraged. A growing number of constituencies acknowledge the urgency of the reform, and that it must be transformative – revolutionary, if not in name, at least in spirit. The new alliances that are currently formed, the systemic nature of the crisis, and the power of social innovations that provide evidence that alternatives are possible, allow some optimism about the future. In that sense, this book is also timely: it provides us with the intellectual tools needed to transform impatience into action.

Olivier De Schutter

Former UN Special Rapporteur on the right to food (2008–2014)

References

Bates, R. H. (1981). *Markets and states in tropical Africa: The political basis of agricultural policies.* Berkeley, CA: University of California Press.

Bates, R. H. (2005). *Markets and states in tropical Africa: The political basis of agricultural policies.* 2nd edn. Oakland, CA: University of California Press.

BatesR. H., BiaisB., & AzamJ.-P. (2009). Political predation and economic development. *Economics and Politics*, 21(2), 255–277.

Birner, R., & Resnick, D. (2010). The political economy of policies for smallholder agriculture. *World Development*, 38(10), 1442–1452.

Hirschman, A. O. (1991). *The rhetoric of reaction: Perversity, futility, jeopardy.* Cambridge, MA: Harvard University Press.

IPES-Food (International Panel of Experts on Sustainable Food Systems). (2016). *From uniformity to diversity. A paradigm shift from industrial agriculture to diversified agroecological systems.* Brussels: IPES.

IPES-Food (International Panel of Experts on Sustainable Food Systems). (2017). *Too big to feed: Exploring the impacts of mega-mergers, consolidation and concentration of power in the agri-food sector.* Brussels: IPES.

Lipton, M. (1977). *Why poor people stay poor: Urban bias in world development.* Cambridge, MA: Harvard University Press.

Naseem, A., Spielman, D. J. & Omamo, S. W. (2010), Private-sector investment in R&D: A review of policy options to promote its growth in developing-country agriculture. *Agribusiness*, 26, 143–173. doi:10.1002/agr.20221.

Oxfam. (2018). *Ripe for change: Ending human suffering in supermarket supply chains.* London: Oxfam.

Reardon, T. & Berdegué, J.A. (2002). The rapid rise of supermarkets in Latin America. Challenges and opportunities for development. *Development Policy Review*, 20(4), 317–334.

ReardonT., Timmer, C.P., Barrett, C.B., & Berdegué, J.A. (2003). The rise of supermarkets in Africa, Asia, and Latin America. *American Journal of Agricultural Economics*, 85(5), 1140–1146.

Reardon, T., Timmer, C.P., & Minten, B. (2010). Supermarket revolution in Asia and emerging development strategies to include small farmers. *Proceedings of the National Academy of Sciences*. Available at: www.pnas.org/cgi/doi/10.1073/pnas.1003160108

ABBREVIATIONS

AFOLU	agriculture, forestry and other land use
ASFs	animal source foods
CAISAN	Inter-ministerial Chamber of Food and Nutritional Security
CAP	Common Agricultural Policy
CBD	Convention on Biological Diversity
CESCR	Committee on Economic, Social and Cultural Rights
CGRFA	Commission on Genetic Resources for Food and Agriculture
CIMSANS	Center for Integrated Modeling of Sustainable Agriculture and Nutrition Security
Codex	Codex Alimentarius Commission
CONSEA	National Council for Food and Nutrition Security
CSA	community-supported agricultural enterprises
CSR	corporate social responsibility
DALY	disability-adjusted life-years
DG	dietary guideline
EDNP	energy-dense, nutrient-poor
EIU	Economist Intelligence Unit
ENSO	El Niño-Southern Oscillation
FAO	Food and Agriculture Organization
FBSSAN	Brazilian Forum on Food and Nutrition Security and Sovereignty
FCCC	UN Framework Convention on Climate Change
FCFS	Framework Convention on Food Systems
FCR	fast-casual restaurants
FCTC	Framework Convention on Tobacco
FSR	full-service restaurants
GECAFS	global environmental change and food systems
GHG	greenhouse gas
GIAHS	globally important agriculture heritage systems
GMA	Grocery Manufacturers Association

GMOs	genetically modified organisms
GPS	global positioning system
IAASTD	International Assessment of Agricultural Knowledge, Science, and Technology for Development
ICN	International Conference on Nutrition
ICN2	Second International Conference on Nutrition
IUNS	International Union of Nutritional Sciences
LBW	low birth weight
LCA	life cycle assessment
LMICs	low- and middle-income countries
LSR	limited-service restaurants
MAD	minimally acceptable diet
MDGs	Millennium Development Goals
MEU	maximising expected utility
MMCA	marketing mix and choice architecture
MSPs	multi-stakeholder partnerships
NAO	North Atlantic Oscillation
NCD	non-communicable disease
NGO	non-governmental organisation
NRA	National Restaurant Association
PPPs	public-private partnerships
QSR	quick-service restaurant
ReFED	Rethinking Food Waste through Economics and Data
RSPO	Roundtable on Sustainable Palm Oil
SDGs	Sustainable Development Goals
SDI	Sustainable Development Indicator
SFS	Sustainable Food Systems Programme
SSB	sugar-sweetened beverages
SUSFANS	SUStainable Food And Nutrition
TFC	transnational food corporation
TNFRC	transnational food retail corporation
UK	United Kingdom
UMIC	upper middle-income country
UN	United Nations
UNEP	United Nations Environmental Programme
UNSD	United Nations Statistics Division
USA	United States of America
WCED	World Commission on Environment and Development
WHO	World Health Organization
WMO	World Meteorological Organization
WTO	World Trade Organization

AN INTRODUCTION TO HEALTHY AND SUSTAINABLE FOOD SYSTEMS

Mark Lawrence and Sharon Friel

Humanity is facing an existential threat as the impacts of its activities exceed planetary boundaries. Modern industrialised food systems are major contributors to this threat through their profligate use of finite resources, including land, energy and freshwater (Steffen et al., 2015) and degradative impacts on the environment, including greenhouse gas emissions (Vermeulen, Campbell, & Ingram, 2012), biodiversity loss (FAO, 2019) and food waste (FAO, 2011). In turn, these environmental harms are affecting food yields, quality and safety as well as the macro- and micro-nutrient composition of certain staple foods (Ebi, Campbell-Lendrum, & Wyns, 2018).

Modern industrialised food systems are also associated with poor public health outcomes. Dietary risk factors are leading contributors to the global burden of disease (Afshin et al., 2019). In particular, dietary imbalances are associated with a number of non-communicable diseases (NCDs), such as cardiovascular disease, and certain cancers and diabetes and dietary excesses are associated with nearly 2 billion adults being overweight or obese (Afshin et al., 2019). At the same time, dietary inadequacies are contributing to 2 billion people suffering from micronutrient deficiencies (FAO, IFAD, UNICEF, WFP, & WHO, 2018) and 821 million people being undernourished. It is estimated that malnutrition in all its forms costs the global economy up to US\$3.5 trillion each year (World Health Organization, 2016).

Healthy and sustainable food systems are prerequisites for human existence. They must provide a sufficient amount, quality and variety of nutritious food while discouraging the proliferation of junk food (ultra-processed food or nutritionally poor, resource-wasteful food) to meet the nutritional and socio-cultural needs of populations now and into the future. To do this, food systems must function in ways that do not undermine the Earth's capacity to provide life-sustaining resources (Niles et al., 2017). However, current food systems are broken (Branca et al., 2019) and their contributions to poor public health outcomes and environmental harms are not only substantial in absolute terms but also inequitable, with those who have contributed minimally to the problems often being most affected and least able to respond (Friel, 2019).

In this book we adopt the UN's High Level Panel of Experts on Food Security and Nutrition's definition of a food system as being an entity that "gathers all the elements (environment, people, inputs, processes, infrastructures, institutions, etc.) and activities that relate to the production, processing, distribution, preparation and consumption of food and the outputs of these activities, including socio-economic and environmental outcomes" (HLPE, 2014). And a *sustainable* food system is one that "delivers food security and nutrition for all in such a way that the economic, social and environmental bases to generate food security and nutrition for future generations are not compromised" (HLPE, 2014). Health is implicit in this food system definition through its reference to delivering food security and nutrition outcomes.

The evolution of modern humans began about 2.5 million years ago (Harari, 2015), and over approximately 100,000 generations since that time humans have survived, thrived and evolved, all the while being nurtured by food systems of various forms. Though the health and sustainability qualities of those food systems have varied over time and by place, it is self-evident they have persisted sufficiently to support the endurance of humans to the present time and across the globe. Today, it is multiple interrelated social, economic, demographic, political and technological developments that are rendering relationships between food systems and human existence untenable. Fundamentally, the extent and pace of these developments clash with two immutable realities: the physical limits of the planet's environmental boundaries (Steffen et al., 2015); and the nutritional requirements of the human body, which have evolved over millions of years (Eaton, Eaton III, Konner, & Shostak, 1996). Unless significant and prompt action is taken, the adverse impacts resulting from the gap between policy and human behaviour practices and fixed realities are destined to be exacerbated as the global population approaches an estimated 10 billion people by 2050 (UN DESA, 2017).

After approximately 100,000 generations of human existence, whether there will be sufficient, nutritious, safe and affordable food to continue to nurture humanity into the future will be determined by the actions of our generation.

Global policies and actions to promote healthy and sustainable food systems

The body of evidence associated with the challenges to healthy and sustainable food systems is growing rapidly. Consequently, the agenda has begun to receive significant policy attention from UN, national, and local government agencies as well as from researchers, practitioners, civil society and the private sector. Notable global policy developments in recent times have been:

1. *2014: The Second International Conference on Nutrition's Rome Declaration on Nutrition*: the ICN2, co-organized by the Food and Agriculture Organization of the United Nations (FAO) and the World Health Organization (WHO), held in Rome, in November 2014, adopted the Rome Declaration on Nutrition and its companion Framework for Action (FAO & WHO, 2015). The Framework for Action sets out 60 voluntary recommendations for policies and actions necessary to achieve the objectives of ending all forms of malnutrition and providing sustainable food systems delivering healthy diets to all. Subsequently, the Framework has been supported with a follow-up resource guide for countries, based on the policy recommendations of the ICN2 and entitled, *Strengthening Nutrition Action* (FAO & WHO, 2018).
2. *2015: The UN Agenda for Sustainable Development and Sustainable Development Goals*: In September 2015, world leaders adopted the 2030 Agenda for Sustainable Development and its associated Sustainable Development Goals (SDGs) at the UN

General Assembly. The SDGs set out a roadmap for achieving equitable development and global prosperity by 2030. Most of the goals and targets directly or indirectly impact nutrition and, conversely, investing in and acting on food systems will help achieve the SDGs. Of particular relevance to this book is SDG12, "Sustainable consumption and production", being implemented through the Sustainable Food Systems Programme of the One Planet Network which itself is implementing the 10-year Framework of programmes on sustainable consumption and production (UN DESA, 2014).

3. *2016: The UN Decade of Action on Nutrition (2016–2025)*: In April 2016, the UN General Assembly proclaimed the period from 2016 to 2025 the UN Decade of Action on Nutrition (UN, 2016) with the UN Resolution on the UN Decade of Action on Nutrition. The aim of the Decade of Action on Nutrition is to have countries and their partners commit to and act on nutrition objectives: (a) to implement the ICN2 commitments; (b) to achieve the Global Nutrition and diet-related NCD targets by 2025 (WHO, 2010; 2014); and (c) to achieve the SDGs by 2030. The Decade of Action on Nutrition activities are centred on six cross-cutting Action Areas that are used to cluster the 60 ICN2 Framework for Action recommendations. The first of these Action Areas is "Sustainable, resilient food systems for healthy diets" (FAO & WHO, 2018).

4. *2019: The EAT-Lancet Commission report on healthy diets from sustainable food systems, and the Lancet Commission report on the Global Syndemic of Obesity, Undernutrition, and Climate Change*: In 2019, two landmark Lancet Commission reports were published, each including analyses of the causes of and solutions to topics related to healthy and sustainable food systems. First, the EAT-Lancet report on healthy diets from sustainable food systems (Willett et al., 2019) proposes dietary modelling-informed targets for healthy diets and sustainable food systems that are designed to help achieve the SDGs and the Paris Climate Agreement and to be universal for all food cultures and production systems. The report recommends that to feed 10 billion people in 2050, dietary patterns typically should consist of a diverse range of plant-based foods, low amounts of animal-based foods, unsaturated fats, and small amounts of refined grains, processed foods and added sugars, in amounts appropriate for a healthy weight (Willett et al., 2019).Second, the Report of the Lancet Commission on Obesity demonstrates that the pandemics of obesity, undernutrition, and climate change represent the paramount challenge for humans, the environment and our planet (Swinburn et al., 2019). These interacting pandemics represent the Global Syndemic with common, underlying drivers in the food, transport, urban design, and land use systems. The Lancet report proposes nine recommendations to mitigate these three pandemics simultaneously.

5. *2019: Climate Change and Land: an IPCC special report on climate change, desertification, land degradation, sustainable land management, food security, and greenhouse gas fluxes in terrestrial ecosystems*: In August 2019, the Intergovernmental Panel on Climate Change released its Special Report on Climate Change and Land (IPCC, 2019). Its chapter on food security uses a food systems approach to examine how climate change affects food and nutrition security. This comprehensive chapter addresses the supply-side and demand-side options available for food systems to adapt and mitigate and the synergies and trade-offs associated with these options

Why healthy and sustainable food systems?

There is no one universal cause of, nor one silver bullet solution to, the food-related public health and environmental sustainability problems confronting humankind. Instead the formulation of effective and safe policy and action responses to these problems faces multiple challenges. First, there is the challenge of the complexity and sheer size of these problems involving multiple drivers, actors and places. Second, there is the challenge that among these drivers, actors and places, there are multiple dynamic non-linear interactions. Third, contexts can play a significant role in shaping the nature and scope of the problem and potential solution. For instance, although consensus is emerging around the characteristics of a healthy and sustainable diet, the generalisability of the dietary advice is conditional on many contextual factors that affect how foods are produced, processed, distributed and consumed in different places around the world. Fourth, food's integral role in economies means that politics, particularly involving actors whose interests align with maintaining the status quo, is inevitable in formulating policy activities to transform food systems (Lawrence, Friel, Wingrove, James, & Candy, 2015).

These challenges highlight why a healthy and sustainable food systems perspective provides a fit-for-purpose approach to analysing causes and identifying solutions to the problems. A systems perspective provides the means to see all drivers, actors, places, contexts and circumstances (as well as all their inter-relationships) associated with food supply and food demand as a whole rather than thinking of them operating in isolation from each other. Systems thinking enables analysis of multiple dynamic non-linear interactions among those factors affecting food-related problems and to identify how and where to intervene effectively, taking into account potential trade-offs, to tackle those problems (Peters, 2014). Also there are synergies to be leveraged and co-benefits to be gained from such food systems' interventions because they can contribute simultaneously to health and sustainability outcomes (Tirado, 2015; Global Panel on Agriculture and Food Systems for Nutrition, 2016; Niles et al., 2018; Parsons & Hawkes, 2018).

Figure 0.1 provides a conceptual framework for thinking about the structure and operation of a food system. The framework sets out an overarching coherent perspective to the system's multiple structural components that at its core extend across food supply chains, food environments and consumer behaviour and how these lead to diets and ultimately nutrition and health outcomes and social, economic and environmental impacts. These structural components are themselves underpinned by political, programme and institutional actions that also are linked to the SDGs. And overlaying the core structural components are the following drivers:

- biophysical and environmental;
- innovation, technology and infrastructure;
- political and economic;
- socio-cultural; and demographic.

The framework also illustrates the intricate operations of the system in terms of the many inputs and outputs and multiple relationships among its structural components. Critically, those relationships are not simply a series of linear connections between system

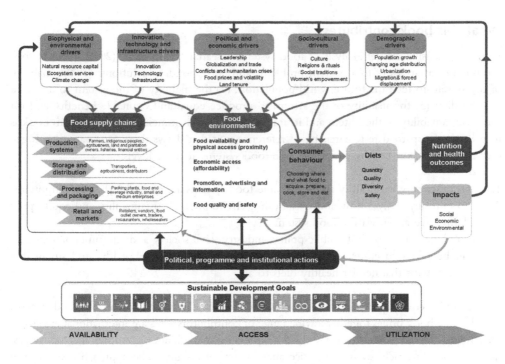

FIGURE 0.1 Conceptual framework of the structure and operation of a food system
Source: FAO (2017).

components. Instead the relationships are characterised by multiple interactions among component parts and so are continuously changing and influencing one another through non-linear pathways and feedback mechanisms. Therefore, any attempt to understand a food system simply by looking at its individual parts is limited because parts rarely operate in isolation. Rather, there is a need to think of the whole food system as being greater than the sum of its individual parts.

The framework presented in Figure 0.1 not only helps us understand the structure and operation of a food system, but also it serves as a heuristic device for strategically planning and evaluating policies and actions designed to promote healthy and sustainable food systems. It can help us analyse the underlying causes of a problem, and in certain instances the "causes of the causes" of a problem, and therefore identify where to intervene in the system and predict the consequences of that intervention throughout the system. For instance, overconsumption of junk food is both a health and sustainability problem. The immediate cause of that problem is located in the consumer behaviour component of the system and therefore the immediate solution is to intervene to change consumer behaviour. However, how accurate is that analysis and how effective is the proposed solution? When viewed from a food systems perspective, the antecedents of this behaviour might be located at several other points within the system. Is junk food more affordable, accessible and/or available than a more nutritious alternative? How and why is this happening? Does the cost of junk food reflect the true health or environmental cost of that food or are such costs externalised? If locally sourced nutritious foods were to replace junk foods, might there be additional benefits, such as supporting local food economies and cultures?

What this book contributes

In their extensive critical analysis of food systems research, Béné et al. (2019) identify four prominent narratives of food system problems and corresponding solutions: (1) the inability of the system to feed the future world population; (2) the inability of the system to deliver a healthy diet; (3) the inability of the system to produce equal and equitable benefits; and (4) the unsustainability of the system and its impact on the environment. The aim of this book is to provide an up-to-date research-based reference text that draws these four narratives together by focusing on healthy and sustainable food systems at three levels:

1. To describe what healthy and sustainable food systems are and why they are important.
2. To critically analyse how and why health, environmental sustainability and equity problems have arisen via the food system.
3. To identify the political, public policy, industry, civil society and consumer actions that can be taken to ensure sustainable food systems that achieve healthy and sustainable food systems that deliver healthy diets to all.

The topics covered in the book are priorities for a healthy and sustainable food systems agenda. The book brings together a wide range of contributors who are international experts in their field. Their experience is derived from a plurality of disciplines, countries and topic areas, thereby providing rich research, practice and contextual insights. The approach taken in the book is innovative in two key ways: (1) it links health, environmental sustainability and equity dimensions; and (2) it challenges the dominance of a "reductionist" (nutrient) worldview, i.e. a focus on changing people's consumption of certain nutrients as a means to tackle nutrition problems, that pervades much nutrition policy discourse and reorients to a "holistic" (foods, diets and food systems) worldview as a basis to inform nutrition policy activities.

The structure of the book

The book is divided into four integrated Parts. Each Part consists of chapters based on an evidence-informed approach to the topic by drawing on recent authoritative global reports and/or peer-reviewed literature.

Part I, "Overarching dimensions of healthy and sustainable food systems", explains the nature and scope of the challenges confronting food systems. It consists of three chapters that set out the core topics for the overall themes of the book, written by leading international experts in each of these topics:

1. *Health*: Based on the findings of the latest Global Nutrition Report and prepared by the co-editors of the Report (Chapter 1).
2. *Sustainability*: Prepared by the Chair of the International Union of Nutritional Sciences Task Force on Sustainable Diets (Chapter 2).
3. *Equity*: Led by a member of the Project Team for the Nutrition and Food Systems Report of the UN's High Level Panel of Experts/Committee on World Food Security (Chapter 3).

Part II, "The food system", identifies the components, the actors and the inter-relationships within food systems. This Part starts with a scene-setting chapter that provides an overview of different concepts and models for food systems as a coherent whole (Chapter 4). Then each of the remaining five chapters provides an in-depth analysis of one of the following food system components: food production (Chapter 5); food manufacturing (Chapter 6); food retail and distribution (Chapter 7); the food services sector (Chapter 8); and food consumption (Chapter 9). We are aware of the potential contradiction of organising Part II as a linear sequence of the constituent parts of the food system when otherwise we emphasise the importance of thinking about food systems as joined-up entities in which the whole is more than the sum of its parts. However, organising as separate chapters affords the opportunity to undertake a detailed examination of the parts and the integration is addressed in this chapter and the Conclusion, as well as the dedicated chapter on food systems as a whole at the start of this Part (Chapter 4).

Part III, "Healthy and sustainable diets", analyses the characteristics of a healthy and sustainable diet. The Part starts with a scene-setting chapter (Chapter 10) that provides an overview of what a healthy and sustainable diet should be. Then each of the remaining four chapters provides an in-depth analysis of one of the following commonly identified challenges to a healthy and sustainable diet: overconsumption (Chapter 11); excessive animal product consumption (Chapter 12); excessive junk food consumption (Chapter 13); and food waste (Chapter 14).

Part IV, "Creating healthy and sustainable food systems: politics, policy, people and practitioners", examines political, policy, people and practitioner activities to help transform the current food system into a healthy and sustainable food system. Despite much knowledge about the problem and awareness of the need for transformation, there is general inertia regarding meaningful action by policy-makers and behaviour change by the population. The Part commences with a chapter that frames the food system from a political economy perspective that explains why planning for change needs to extend beyond changes to the health sector to other sectors, such as agriculture, other systems, such as the economic system, and other actors, such as philanthropists (Chapter 15). Then each of the remaining three chapters provides an in-depth analysis of how change can be achieved in one of the following settings: policy actions (Chapter 16), people's practices (Chapter 17); and practitioners' advocacy (Chapter 18).

The Conclusion provides a discussion of the main issues raised throughout the book, the lessons learned and a view to the future for promoting healthy and sustainable food systems.

References

Afshin, A., Sur, P. J., Fay, K. A., Cornaby, L., Ferrara, G., Salama, J. S., ... Murray, C. J. L. (2019). Health effects of dietary risks in 195 countries, 1990–2017: A systematic analysis for the Global Burden of Disease Study 2017. *The Lancet*. doi:10.1016/S0140-6736(19)30041-8.

Béné, C., Oosterveer, P., Lamotte, L., Brouwer, I. D., de Haan, S., Prager, S. D., ... Khoury, C. K. (2019). "When food systems meet sustainability – Current narratives and implications for actions." *World Development*, 113: 116–130.

Branca, F., Lartey, A., Oenema, S., Aguayo, V., Stordalen, G. A., Richardson, R., ... Afshin, A. (2019). Transforming the food system to fight non-communicable diseases. *BMJ*, 364, 1296. doi:10.1136/bmj.l296.

Eaton, S. B., EatonIII, S. B., Konner, M. J., & Shostak, M. (1996). An evolutionary perspective enhances understanding of human nutritional requirements. *Journal of Nutrition*, 126, 1732–1740.

Ebi, K., Campbell-Lendrum, D., & Wyns, A. (2018). The 1.5 health report: Synthesis on health and climate science in the IPCC SR1.5. Available at: www.who.int/globalchange/181008_the_1_5_healthreport.pdf

FAO. (2011). *Global food losses and food waste: Extent, causes and prevention*. Rome: FAO.

FAO (2017). Nutrition and food systems: A report by the High Level Panel of Experts on Food Security and Nutrition of the Committee on World Food Security. Rome: FAO. Available at: www.fao.org/3/a-i7846e.pdf

FAO. (2019). The state of the world's biodiversity for food and agriculture. Available at: www.fao.org/3/CA3129EN/CA3129EN.pdf

FAO, IFAD, UNICEF, WFP, & WHO. (2018). The state of food security and nutrition in the world 2018: Building climate resilience for food security and nutrition. Available at: www.fao.org/3/I9553EN/i9553en.pdf

FAO & WHO. (2015). Second International Conference on Nutrition: Report of the Joint FAO/WHO Secretariat on the Conference. Available at: www.who.int/nutrition/topics/WHO_FAO_announce_ICN2/en/index2.html

FAO & WHO. (2018). Strengthening nutrition action: A resource guide for countries based on the policy recommendations of the Second International Conference on Nutrition (ICN2). Available at: www.who.int/nutrition/publications/strengthening-nutrition-action/en

Friel, S. (2019). *Climate change and the people's health.* New York:Oxford University Press.

Global Panel on Agriculture and Food Systems for Nutrition. (2016). Food systems and diets: Facing the challenges of the 21st century. Available at: www.glopan.org

Harari, Y. N. (2015). *Sapiens: A brief history of humankind.* New York: Harper.

HLPE. (2014). Food losses and waste in the context of sustainable food systems. Rome: HLPE.

IPCC. (2019). Climate change and land. Available at: www.ipcc.ch/report/srccl

Lawrence, M. A., Friel, S., Wingrove, K., James, S. W., & Candy, S. (2015). Formulating policy activities to promote healthy and sustainable diets. *Public Health Nutrition,* 18(13): 2333–2340.

Niles, M. T., Ahuja, R., Barker, T., Esquivel, J., Gutterman, S. ... Vermeulen, S. (2018). Climate change mitigation beyond agriculture: A review of food system opportunities and implications. *Renewable Agriculture and Food Systems,* 33(3): 297–308. doi:10.1017/S1742170518000029.

Niles, M. T., Ahuja, R., Esquivel, M., Mango, N., Duncan, M., Heller, M., & Tirado, C. (2017). Climate change and food systems: Assessing impacts and opportunities. Washington, DC: Meridian Institute. Parsons, K. & Hawkes, C. (2018). Connecting food systems for co-benefits: How can food systems combine diet-related health with environmental and economic policy goals?Copenhagen, Denmark: WHO.

Peters, D. H. (2014). The application of systems thinking in health: Why use systems thinking? *Health Research Policy and Systems,* 12(1), 51. doi:10.1186/1478-4505-12-51.

Steffen, W., Richardson, K., Rockström, J., Cornell, S. E., Fetzer, I., Bennett, E. M., ... Sörlin, S. (2015). Planetary boundaries: Guiding human development on a changing planet. *Science,* 347(6223), 1259855. doi:10.1126/science.1259855 %J Science.

Swinburn, B. A., Kraak, V. I., Allender, S., Atkins, V. J., Baker, P. I., Bogard, J. R., ... Devarajan, R. (2019). The global syndemic of obesity, undernutrition, and climate change: The Lancet Commission report. *The Lancet,* doi:10.1016/S0140–6736(18)32822–32828.

Tirado, C. (2015). Sustainable food systems and health: The convenient truth of addressing climate change while promoting health. Available at: www.unscn.org/files/Announcements/EXE_2_Sustainable_Food_systems_and_health.pdf

UN (United Nations). (2016). Decade of action on nutrition. Available at: www.who.int/nutrition/GA_decade_action/en/

UN DESA. (2014). The 10-Year Framework of Programmes on sustainable consumption and production patterns (10YFP). Available at: https://sustainabledevelopment.un.org/content/documents/1444HLPF_10YFP2.pdf

UN DESA. (2017). World population prospects 2017. Available at: https://population.un.org/wpp/

Vermeulen, S. J., Campbell, B. M., & Ingram, J. S. I. (2012). Climate change and food systems. *Annual Review of Environment and Resources,* 37(1), 195–222. doi:10.1146/annurev-environ-020411-130608.

WHO. (2010). Diet-related voluntary global NCD targets. Available at: www.who.int/nmh/ncd-tools/definition-targets/en/

WHO. (2014). Global nutrition targets 2025. Available at: www.who.int/nutrition/global-target-2025/en/

WHO. (2016). Malnutrition in the crosshairs. Available at: www.who.int/nutrition/pressrelease-FAO WHO-symposium-malnutrition/en/

Willett, W., Rockström, J., Loken, B., Springmann, M., Lang, T., Vermeulen, S., ... Murray, C. J. L. (2019). Food in the Anthropocene: The EAT-Lancet Commission on healthy diets from sustainable food systems. *The Lancet.* doi:10.1016/S0140–6736(18)31788–31784.

PART I

Overarching dimensions of healthy and sustainable food systems

1

HEALTH

Corinna Hawkes and Jessica Fanzo

Introduction

Every human being has the right to adequate, nutritious food. The realisation of this right around the world will not be achieved without food systems that ensure optimal nutrition for everyone, now and into the future. Food systems are meant to provide food that is healthy, of sufficient quality and quantity, affordable, safe and culturally acceptable. However, something has gone wrong, and what we are left with is a high burden of malnutrition in all its forms (undernutrition, micronutrient deficiencies, overweight and obesity) which affects every country on the planet.

With urbanisation and globalisation, economic growth, and food industry consolidation, the length of the food supply chains has increased, and food environments have become more complex. Bold policies, initiatives and investments are needed to shape food systems that contribute to improved nutrition and ensure that food is produced, distributed and consumed in a sustainable manner that protects the right to adequate food for all. This chapter provides an overview of the importance of diets and food systems in shaping nutrition.

Malnutrition and ill-health

Malnutrition, in all its forms (Figure 1.1), is to blame for a significant proportion of global ill-health. Child and maternal malnutrition have been identified as the world's leading cause of human mortality and years of healthy life lost (or disability-adjusted life-years, DALY) with sub-optimal diets, estimated to be the second top risk factor (Gakidou et al., 2017) (Figure 1.2).

Malnutrition affects people's health by: (1) impacting negatively on physical and cognitive development; (2) compromising the immune and cellular systems; (3) increasing susceptibility to communicable and non-communicable diseases and associated risk factors; and (4) restricting the attainment of human potential and reducing productivity (Black et al., 2008). Young children are particularly susceptible to malnutrition. As of 2017, 151 million children under the age of 5 suffer from stunting – they do not grow tall enough for their age. Wasting affects 51 million children under the age of 5 (UNICEF et al., 2018). Another indicator of

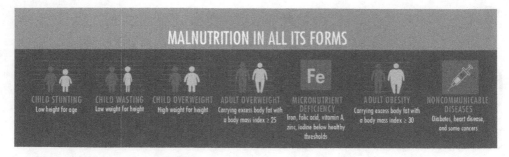

FIGURE 1.1 Malnutrition in all its forms
Source: IFPRI (2016).

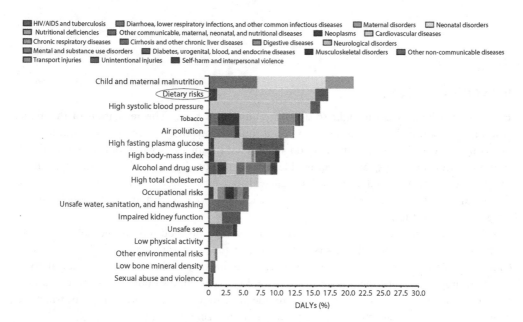

FIGURE 1.2 Major risk factors for global morbidity and mortality
Source: Gakidou et al. (2017).

poor nutritional status is low birth weight (LBW), defined as live births in a given population and over a given time period that, with birth weight of less than 2.5 kg, places infants at increased risk of morbidity and mortality. Estimates suggest that 20 million newborn babies have LBW (DI, 2018). In addition, it is estimated that 38.3 million children under the age of 5 are overweight (UNICEF et al., 2018).

Micronutrient deficiencies, in particular, Vitamin A, iodine, iron and zinc, affect billions of people. Although the estimates of the true extent of the problem are incomplete, the link between deficiencies and disease is well established (Allen de Benoist, Dary, & Hurrell, 2006). Iodine deficiency is associated with goitre and can compromise mental health, leading to reduced intellectual capacity. Vitamin A deficiency is associated with visual impairment and increased risk of diarrhoeal disease and measles. Deficiencies affect a whole range of further problems for growth and development, including birth defects, growth impairment, reduced cognitive function and greater vulnerability to infectious diseases. Iron deficiency is one cause of anaemia, which is associated with maternal and child mortality, poor physical performance, and chronic kidney and heart disease (Lopez, Cacoub, Macdougall, & Peyrin-Biroulet, 2016). Anaemia prevalence in girls and women aged 15–49 is 32.8 per cent and among pregnant women, 40.1 per cent in 2016 (DI, 2018). Currently, millions of women are too thin; 9.7 per cent of women and 5.7 per cent of adolescent girls are underweight. All forms of women's undernutrition affect their health (Fox et al., 2018), and if during pregnancy, contributes to foetal growth restriction, in turn, increasing the risk of infant deaths and among those who survive, stunting (Black et al., 2013).

At the same time, a staggering 2 billion adults are overweight, 678 million with obesity. Data on the prevalence of overweight adults (age 18+ years) show an increase from 35.7 per cent in 2010 to 38.9 per cent in 2016. Obesity prevalence in adults also shows an increase from 11.2 per cent in 2010 to 13.1 per cent in 2016. Globally, women have a higher prevalence of both overweight and obesity compared to men (DI, 2018). Obesity is a risk factor for a wide range of non-communicable diseases. Diet-related non-communicable diseases are a leading contributor to this mortality and morbidity, notably heart diseases, diabetes and some cancers. In total, "NCDs were responsible for 41 million of the world's 57 million deaths (71 per cent) in 2016, of which diet was one of the four leading risk factors" (WHO, 2018). Some 15 million of these deaths were premature (within the ages of 30–70 years). Some 78 per cent of all NCD deaths occur in low- and middle-income countries. Of these, 85 per cent are premature deaths.

Countries experience multiple burdens of these different forms of malnutrition. Data analysed by the 2018 Global Nutrition Report show that 88 per cent of the 141 countries with consistent data on three forms of malnutrition – childhood stunting, anaemia in women of reproductive age and overweight adults – experience a high level of at least two types of malnutrition, with 29 per cent (41 countries) having high levels of all three (DI, 2018). Most of these 41 countries are in Africa. When thinness among women is added, 23 per cent – almost one quarter of countries – have high burdens of four forms of malnutrition.

In individuals, estimates suggest that 1.9 per cent (8.23 million children under the age of 5) experience conditions associated with both deficiency (stunting) and excess (overweight) at the same time (DI, 2018). Almost 4 per cent of under-fives globally are both stunted and wasted – 15.95 million children. While the physiological mechanisms leading to this are not well understood, important evidence indicates that these children are at an elevated risk of mortality comparable to that associated with severe wasting (McDonald et al., 2013). Different forms of malnutrition can overlap in individuals and households (Tzioumis & Adair, 2014). Studies have shown that some households contain both overweight parents and undernourished children. The prevalence of these "double burden" households varies considerably (Tzioumis & Adair, 2014; Wojcicki, 2014). In Asia, for example, the prevalence of double burden households ranges from 5.0 per cent in Vietnam to 30.6 per cent in Indonesia (Rachmi, Li, & Baur 2018).

The link between diets and malnutrition

The burden of ill-health caused by malnutrition is directly linked to the food system because what people eat is a common cause of malnutrition in all its forms. Other factors also matter, including breastfeeding, access to clean water and physical activity. However, eating the right diets to meet nutrient needs is necessary, albeit not sufficient. Diets that promote good nutrition and health outcomes can be termed "healthy diets". There is no one single diet that promotes good health, but to avoid malnutrition and related health outcomes, a person must meet their needs for essential macronutrients (proteins, fats and carbohydrates, including dietary fibres) and micronutrients (vitamins, minerals and trace elements), which vary with their gender, age, physical activity level and physiological state. Conversely, healthy diets do not include excessive amounts of dietary energy, nor nutrients that have negative health outcomes when consumed in excess, such as trans and saturated fats, added sugars, salt. Available scientific evidence has led to recommendations on the general dietary patterns that promote health (Box 1.1).

BOX 1.1 A HEALTHY DIET

Based on the available scientific evidence on the link between diet, malnutrition and diseases, The World Health Organization (WHO, 2015a) recommend the following as a diet that prevents malnutrition in all its forms and diet-related non-communicable diseases:

- High in fruits, vegetables, legumes (e.g. lentils, beans), nuts and whole grains (e.g. unprocessed maize, millet, oats, brown rice).
- Intake of animal source foods (dairy, meat, eggs, fish and shellfish, etc.) in moderation, and limit processed meats.
- Low intake of refined sugars that are added to foods or drinks by the manufacturer, cook or consumer, and concentrated sugars naturally present in honey, syrups, fruit drinks and fruit juice concentrates.
- Substitute unsaturated fats or vegetable oils (e.g. found in fish, avocado, nuts, sunflower, canola and olive oils) in place of saturated fats (e.g. found in fatty meat, butter, palm and coconut oil, cream, ghee and lard). Industrial trans fats, or partially hydrogenated oils (found in processed food, fast food, snack food, fried food, baked goods, margarines and spreads), are not part of a healthy diet.

Whatever form they take, to promote health, diets must be sufficient and balanced in terms of quantity, quality and safety, each of which is described below:

Quantity

The first consideration is quantity. For optimal nutrition, diets must be adequate in energy (in the form of calories) to maintain life, support physical activity and maintain a healthy body weight, but without excessive consumption of dietary energy. If dietary energy intake exceeds energy expenditure, overweight and obesity can potentially ensue. Everyone requires different amounts of energy each day, depending on age, sex, size and activity level. When insufficient energy is consumed, hunger ensues. Even temporary periods of hunger can be debilitating to longer- term human growth and development. Acute hunger is when lack of food is short-term and is often caused by shocks, whereas chronic hunger is a constant or recurrent lack of food (Webb et al., 2006). The term undernourishment defines insufficient food intake to continuously meet dietary energy requirements with the Food and Agricultural Organization (FAO) further defining hunger as the consumption of less than 1600–2000 calories per day.

Quality

The second consideration is *quality* – the types of foods consumed and their diversity. Dietary diversity is a vital element of diet quality – the consumption of a variety of foods across and within food groupings including vegetables, fruits, whole grains and cereals, dairy foods and animal- and plant-based protein foods, while limiting foods and beverages high in saturated and trans fats, added sugars and salt. Fibre, legumes, omega-3 fatty acids, and polyunsaturated fatty acids, are other dietary elements that contribute positively to health. Consuming in this way more or less guarantees an adequate intake of essential nutrients and important non-nutrient factors. Research has demonstrated a strong association between dietary diversity and diet quality, and nutritional status of children and women (Arimond & Ruel, 2004; Jones, 2017). It is also clear that household dietary diversity is a sound predictor of the micro-nutrient (vitamins and minerals) density of the diet, particularly for young children (Girard, Self, McAuliffe, & Olude, 2012). Consuming inadequate amounts of nutrient-dense foods – particularly fruits, vegetables, whole grains, and nuts and seeds – is a leading contributor to the global burden of disease (see Figure 1.2) (Gakidou et al., 2017).

However, diversity in and of itself is not sufficient if the diet includes too many foods high in fats, sugars and salt, leading to obesity and non-communicable diseases (NCDs). The quality of diets thus also depends on limiting foods and beverages high in saturated and trans fats, added sugars and salt. Diets high in red meat, processed meat (smoked, cured, salted or chemically preserved), sugar-sweetened beverages, trans fats and sodium detract from diet quality and health. Minimally processed whole grains with higher dietary fibre content promote health relative to refined grains (e.g. starchy white breads). There are healthy sources of fats including monounsaturated and polyunsaturated fats that lower risk of NCDs, including olive oil, canola and sunflower oil, as well as fats found in certain foods like seeds and fish. Unhealthy fats are trans fats, made from partially hydrogenated oil and less so but still not with minimal harm, saturated fats found in coconut and palm oils, red meats, butter and cheese (Hu, 2010).

Foods undergo various forms of processing. This includes milling brown rice into white and wholewheat flour into white, pasteurisation and fermentation of milk, cutting up, canning and freezing vegetables, and manufacturing foods that are ready to eat or ready to heat from a range of different ingredients, including preservatives and emulsifiers. These processing methods can help to increase food availability, extend seasonality through the "hunger gap" and make food safer to eat (Global Panel on Agriculture and Food Systems for Nutrition, 2016). Yet a significant proportion of industrially-processed, packaged foods available in the marketplace are high in fats, sugars and salt. An analysis published in the 2018 *Global Nutrition Report* found that 23,013 packaged food products sold by 21 of the world's largest food and beverage manufacturers in nine countries were of relatively low nutritional quality (DI, 2018).

Safety

The third consideration is *safety*. Food safety refers to "all those biological, chemical and physical hazards, whether chronic or acute, that may make food injurious to the health of the consumer" (FAO & WHO, 2003). It refers to ways to prevent foodborne diseases, arising from food contamination during production, processing, storage, transport and distribution of food, as well as in the household. It also refers to the standards and controls that are in place to protect consumers from unsafe foods. Food safety and nutrition are closely associated because unsafe food (contaminated with pathogens or chemicals) can spur on foodborne diseases which lead to a potential vicious cycle of diarrhoea and malnutrition (WHO, 2015b).

Current status of diets

Globally comparable data on what people eat contains many gaps in terms of quantity, quality and safety. However, what is available (often modelled estimates from national surveys) provides an indication of why the world faces such a high burden of malnutrition in all its forms. The problem starts in infancy. Fewer than one in five children (16 per cent) aged 6–24 months eat what is defined as a "minimally acceptable diet" (MAD). This is the proportion of children aged 6–23 months who receive a minimum acceptable diet (apart from breast milk). Because appropriate feeding of children 6–23 months is multi-dimensional, it is important to have a composite indicator that tracks the extent to which multiple dimensions of adequate child feeding are being met. The MAD indicator combines standards of dietary diversity and feeding frequency with breastfeeding status. The indicator thus provides a useful way to track the progress of simultaneously improving the key quality and quantity dimensions of children's diets. Only two-thirds (69 per cent) of infants aged 6–8 months eat any solid food at all, and more than half (51 per cent) of children aged 6–24 months do not get the recommended minimum number of meals. While there are significant differences between rural and urban areas, and across all wealth groups, the diets of infants and young children remain inadequate in all countries (UNICEF et al., 2018).

The dietary constraints continue into childhood and adolescence. Around one-third of young people aged 10–17 do not eat fruit daily, with 14 per cent not eating vegetables. Yet 44 per cent of children report consuming soda every day (DI, 2018). The prevalence of inadequate intake of iron, zinc, calcium, vitamin D, folate, thiamine and riboflavin among 10–20-year-old adolescent girls in low- and middle-income countries is estimated at over 50 per cent (Keats et al., 2018).

Adult diets show a mixed picture. There are widespread differences between countries and contexts. Fruit consumption is higher in high-income regions as compared with low-income regions, whereas vegetable consumption is lower in high-income regions. Consumption of seafood is relatively low globally, with the highest consumption in South-East Asia (Figure 1.3, Panel A). Dairy consumption is highest in North America and the EU-15. The term EU-15 refers to the 15 Member States of the European Union as of 31 December 2003. Red meat consumption is similar in East Asia, Latin America, North America and EU-15. Trans fat intake is highest in South Asia, whereas the consumption of sugar-sweetened beverages (SSBs) is highest in Latin America and North America (Figure 1.3, Panel B).

Diets and food systems

A broad range of social, economic, demographic, and psychological factors influence the diets that people eat. These factors operate within the context of an overarching determinant - the "food system". The food system encompasses everything and everybody involved in producing, storing, packing, processing, distributing, consuming and disposing of food (FAO, 2013). This includes the chain of processes, institutions and people through which food

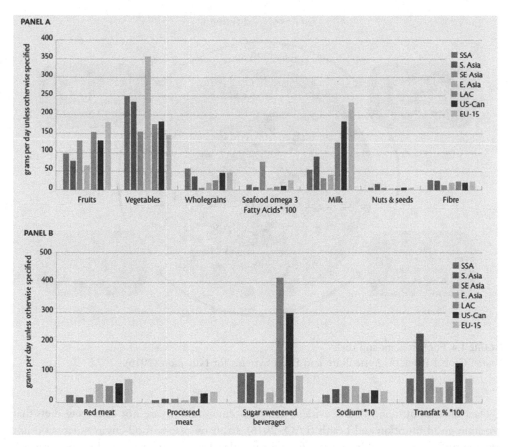

FIGURE 1.3 Intake of key foods and diet components, by region, 2016
Source: Global Panel on Agriculture and Food Systems for Nutrition (2016).

travels from farm to fork and beyond – the production of agricultural inputs, agricultural production (arable, livestock, fish, horticulture); distribution, transport, storage and trade; food processing and other forms of transformation, food retailing and other forms of provisioning (Figure 1.4).

The way food systems function – including what is produced, how these products are transformed through food supply chains, the way that economic value is generated, gained and lost – influences which foods are available, what they cost, and how they are marketed. That is, they influence *food environments*, the foods available to people as they go about their everyday lives, and their nutritional quality, safety, price and promotion (FAO, 2016; HLPE, 2017). Food environments play an important role in shaping diets because they provide the choices from which people make decisions about what to eat; they constrain and signal what people can acquire and, as a consequence, influence the decisions people make about what they eat (Story, Kaphingst, Robinson-O'Brien, & Glanz 2008; Herforth & Ahmed, 2015; HLPE, 2017). While individual and household circumstances also play an important role in the decisions people make about what to eat, food environments circumscribe how income can be spent on food (Herforth & Ahmed, 2015) and contribute to shaping people's food preferences, attitudes and beliefs and, therefore, food cultures more broadly (Hawkes et al., 2015).

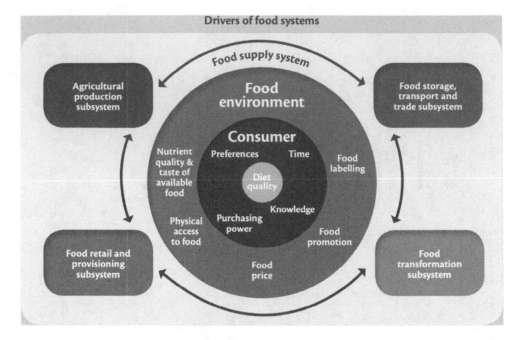

FIGURE 1.4 Food systems and diets
Source: Global Panel on Agriculture and Food Systems for Nutrition (2016).

Data on malnutrition make it evident that food environments are not delivering diets that promote good nutrition and health (FAO, 2016). In many places, food environments do not provide sufficient, affordable and safe food for people's basic nutrient needs. In other places – even in the same places – they are driving unhealthy diets and excessive food intake, leading to obesity and other risk factors for NCDs. Food environments also include unsafe foods, especially in low- and middle-income countries, leading to high rates of foodborne diseases, mainly through microbial pathogens (FAO, 2016).

Food environments have, over time, been shaped by the food systems of which they are part. Historically, the policies and processes that affect food systems have not had the objective of creating food environments that deliver healthy diets for all. Rather, the focus has been on delivering *enough dietary energy* to meet the needs for a growing population (World Bank, 2014). The context has been concerns about scarcity – hunger, famines and fears the food supplies will run out. Throughout, "food security" has been the dominant objective of food system policies (Pinstrup-Andersen & Watson, 2011). For example, the Depression-induced farm crisis in the United States and food shortages in war-torn Europe in the 1930s led to policy prescriptions designed to incentivise farmers to produce more (Lang & Heasman, 2015). Technologies to improve yields, such as breeding new varieties of crops and livestock, intensive irrigation, and fertilisers and pesticides. were developed and adopted. In the 1970s, famines in the developing world stimulated world leaders to convene the first World Food Conference in 1974, which produced the first ever definition of food security as "availability at all times of adequate world food supplies". Crop breeding programmes initially funded in the 1940s took off in Latin America and Asia, to become the "Green Revolution".

The intense focus on the agricultural element of food systems was successful in its objective of increasing supplies of dietary energy, with world food supplies keeping up with population growth (World Bank, 2008). It is estimated that between 1960 and 2000, "yields for all developing countries rose 208% for wheat, 109% for rice, 157% for maize, 78% for potatoes, and 36% for cassava" (Pingali, 2012). Europe and North America experienced food surpluses. Globally, food prices fell. The global standard adopted to measure success was the prevalence of undernourishment. The prevalence of under-nourishment fell in the late 1960s, a trend that continued until 2014 (FAO, 2010; 2015).

Yet many problems remained. Progress in increasing foods available for growing populations remained highly uneven between regions, countries and populations (FAO, 2015). It became evident that hunger was not just a problem of enough food, but the economic ability to access that food (Sen, 1982), leading to a redefinition of food security in 1983 to "ensuring that all people at all times have both physical and economic access to the basic food that they need" (FAO, 2006). The focus on dietary energy had also sidelined the importance of other aspects of diet. For example, while the Green Revolution is credited with boosting overall calorie consumption from basic cereals – rice, wheat – it did little to improve dietary diversity and micronutrient malnutrition, and may have even worsened trends (Pingali, 2012). And there was no focus at all on the emergence of overweight and obesity as a threat to the gains made to undernourishment.

At the same time, the global food system was undergoing a remarkable transformation. The strategy underpinning food systems – state intervention to encourage production – underwent a structural shift to enable and encourage markets to flourish (Hawkes, Friel, Lobstein, & Lang, 2012). In what is commonly termed "globalisation", governments put policies into place to liberalise trade, privatise state-run institutions and reduce barriers to cross-border investment (Hawkes & Murphy, 2010). Power shifted to the "middle of the chain" – the food processors, manufacturers, caterers and retailers that move farm products through the market (Reardon, 2015). These private food companies consolidated to become huge transnational corporations responsible for growth, distributing and processing and retailing (IPES-Food, 2017). Supply chains became more tightly coordinated, increasing the ability of these industries to control the price they paid to farmers, introduce technologies that prolonged shelf-life, and to process farm produce into highly differentiated products that consumers were willing to pay more for. With this consumer pull, food companies also had a clear incentive not just to meet demand, but to mobilise and create it through product innovation and marketing (Hawkes, 2012). With the ready availability of grains and technology, food companies generated a diversity of palatable, packaged foods high in refined carbohydrates, sugars and fats and heavily promoted them. The result is a double-edged sword – residual inadequacy of dietary diversity among populations at risk of undernutrition, rising consumption of industrially-manufactured, packaged foods high in refined carbohydrates depleted of fibre, sugars, unhealthy fats and salt, but accompanied by various positive trends, such as more readily available fruits and vegetables to those who could afford it (Popkin & Reardon, 2018). It has become what has been termed a "distorted" food system that failed to put quality protein and diversity into the diets of the poor while "succeeding" in feeding people large quantities of dietary energy, refined carbohydrates and packaged foods high in sugars, fats and salt (Popkin, 2014; Global Panel on Agriculture and Food Systems for Nutrition, 2016).

Conclusion

In 2015, the 193 Member States of the United Nations adopted the Sustainable Development Goals as the global agenda driving development. It included a target (2.2) to end malnutrition in all its forms by 2030. Redesigning food systems for better diets, nutrition and health will be crucial if the world is to meet this ambitious goal. The first step is the recognition that the food system exists not just to feed the world, but to nourish it (Haddad et al., 2016). Major transformations will be needed to reorient the food system towards the production, distribution, processing and sale of foods aligned with healthy diets. The impact would be to improve the health and well-being of billions of people.

References

Allen, L., de Benoist, B., Dary, O., & Hurrell, R. (2006). Guidelines on food fortification with micronutrients. Rome: World Health Organization and Food and Agriculture Organization of the United Nations.

Arimond, M. & Ruel, M. T. (2004). Dietary diversity is associated with child nutritional status: evidence from 11 demographic and health surveys. *The Journal of Nutrition*, 13410), 2579–2585.

Black, R. E., Allen, L. H., Bhutta, Z. A., Caulfield, L. E., De Onis, M., Ezzati, M., … Rivera, J. Maternal and Child Undernutrition Study Group. (2008). Maternal and child undernutrition: Global and regional exposures and health consequences. *The Lancet*, 371(9608), 243–260.

Black, R. E., Victora, C. G., Walker, S. P., Bhutta, Z. A., Christian, P., De Onis, M., … Uauy, R. (2013). Maternal and child undernutrition and overweight in low-income and middle-income countries. *The Lancet*, 382(9890), 427–451.

DI (Development Initiatives). (2018). *Global nutrition report: Shining a light to spur action on nutrition.* Bristol, UK: Development Initiatives.

FAO. (2006). Policy brief: food security. Rome: FAO. Available at: www.fao.org/fileadmin/templates/faoitaly/documents/pdf/pdf_Food_Security_Concept_Note.pdf

FAO. (2010). The state of food insecurity in the world: Addressing food insecurity in protracted crises. Rome: FAO. Available at: www.fao.org/3/a-i1683e.pdf

FAO. (2013). The state of food and agriculture: Food systems for better nutrition. Rome: FAO. Available at: www.fao.org/docrep/018/i3300e/i3300e00.htm

FAO. (2015). The state of food insecurity in the world 2015: Meeting the 2015 international hunger targets: Taking stock of uneven progress. Rome: FAO. Available at: www.fao.org/3/a-i4646e.pdf

FAO. (2016). Influencing food environments for healthy diets. Rome: FAO. Retrieved from: www.fao.org/3/a-i6484e.pdf

FAO & WHO. (2003). Assuring food safety and quality: Guidelines for strengthening national food control systems. Rome: FAO.

Fox, E. L., Davis, C., Downs, S. M., Schultink, W. & Fanzo, J. (2018). Who is the woman in women's nutrition? A narrative review of evidence and actions to support women's nutrition throughout life. *Current Developments in Nutrition*, 3(1).

Gakidou, E., Afshin, A., Abajobir, A. A., Abate, K. H., Abbafati, C., Abbas, K. M., … Abu-Raddad, L. J. (2017). Global, regional, and national comparative risk assessment of 84 behavioural, environmental and occupational, and metabolic risks or clusters of risks, 1990–2016: A systematic analysis for the Global Burden of Disease Study 2016. *The Lancet*, 390(10100), 1345–1422.

Girard, A.W., Self, J. L., McAuliffe, C. & Olude, O. (2012). The effects of household food production strategies on the health and nutrition outcomes of women and young children: A systematic review. *Paediatric and Perinatal Epidemiology*, 26, 205–222.

Global Panel on Agriculture and Food Systems for Nutrition (GLOPAN). (2016). Food systems and diets: Facing the challenges of the 21st century. Available at: www.glopan.org

Haddad, L., Hawkes, C., Webb, P., Thomas, S., Beddington, J., … Flynn, D. (2016). A new global research agenda for food. *Nature News*, 540(7631), 30.

Hawkes, C. (2012). Food policies for healthy populations and healthy economies. *BMJ*, 344, e2801.

Hawkes, C., Friel, S., Lobstein, T. & Lang, T. (2012). Linking agricultural policies with obesity and noncommunicable diseases: A new perspective for a globalising world. *Food Policy*, 37(3), 343–353.

Hawkes, C. & Murphy, S. (2010). An overview of global food trade. In: C. Hawkes, C. Blouin, S. Henson, N. Drager, & L. Dubé (eds), *Trade, food, diet and health: Perspectives and policy options*. Oxford: Wiley-Blackwell, pp. 16–32.

Hawkes, C., Smith, T. G., Jewell, J., Wardle, J., Hammond, R. A., … Kain, J.,(2015). Smart food policies for obesity prevention. *The Lancet*, 385(9985), 2410–2421.

Herforth, A. & Ahmed, S. (2015). The food environment, its effects on dietary consumption, and potential for measurement within agriculture-nutrition interventions. *Food Security*, 7(3), 505–520.

HLPE. (2017). Nutrition and food systems: A report by the High Level Panel of Experts on Food Security and Nutrition of the Committee on World Food Security. Rome: HLPE.

Hu, F. B. (2010). Are refined carbohydrates worse than saturated fat? *American Journal of Clinical Nutrition*, 91(6), 1541–1542.

IFPRI. (2016). Global nutrition report 2016: From promise to impact: Ending malnutrition by 2030. Washington, DC: International Food Policy Research Institute.

IPES-Food. (2017). Too big to feed: Exploring the impacts of mega-mergers, consolidation, and concentration of power in the agri-food sector. Available at: www.ipes-food.org

Jones, A. D. (2017). Critical review of the emerging research evidence on agricultural biodiversity, diet diversity, and nutritional status in low- and middle-income countries. *Nutrition Reviews*, 75(10), 769–782.

Keats, E., Rappaport, A., Shah, S., Oh, C., Jain, R., & Bhutta, Z. (2018). The dietary intake and practices of adolescent girls in low- and middle-income countries: A systematic review. *Nutrients*, 10(12), 1978.

Lang, T., & Heasman, M. (2015). *Food wars: The global battle for mouths, minds and markets*. 2nd edn. London: Routledge.

Lopez, A., Cacoub, P., Macdougall, I. C., & Peyrin-Biroulet, L. (2016). Iron deficiency anaemia. *The Lancet*, 387(10021), 907–916.

McDonald, C. M., Olofin, I., Flaxman, S., Fawzi, W. W., Spiegelman, D., Caulfield, L.E., … Danaei, G. Nutrition Impact Model Study. (2013). The effect of multiple anthropometric deficits on child mortality: Meta-analysis of individual data in 10 prospective studies from developing countries. *American Journal of Clinical Nutrition*, 97(4), 896–901.

Pingali, P.L. (2012). Green Revolution: Impacts, limits, and the path ahead. *Proceedings of the National Academy of Sciences*, 109(31), 12302–12308.

Pinstrup-Andersen, P. & WatsonII, D. D. (2011) *Food policy for developing countries: The role of government in global, national, and local food systems*. Ithaca, NY: Cornell University Press.

Popkin, B. M. (2014). Nutrition, agriculture and the global food system in low and middle income countries. *Food Policy*, 47, 91–96.

Popkin, B. M. & Reardon, T. (2018). Obesity and the food system transformation in Latin America. *Obesity Reviews*, 19(8): 1028–1064. Rachmi, C. N., Li, M. & Baur, L.A., (2018). The double burden of malnutrition in Association of South East Asian Nations (ASEAN) countries: A comprehensive review of the literature. *Asia Pacific Journal of Clinical Nutrition*, 27(4), 736.

Reardon, T., (2015). The hidden middle: The quiet revolution in the midstream of agrifood value chains in developing countries. *Oxford Review of Economic Policy*, 31(1), 45–63.

Sen, A. (1982). The food problem: Theory and policy. *Third World Quarterly*, 4(3), 447–459.

Story, M., Kaphingst, K. M., Robinson-O'Brien, R. & Glanz, K. (2008). Creating healthy food and eating environments: Policy and environmental approaches. *Annual Review of Public Health*, 29, 253–272.

Tzioumis, E. & Adair, L.S. (2014). Childhood dual burden of under- and overnutrition in low- and middle-income countries: A critical review. *Food and Nutrition Bulletin*, 35(2),230–243.

UNICEF (United Nations Children's Fund), World Health Organization, International Bank for Reconstruction and Development &The World Bank. (2018). Levels and trends in child malnutrition: Key findings of the 2018 Edition of the Joint Child Malnutrition Estimates. Geneva: World Health Organization.

Webb, P., Coates, J., Frongillo, E.A., Rogers, B. L., Swindale, A., & Bilinsky, P. (2006). Measuring household food insecurity: Why it's so important and yet so difficult to do. *The Journal of Nutrition*, 136(5), 1404S–1408S.

WHO. (2015a). Healthy diets. Fact sheet. Geneva:WHO. Available at: www.who.int/nutrition/publica tions/nutrientrequirements/healthydiet_factsheet394.pdf

WHO. (2015b). Food Safety. Fact sheet. Geneva:WHO. Available at: www.who.int/news-room/fa ct-sheets/detail/food-safety

WHO. (2018). Noncommunicable diseases country profiles 2018. Geneva:WHO. Available at: www. who.int/nmh/publications/ncd-profiles-2018/en/

Wojcicki, J.M. (2014). The double burden household in Sub-Saharan Africa: Maternal overweight and obesity and childhood undernutrition from the year 2000: results from World Health Organization Data (WHO) and Demographic Health Surveys (DHS). *BMC Public Health*, 14(1), 1124.

World Bank. (2008). World development report 2008: Agriculture for development. Washington, DC: World Bank.

World Bank. (2014). Learning from World Bank history. Agriculture and food-based approaches for addressing malnutrition. World Bank Report No. 88740-GLB. Washington, DC: World Bank.

2

SUSTAINABILITY

Barbara Burlingame

Introduction

Sustainability is the ubiquitous descriptor for almost everything that is done in research, policies, programmes and interventions, regardless of the sector or discipline. Almost all initiatives undertaken in the United Nations (UN) system, and by national and local governments, civil society and the private sector, have sustainability as a fundamental aim. A quick search of the food, agriculture and nutrition scientific literature over time shows exponential increases in "sustainable" and its variants as keywords.

For the purpose of this chapter, sustainable in the context of a food system is confined to environmental sustainability. Furthermore, the assumption is that, in order to be sustainable, a food system must be healthy. In order to more comprehensively incorporate "healthy" as both a human concern and environmental concern, sustainable diets will also be discussed. And as is the case with sustainable food systems, the assumption for sustainable diets is that it is also, by definition, healthy (FAO, 2012). It is worth noting that the reverse is not necessarily true, i.e. while a sustainable diet is necessarily a healthy diet, a healthy diet, by conventional definitions, is not necessarily a sustainable diet.

Throughout the 1950s, a huge body of scientific research developed, showing that food systems as products of industrial agriculture are not sustainable, contributing to both human morbidity and mortality and environmental damage (Gannon, Link, & Decker,1959; Chichester, 1965). Since the 1960s, public awareness of these dangers has increased, fuelled by best-selling books such as *Silent Spring* (Carson, 1962) and *Diet for a Small Planet* (Lappé, 1971).

Modern, resource-intensive food systems, requiring high chemical inputs for ever-increasing production yields, were named the Green Revolution. For all its successes in increasing the supply of starchy staple foods and contributing to improved food security as measured by dietary energy supply, the unsustainability of the Green Revolution was obvious to many, as it was related to, among other things, environmental degradation and biodiversity loss.

The United Nations steps up

The UN had been active in preparing initiatives to address the numerous environmental catastrophes that had occurred or that were looming. In 1972, the first UN Conference on the Human Environment was held in Stockholm (UN, 1972). The meeting agreed upon a Declaration, i.e. the Stockholm Declaration, containing 26 principles concerning the environment and development, along with an Action Plan itemising 109 recommendations, and a Resolution. Significantly, it also resulted in the agreement to create the United Nations Environment Programme. The word *sustainability* is not used in the document, but the essence of the concept is illustrated throughout. Urgency of action was conveyed, and yet the principles and recommendations nearly 50 years ago are still to be effectively addressed by global leaders and other stakeholders.

Just two years later, in 1974, the first UN World Food Conference was held in Rome. It made few statements about resource exploitation and environmental sustainability, and addressed agriculture for its role in increasing economic development. Nevertheless, it recognised the central role of climate in world food production and in its Universal Declaration on the Eradication of Hunger and Malnutrition, stated that, "the effort to increase food production should be complemented by every endeavour to prevent wastage of food in all its forms", and "to assure the proper conservation of natural resources being utilized, or which might be utilized, for food production, all countries must collaborate in order to facilitate the preservation of the environment, including the marine environment" (UN, 1975).

There were many UN-led initiatives in the 1970s with direct relevance to sustainable food systems. In addition to the Human Environment Conference and the World Food Conference mentioned above, there was the 1976 UN World Water Conference in Mar del Plata, Argentina (UN, 1979); the 1976 UN Conference on Desertification, New York (UN, 1978); and the 1979 First World Climate Conference, Geneva (WMO, 1979). Environmental sustainability and sustainable food systems, directly and indirectly, were the goal of each of these, but the term was never used directly.

The first significant attempt at defining sustainability *per se* came in the form of the 1987 UN report, *Our Common Future*, often referred to as the Brundtland Report (WCED, 1987). The sustainable development framework it presented brought the environment and natural resource issues into clear focus. It defined sustainability as sustainable development, and sustainable development as "development that meets the needs of the present without compromising the ability of future generations to meet their own needs". Food security and human nutrition were specifically addressed, the former with its own chapter and the latter with mentions throughout the report. Sustainable food systems were not a term used; however, as a concept they were widely covered with statements such as, "increased food production should not be based on ecologically unsound production policies and compromise long-term prospects for food security".

Around the same time as the Brundtland Report, some others in the field of nutrition were pursuing the idea of sustainability of diets. Gussow and Clancy (1986) published an article, "Dietary guidelines for sustainability", in which they argued the following:

> Information on the relationship between human health and food choices is not a sufficient basis for nutrition education. In our time, educated consumers need to make food choices that not only enhance their own health but also contribute to the protection of

our natural resources. Therefore, the content of nutrition education needs to be broadened and enriched not solely by medical knowledge, but also by information arising from disciplines such as economics, agriculture, and environmental science.

A few years later, planning was underway for the joint FAO/WHO International Conference on Nutrition (ICN),[1] to be held in Rome in 1992. For scientists in health, agriculture, environment, and other relevant disciplines, and for many civil society organisations, hopes were high for nutrition to embrace sustainable food systems. Indeed, from the inaugural statements and main report, to the World Declaration and Plan of Action for Nutrition, sustainable agriculture, environmentally sound sustainable development and the protection of biodiversity featured prominently (FAO & WHO, 1992).

While countries were in the process of preparing their post-ICN National Plans of Action for Nutrition, the International Union of Nutritional Sciences (IUNS) adopted the theme, "Nutrition in a Sustainable Environment" (Wahlqvist. Truswell, Smith, & Nestel, 1994) for its 1993 International Congress of Nutrition (IUNS-ICN), in the hope of maintaining the momentum from the FAO and WHO-ICN. Almost prescient to the future decades of activity in nutrition, the FAO presentation at the IUNS-ICN on the follow-up to the FAO and WHO ICN, mentioned nothing about environmental sustainability, sustainable food systems or the protection of ecosystems and biodiversity, in spite of these elements being emphasised in both, i.e. the theme of the IUNS-ICN and the report of the FAO and WHO-ICN.

The Food and Agricultural Organisation's (FAO) aim was to improve food security, the metric for which was dietary energy supply, or quantity of food expressed as kcal per person per day. This aim was enhanced by intensive food systems and short-term horizons, e.g. yearly reporting of progress until 2017 in the flagship publication, *State of Food Insecurity in the World* (FAO, 1999), and achieving the Millennium Development Goal 1C, the hunger target, by 2015. The World Health Organization (WHO) was concerned with disease burdens, and therefore the environmental issues were more related to sanitation than ecosystems. For the remainder of the 1990s and into the 2000s, attempts to address healthy and sustainable food systems in nutrition were thwarted because of low priority, and funding was largely directed to other areas.

Some sectors were absent from the UN agency mix addressing nutrition, the environment sector being the most important lacuna. Thus, it was transformational when the environment sector, strongly led by the Convention on Biological Diversity (CBD), proposed and ushered through its processes the Cross-cutting Initiative on Biodiversity for Food and Nutrition in 2006 (CBD, 2006). The FAO was requested to take charge, in collaboration with Bioversity International, and their workplans included activities to address nutrition in the context of biodiversity and environmental sustainability (Toledo & Burlingame, 2006; Burlingame, Charrondiere, & Mouille, 2009), diets and nutrients as ecosystem services (Halwart et al., 2006; CGRFA, 2013), biodiversity to improve micronutrient intakes (Burlingame, Charrondiere, & Halwart, 2006; Burlingame & Dernini, 2011; Lacirignola et al., 2012), traditional food systems of indigenous peoples (Kuhnlein, Erasmus, & Spigelski, 2009; Kuhnlein, Erasmus, Spigelski, & Burlingame, 2013), nutrient composition of neglected and underutilised species (FAO, INFOODS, & Bioversity International, 2008; 2010; Lutaladio, Burlingame, & Crews, 2010; Charrondiere, Stadlmayr, Nilsson, & Burlingame, 2010; et al., 2012; FAO/INFOODS, 2017), greenhouse gases, livestock industries and protein (Steinfeld & Gerber, 2010; Gerber et al., 2013; Burlingame, 2015), agro-ecology and organic production methods

(Meybeck, Redfern, Paoletti, & Strassner, 2015), and metrics and models for characterising sustainable diets (Meybeck et al., 2015).

Several regional and global scientific conferences and symposia were convened to share research and interventions linking the field of nutrition with environmental sustainability. One of these was the International Scientific Symposium on Biodiversity and Sustainable Diets, in 2010 organised by the FAO in collaboration with Bioversity International (FAO, 2012). A consensus definition for sustainable diets was developed by a working group at the symposium in an attempt to capture the fundamentals of sustainable food systems for human and environmental health. It was then adopted by the delegates in the final plenary session:

> Sustainable Diets are those diets with low environmental impacts which contribute to food and nutrition security and to healthy life for present and future generations. Sustainable diets are protective and respectful of biodiversity and ecosystems, culturally acceptable, accessible, economically fair and affordable; nutritionally adequate, safe and healthy; while optimizing natural and human resources.
>
> *(FAO, 2012)*

Another significant initiative taking place, co-sponsored by the World Bank and FAO, was the International Assessment of Agricultural Knowledge, Science, and Technology for Development (IAASTD). This global consultative process, which ran from 2002 to 2009, was charged with reviewing the sustainability of agriculture and food systems and recommending options for action to governments, international agencies, academia, research organisations and other decision-makers around the world. Its 600-page final report documents the necessity to adopt new national, regional and international agreements

> to support further shifts towards ethical, equitable and sustainable food and agriculture systems in response to the urgent challenges such as those posed by the declining availability of clean water and competing claims of water, loss of biodiversity, deforestation, climate change, exploitative labour conditions.
>
> *(IAASTD, 2009)*

The report draws heavily on lessons from the past with implications for the future.

The Sustainable Development Goals (SDGs) are the culmination of efforts dating as far back as the creation of the UN itself, but they are a direct outcome of the United Nations Conference on Sustainable Development, Rio+20, in 2012. During Rio+20, the Secretary-General of the UN, Ban Ki Moon put forward the Zero Hunger Challenge, with five pillars. The central pillar of this aspirational challenge was, "all food systems are sustainable". As the SDGs were being negotiated, Zero Hunger re-emerged as SDG 2. Its short title is Zero Hunger, while its long title is "End hunger, achieve food security and improved nutrition and promote sustainable agriculture". Just as sustainable food systems was the theme running through every aspect of Rio +20, so do sustainable food systems feature, directly and indirectly, in all the SDGs.

Also emerging from Rio+20 is the Sustainable Food Systems Programme (SFS), part of the 10-Year Framework of Programmes on Sustainable Consumption and Production. This Programme aims to promote sustainability all along the food value chain, bringing together existing initiatives and partnerships working in related areas. It focuses on priority activities such as sustainable diets and the reduction of food losses and waste (UNEP, 2018).

Core indicators of sustainable food systems

There are many variations in definitions, conceptual frameworks, typologies, metrics and models for developing or selecting indicators in the context of sustainable food systems. Indicator development requires a classification system of increasing levels of disaggregation. For example, the 17 *goals* of the SDGs are disaggregated into 169 *targets*, which are further disaggregated into 232 *indicators*. The Mediterranean Diet as a sustainable food system model presents four "thematic areas", which are then disaggregated into 27 indicators (Dernini et al., 2016; Donini et al., 2016). Chaudhary et al. (2018) propose seven "domains" which disaggregate into 25 indicators, while Nugent et al. (2015) propose four "outcomes" which disaggregate into 13 indicators. The Food Sustainability Index (EIU, 2016) classifies 58 indicators under three "pillars". Table 2.1 shows a selection of indicator classifications from these five sources.

Nutrition appears specifically in all five classifications, explicitly and singly as "nutrition" and "nutrition challenges", or combined with health status; or further disaggregated into hunger and malnutrition, as is the case with the SDGs. Under Thematic Areas, it is spread between biochemical characteristics and clinical aspects, and also included within food quality, as in nutrient content of foods and diets. Environment also appears specifically in all classifications; again explicitly by name in three classifications or implied within sustainable production and sustainable agriculture in the other two. Biodiversity appears explicitly in the SDG targets, whereas it is represented in the indicators for the other four, variously under the classifications environment, food quality, food consumption diversity and sustainable agriculture. Food affordability shows up as a specific classification element in two sources. Classifications unique to only one source include socio-cultural well-being, food safety and lifestyle.

The choice of indicators for any given purpose must be based on commonly agreed criteria, e.g. relevant, methodologically sound, measurable, monitorable, outcome-focused, easy to interpret and communicate (UNSD, 2015). The greatest limitation related to indicators is lack of availability of sound data sets, which suggests that data generation should be a priority in order to have robust indictors.

TABLE 2.1 A selection of sustainable food systems indicator classifications

Domains (Chaudhary et al., 2018)	Targets (SDG 2-only)	Thematic areas (Dernini et al., 2016; Donini et al., 2016)	Outcomes (Nugent et al., 2015)	Pillars (EIU, 2016)
Nutrition	Hunger	Biochemical characteristics	Food affordability	Food loss and waste
Environment	Malnutrition	Food quality	Food consumption diversity	Sustainable agriculture
Food affordability and availability	Food productivity and incomes	Environment	Health and nutrition status	Nutritional challenges
Sociocultural well-being	Sustainable and resilient food production and agricultural practices	Lifestyle	Environmental sustainability	
Resilience	Biodiversity	Clinical aspects		
Food safety				
Waste				

Examples of effective action

In spite of the lack of progress globally in redressing the problems, big and small, there are examples of some successes in policies and actions. There is a large body of basic and applied research showing that food systems can be designed and managed sustainably – including agriculture production systems, where arguably most of the environmental damage takes place. Research has shown that sustainable agriculture in different parts of the world can produce enough food to support the global population, without the need to bring more land into agricultural production (Pretty, Morison, & Hine, 2003).

Agro-ecology, i.e. applying ecological concepts and principles to agricultural production systems (Gliessman, 2007), is an appropriate overarching approach to achieve sustainability. It applies to a number of practices that maintain and enhance biodiversity, build soil fertility, minimise agro-chemical inputs and maximise efficiencies in natural resource use. Additionally, agro-ecology promotes diversification within the system, which is estimated to improve yields between 20 and 60 per cent higher than monocultures (Koohafkan & Altieri, 2010). The different agro-ecological approaches, e.g. organic agriculture, endeavour to maintain productivity while restoring ecosystem health, and enhance food security and nutrition – without which, food systems, per se, would not be sustainable.

Europe plays a valuable leadership role in encouraging sustainable food systems, including production systems, through legislation. The 2013 Common Agricultural Policy (CAP) built in a number of aspects of sustainability. For example, these reforms made direct payments to farmers conditional on diversifying crops, maintaining permanent grassland, and dedicating 5 per cent of arable land to ecologically beneficial elements. Under these rules, farmers receiving payments help conserve the environment and contribute to addressing greenhouse gas (GHG) emissions by the following means:

- making soil and ecosystems more resilient by growing a greater variety of crops;
- conserving soil carbon and grassland habitats associated with permanent grassland;
- protecting water and habitats by establishing ecological focus areas.

Built on the CAP are the European regulations for organic foods. The EU recognises the role of organic systems to deliver public goods contributing to the protection of the environment and animal welfare, along with other benefits to consumers and for rural development (EU, 2018a). At the start of 2018, Europe had approximately 306,500 organic operators (i.e. farmers, processors and importers), and certified organic land represented almost 7 per cent of the EU agriculture land, with seven EU Member States already exceeding 10 per cent. Organic retail sales amounted to €30.7 billion, with an annual growth of 12 per cent (EU, 2018a), which is considered unprecedented in the rest of the agri-food sector. In addition to legislation, the European Parliament also provides advocacy for organic foods with a series of infographics aimed at consumers. One such infographic, reproduced as Figure 2.1, illustrates four key principles of organic food production: (1) the use of chemical pesticides and synthetic fertilisers is banned; (2) antibiotics (for animals) are severely restricted; (3) genetically modified organisms (GMOs) are not allowed; and (4) crops are rotated (EU, 2018b).

Cuba provides another example of sustainable food systems. Since the late 1990s, Cuba has changed its agricultural system from industrial to agro-ecological. The Cuban government promotes agro-ecology now as the farming standard (Febles-González et al., 2011).

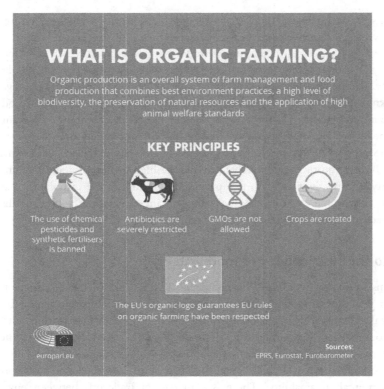

FIGURE 2.1 Example of an advocacy campaign by the European Parliament to encourage sustainable and healthy food systems
Source: EU (2018b).

Regardless of the type of land ownership, agriculture in Cuba is oriented towards agro-ecology and sustainable food production (Palma, 2015). Small-holder family farms in Cuba practising agro-ecology account for as much as, or more than, 65 per cent of the domestic food supply (Altieri & Toledo, 2011; Rosset, Sosa, Jaime, & Lozano, 2011). Agro-ecology is also practised in urban agriculture in which 40 per cent or more of households are actively engaged. Due in large part to the success of its food systems, Cuba was one of only eight countries to meet two key conditions for sustainable development, that is, high human development while keeping their ecological footprint lower than 1.7 global hectares per person (GFN, 2015).

Other examples of success include the following:

- The Brazilian National Plan for Agroecology and Organic Production supports organic and agro-ecological production for its sustainable development. Ten government ministries participate. Its goal is to promote the transition to sustainable production systems for family farmers, agrarian reform settlers, fishermen and fish farmers, traditional populations and rural youth; to develop and provide technological innovation and training with an emphasis on agro-ecology; to support the promotion and marketing of organic and agro-ecological products; and increase the share of organic and agro-ecological products in local markets. Biodiversity for food and nutrition is a key feature (Brazilian Ministry of Agrarian Development, 2013).

- In Malawi, permaculture-based solutions are focusing on local sources of plant foods to provide a year-round, highly nutritious diet, along with neglected and underutilised animal diversity. Community-level movements, e.g. Never Ending Food (2018), are reviving traditional knowledge to instil cultural pride in the use of resilient and adapted local food resources.
- In China, the ancient rice-fish farming system illustrates important ecosystem synergies and the value in safeguarding "Globally Important Agriculture Heritage Systems" (GIAHS) as part of sustainable food systems. In rice-based aquatic ecosystems, it is the fish and other aquatic organisms that provide the high quality protein, vitamins, minerals and fatty acids to the diet, with rice providing the bulk of the carbohydrate and dietary energy. Environmental sustainability is also enhanced with the natural fertilisation and the insect management from the aquatic animals (Burlingame et al., 2006).

Threats to the sustainability of food systems

Food systems around the world are not sustainable. This is acknowledged on many fronts. Climate change is an issue that looms large over all aspects of sustainability, threatening food systems, and indeed all systems of life. Agriculture contributes disproportionately to climate change. For example, consumption and production of products of the livestock industries need to be addressed in the context of climate change, specifically, GHG emissions and land use.

For all food systems, it is a challenge to find a balance between agricultural productivity and environmental sustainability. There is a myriad of trade-offs between environmental outcomes and other food system outcomes. As with climate change, livestock production and consumption bring to light the complexity of the subject. For consumption, meat and dairy provide high quality protein and micronutrients, yet they have a role in diet-related chronic disease aetiology. For production, natural grazing lands are significant repositories of biodiversity, with livestock as a positive contributing synergistic component (e.g. manure), yet GHG emissions are high, even from extensive livestock systems (Steinfeld, 2006).

Among the materials reviewed, the IAASTD report provides the most detailed and comprehensive evidence of threats to the sustainability of food systems, from climate and ecosystem services to food production and consumption (IAASTD, 2009).

Some key threats can be summarised as follows:

- Local food systems, known to sustain livelihoods at micro level, are currently challenged by globalised food systems.
- Agro-biodiversity is threatened by monoculture agriculture and intensive farming and livestock systems, and the associated agro-chemical inputs needed for their support.
- The focus of industrial food processing achieves improved shelf-life, but with concomitant poorer health and nutrition outcomes.
- Agricultural production and trade policies have influenced negative trends in global nutrition, health and livelihoods.

Relevant indicators for monitoring depend on underlying data sets. The absence of high quality data should also be regarded as a threat to sustainable food systems.

Conclusion

Given the plethora of recommendations, commitments, declarations, calls for action, ratified treaties, and universally agreed goals and targets, it is not helpful to create more. Indeed, efforts should be put into reviewing the past to inform the future. In spite of many decades of urgent calls for action, progress on making food systems healthy and sustainable has been unconscionably slow, and even retrograde on some issues, since the 1972 UN Conference on the Human Environment. There seems little reason to be optimistic.

Nevertheless, some see reasons for optimism in the 2030 Agenda for Sustainable Development, with the tag line "people, planet and prosperity". Indeed, nearly every nation has pledged its commitment to the SDGs. The ambitious agenda covers a wide swath of development issues, from universal peace to poverty eradication; from gender equality to corruption and violence. "Healthy and sustainable food systems" will feature greatly in the monitoring and reporting on SDG 2 and SDG 12. How effectively this topic is integrated into all other SDGs will, in large part, determine the degree of success.

Note

1 ICN, the International *Conference* on Nutrition, held by FAO and WHO in 1992 and again in 2014, should not be confused with the ICN, the International *Congress* of Nutrition, which is the official conference of the International Union of Nutritional Sciences and has been held roughly every four years since 1946.

References

Altieri, M. A. & Toledo, V. M. (2011). The agroecological revolution in Latin America: rescuing nature, ensuring food sovereignty and empowering peasants. *The Journal of Peasant Studies*, 38, 587–612. doi:10.1080/ 03066150.2011.582947

Brazilian Ministry of Agrarian Development. (2013). National plan for agroecology and organic production. Available at: www.mda.gov.br/sitemda/sites/sitemda/files/user_arquivos_19/Mont_cartilha_planapo_ingles.pdf

Burlingame, B. (2015). Plant and animal protein ratio. In A. Meybeck, S. Redfern, F. Paoletti, & C. Strassner (eds), *Assessing sustainable diets within the sustainability of food systems*. Rome: FAO. Available at: www.fao.org/3/a-i4806e.pdf (accessed May 2018).

Burlingame, B., Charrondiere, R., & Halwart, M. (2006). Basic human nutrition requirements and dietary diversity in rice-based aquatic ecosystems. *Journal of Food Composition and Analysis*, 19(6–7), 770.

Burlingame, B., Charrondiere, U.R. & Mouille, B. (2009). Food composition is fundamental to the cross-cutting initiative on biodiversity for food and nutrition. *Journal of Food Composition and Analysis*, 22(5), 361–365.

Burlingame, B. & Dernini, S. (2011). Sustainable diets: The Mediterranean diet as an example. *Public Health Nutrition*, 14(12A): 2285–2287.

Carson, R. (1962). *Silent spring*. Boston: Houghton Mifflin.

CBD (Convention on Biological Diversity). (2006). Agricultural biodiversity: Cross-cutting initiative on biodiversity for food and nutrition, COP 8 Decision VIII/23. Available at: www.cbd.int/decision/cop/?id=11037

Charrondiere, U. R., Stadlmayr, B., Nilsson, E., Burlingame, B. (2010). FAO/INFOODS Food Composition Database for Biodiversity version 1.0. Rome: FAO. Available at www.fao.org/3/a-i7364e.pdf.

Charrondiere, U.R., Stadlmayr, B., Rittenschober, D., Nowak, V., Nilsson, E., & Burlingame, B. (2012). FAO/INFOODS Food Composition Database for Biodiversity, version 2.0. Rome: FAO. Available at: www.fao.org/docrep/019/i3560e/i3560e.pdf.

Charrondiere, U.R., Stadlmayr, B., Rittenschober, D., Nowak, V., Nilsson, E., & Burlingame, B. (2013). FAO/INFOODS Food Composition Database for Biodiversity, version 2.1. Rome: FAO.

Chaudhary, A., Gustafson, D., & Mathys, A. (2018). Multi-indicator sustainability assessment of global food systems. *Nature Communications*, 9(1), 848. Available at: www.nature.com/articles/s41467-018-03308-7.

Chichester, C. (ed.) (1965). *Research in pesticides*. New York: Academic Press.

CGRFA (Commission on Genetic Resources for Food and Agriculture). (2013). Review of key issues on biodiversity and nutrition. CGRFA-14/13/8. Rome: FAO. Available at: www.fao.org/docrep/m eeting/027/mf917e.pdf.

Dernini, S., Berry, E., Serra-Majem, L., La Vecchia, C., Capone, R., Medina, F., & Trichopoulou, A. (2016). Med Diet 4.0: The Mediterranean diet with four sustainable benefits. *Public Health Nutrition*, 1–9. doi:10.1017/S1368980016003177.

Donini, L., Dernini, S., Lairon, D., Serra-Majem, L., & Burlingame, B. (2016). A consensus proposal for nutritional indicators to assess the sustainability of a healthy diet: The Mediterranean Diet as a case study. *Frontiers in Nutrition and Environmental Sustainability*, 3(37). doi:10.3389/fnut.2016.00037. Available at: www.frontiersin.org/articles/10.3389/fnut.2016.00037/full.

EIU (Economist Intelligence Unit). (2016). Fixing food: Towards a more sustainable food system. Available at: http://foodsustainability.eiu.com/wp-content/uploads/sites/34/2017/03/FIXING-FOOD-TOWARDS -A-MORE-SUSTAINABLE-FOOD-SYSTEM.pdf

EU. (2018a). Briefing EU Legislation in Progress: Organic farming legislation: Revision of EU Regulation on organic production and labelling of organic products. Available at: www.europarl.europa. eu/RegData/etudes/BRIE/2018/614743/EPRS_BRI%282018%29614743_EN.pdf

EU. (2018b). The EU's organic food market: Facts and rules (infographic). Available at: www.europarl. europa.eu/news/en/headlines/society/20180404STO00909/the-eu-s-organic-food-market-facts-and -rules-infographic

FAO. (1999). State of food insecurity in the world. Rome: FAO.

FAO. (2012). Sustainable diets and biodiversity: directions and solutions for policy, research and action. Rome: FAO. Available at: www.fao.org/docrep/016/i3004e/i3004e00.htm.

FAO/INFOODS. (2017). Food composition database for biodiversity, version 4.0 – BioFoodComp4.0. Rome: FAO. Available at: www.fao.org/3/a-i7364e.pdf

FAO/INFOODS/Bioversity International. (2008). Expert consultation on nutrition indicators for biodiversity 1. Food composition. Rome: FAO. Available at: www.fao.org/3/a-a1582e.pdf

FAO/INFOODS/Bioversity International. (2010). Expert consultation on nutrition indicators for biodiversity 2. Food consumption. Rome: FAO. Available at: www.fao.org/docrep/014/i1951e/i1951e.pdf

FAO & WHO. (1992). International Conference on Nutrition. Final Report of the Conference. Food and Agriculture Organization of the United Nations and World Health Organization, Rome. Rome: FAO. Available at: www.ign.org/p142003016.html?from=142002801

Febles-González, J. M., Tolón-Becerra, A., Lastra-Bravo, X., & Acosta-Valdés, X. (2011). Cuban agricultural policy in the last 25 years: From conventional to organic agriculture. *Land Use Policy*, 28(4), 723–735.

Gannon, H., Link, R. P., & Decker, G. C. (1959). Pesticide residues in meat and milk: Storage of dieldrin in tissues and its excretion in milk of dairy cows fed dieldrin in their diet. *Journal of Agricultural and Food Chemistry*, 7, 824–826.

Gerber, P J., Steinfeld, H., Henderson, B., Mottet, A., Opio, C., Dijkman, J., … Tempio, G. (2013). Tackling climate change through livestock: A global assessment of emissions and mitigation opportunities. Rome: FAO. Available at: www.fao.org/3/a-i3437e.pdf

GFN (Global Footprint Network). (2015). Only eight countries meet two key conditions for sustainable development as United Nations adopts Sustainable Development Goals. Available at: www. footprintnetwork.org/2015/09/23/eight-countries-meet-two-key-conditions-sustainable-developm ent-united-nations-adopts-sustainable-development-goals/

Gliessman, S. R. (2007). *Agroecology: The ecology of sustainable food systems*. New York: CRC Press.

Gussow, J. D. & Clancy, K. L. (1986). Dietary guidelines for sustainability. *Journal of Nutrition Education*, 18(1), 1–5.

Halwart, M., Bartley, D., Burlingame, B., Funge-Smith, S., & James, D. (2006). FAO Regional Technical Expert Workshop on aquatic biodiversity, its nutritional composition, and human consumption in rice-based systems. *Journal of Food Composition and Analysis*, 19(6–7), 752–755. doi:10.1016/j.jfca.2006. 03.doi:011.

IAASTD (International Assessment of Agricultural Knowledge, Science, and Technology for Development). (2009). *Agriculture at a crossroads: The global report of the International Assessment of Agricultural Knowledge, Science, and Technology for Development*. Washington, DC: Island Press. Available at: www.fao.org/fileadmin/templates/est/Investment/Agriculture_at_a_Crossroads_Global_Report_IAASTD.pdf

IPES-Food. (2016). From uniformity to diversity: A paradigm shift from industrial agriculture to diversified agroecological systems. Available at: www.ipes-food.org

Koohafkan, P. & Altieri, M. A. (2010). Globally important agricultural heritage systems: A legacy for the future. Rome: FAO. Available at: www.fao.org/fileadmin/templates/giahs/PDF/GIAHS_Booklet_EN_WEB2011.pdf

Kuhnlein, H., Erasmus, B., & Spigelski, D. (2009). Indigenous peoples' food systems: The many dimensions of culture, diversity and environment for nutrition and health. Rome: FAO and CINE.

Kuhnlein, H., Erasmus, B., Spigelski, D., & Burlingame, B. (2013). Indigenous peoples' food and wellbeing: Interventions and policies for healthy communities. Rome: FAO and CINE.

Lacirignola, C., Dernini, S., Capone, R., Meybeck, A., Burlingame, B., Gitz, V., … Belsanti, V. (2012). Towards the development of guidelines for improving the sustainability of diets and food consumption patterns: The Mediterranean Diet as a pilot study. *Options méditerranéennes*, Series B. Paris: International Centre for Advanced Mediterranean Agronomic Studies.

Lappé, F. M. (1971). *Diet for a small planet*. New York:Ballantine Books.

Lutaladio, N., Burlingame, B., & Crews, J. (2010). Horticulture, biodiversity and nutrition. *Journal of Food Composition and Analysis*, 23, 481–485.

Meybeck, A., Redfern, S., Paoletti, F., & Strassner, C. (eds) (2015). Assessing sustainable diets within the sustainability of food systems. Rome: FAO. Available at: www.fao.org/3/a-i4806e.pdf

Never Ending Food. (2018). Available at: www.neverendingfood.org/

Nugent, R., Levin, C., & Grafton, D. (2015). Indicators for nutrition-friendly and sustainable food systems. In *Global Nutrition Report 2015: Actions and accountability to advance nutrition and sustainable development*. Washington, DC: International Food Policy Research Institute. Available at: http://dx.doi.org/10.2499/9780896298835

Palma, I. P., Toral, J. N., Parra Vázquez, M.R., Fuentes, N. F., & Hernández, F. G. (2015). Historical changes in the process of agricultural development in Cuba. *Journal of Cleaner Production*, 96, 77–84.

Pretty, J., Morison, J., & Hine, R. (2003). Reducing food poverty by increasing agricultural sustainability in developing countries. *Agriculture, Ecosystems, & Environment*, 95, 217–234.

Rosset, P. M., Sosa, B. M., Jaime, A. M. R., & Lozano, D. R. Á. (2011). The Campesino-to-Campesino agroecology movement of ANAP in Cuba: Social process methodology in the construction of sustainable peasant agriculture and food sovereignty. *The Journal of Peasant Studies*, 38, 161–191. doi:10.1080/03066150.2010.538584.

Steinfeld, H. (2006). Livestock's long shadow: Environmental issues and options. Rome: FAO. Available at: www.fao.org/docrep/010/a0701e/a0701e.pdf

Steinfeld, H. & Gerber, P. (2010). Livestock production and the global environment: Consume less or produce better? *Proceedings of the National Academy of Sciences of the U.S.A.*, 107(43), 18237–18238.

Toledo, A. & Burlingame, B. (2006). Biodiversity and nutrition: A common path toward global food security and sustainable development. *Journal of Food Composition and Analysis*, 19(6–7), 477–483.

UN. (1972). Report of the first UN Conference on the Human Environment. A/CONF.48/14/Rev.1. 5–16 June 1972, Stockholm. Available at: www.un-documents.net/aconf48-14r1.pdf

UN. (1975). Report of the World Food Conference, Rome, 5–16 November 1974. United Nations, New York. Available at: www.ohchr.org/EN/ProfessionalInterest/Pages/EradicationOfHungerAndMalnutrition.aspx

UN. (1978). United Nations Conference on Desertification. Round-Up, Plan of Action And Resolutions, New York, 29 August–9 September 1977. United Nations, New York. Available at: www.ciesin.org/docs/002-478/002-478.html.

UN. (1979). Report of the UN World Water Conference in Mar Del Plata, Argentina, 14–25 March 1977. United Nations, New York. Available at: www.ircwash.org/sites/default/files/71UN77-161.6.pdf

UNEP. (2018). Sustainable Food Systems (SFS) Programme. Available at: http://web.unep.org/10yfp/programmes/sustainable-food-systems-programme

UNSD (United Nations Statistics Division). (2015). Discussion paper on principles of using quantification to operationalize the SDGs and criteria for indicator selection: EGM on the Indicator Framework. New York: United Nations Statistics Division.

Wahlqvist, M. L., Truswell, A. S., Smith, R., & Nestel, P. J. (eds) (1994). Nutrition in a sustainable environment. *Proceedings of the XV International Congress of Nutrition.* Adelaide: IUNS.

WCED (World Commission on Environment and Development). (1987). *Our common future. Report of the World Commission on Environment and Development*, (ed.) G. H. Brundtland. Oxford: Oxford University Press. Available at: www.un-documents.net/our-common-future.pdf

WMO (World Meteorological Organization). (1979). Proceedings of the World Climate Conference: A Conference of Experts on Climate and Mankind. Geneva: World Meteorological Organization. Available at: https://library.wmo.int/pmb_ged/wmo_537_en.pdf

3

EQUITY

Elisabetta Recine and Nathalie Beghin

Introduction

Reflecting on equity and food systems requires answers to some questions. How are the goods and natural resources that are necessary at all stages of the food system appropriated? And how are they distributed among different sectors of society? Are the goods and wealth that are generated from the food system fairly distributed? Are food systems contributing to greater or less social justice, and facilitation of human rights?

Equity is understood here as the opportunities and conditions of access to resources that different members of society have, not only with regard to monetary resources but also to others of varying natures. In this chapter we focus on how food systems are organised, the resulting access and sharing of resources, and the consequences of these processes that lead to greater equality among individuals, groups and countries. Logically, different outcomes can arise from specific settings and contexts, but in this chapter we will analyse these aspects from the dominant industrial food system model.

The characteristics of hegemonic food systems, based on an agroindustrial production model,[1] have been justified over the decades by the necessity to guarantee the availability of food for both the present and future billions of inhabitants of our planet. This statement is based, among other arguments, on a concept of diet that is essentially biological, where the priority is to ensure the availability of a certain amount of nutrients to meet the caloric needs of populations. According to this approach, food diversity, origin and processes that produce these nutrient needs are secondary considerations. This perspective disregards the perspective of the Human Right to Adequate Food, which states that all human beings must be free from hunger by having access to adequate food – where adequate is understood as the diversity of biological, cultural and environmental aspects involved in food (CESCR, 1999).

Similar to the Right to Adequate Food framework, healthy diets are increasingly considered in a broader picture within the academic literature, by advocacy groups and progressive policy circles. One such angle is that of sustainable diets. These are defined as:

those with low environmental impacts that contribute to food and nutrition security and to healthy life for present and future generations. Sustainable diets are protective and respectful of biodiversity and ecosystems, culturally acceptable, accessible, economically fair and affordable; nutritionally adequate, safe and healthy; while optimizing natural and human resources.

(FAO, 2012)

The operationalising of these comprehensive ideas of equity, equality, health and sustainability is observed, encouragingly, in the Brazilian Dietary Guidelines, which define an adequate and healthy diet as:

a basic human right. This right implies ensuring permanent and regular access, in a socially fair manner, to food and eating ways that satisfy the social and biological requirements of everybody. It also takes into account special dietary needs, and the needs to be culturally appropriate, and allow for differences in gender, race, and ethnicity. Adequate and healthy diet should be physically and financially accessible, and harmonious in quantity and quality, meeting the needs of variety, balance, moderation, and pleasure. Furthermore, it should derive from sustainable practices of production and distribution.

(Brazil Ministry of Health, 2012)

The argument posed in this chapter is that it is no longer possible to think of equity and food systems in a one-dimensional manner: sustainability must always be included. A sustainable food system is one that guarantees food and nutrition security for all in such a way that environmental, economic and social conditions are not compromised for current and future generations. Models of production and consumption of food can generate inequity, thus sustainability is directly related to equity.

Equity, society and the global food system

Equity is a concept derived from the theoretical framework of social justice, considering that basic needs of each human being should be fulfilled. It is important to highlight that in this chapter we use equity of *opportunities* rather than *outcomes*, which focuses on how the capability to access necessities like food is distributed within and between groups. Equity is therefore promoted when measures are taken to reduce the unfairness of opportunity to access goods and services. The reduction of inequities leads progressively to a reduction in inequalities, differences and disparities in people's living conditions, including access to nutritious foods (Norheim & Asada, 2009).

Poor diets and food and nutrition insecurity are, therefore, related to unequal and/or unfair access to food, land and territories, culture, health, education, employment, environment and other basic rights. To identify how inequity in relation to food systems generates such inequalities, it is necessary to analyse these elements from a global, regional, national or local perspective, depending on the objective. This chapter will not develop a comprehensive analysis of these elements, but will present only some aspects.

Food systems comprise the different elements of the food supply chain, food environments and consumer behaviour. These elements – which are influenced by biophysical and environmental, innovation, technology and infrastructure, political, economic, demographic and socio-cultural drivers – shape diets and determine the final nutrition, health, economic and social outcomes of food systems (HLPE, 2017). The evidence indicates that equitable food systems are not the norm.

Considering the characteristics and the practices of the dominant food systems, it is concluded that it produces huge inequalities. The challenges to understanding the food system drivers seem to centre not so much on "what to do" but mainly on "how to do it", because the concentration of economic and political power is the central determining factor of inequalities in food systems, and is generated by it. This analysis can either be done by going through the stages of the food system or by analysing the four dimensions of food security: (1) availability; (2) access; (3) utilisation; and (4) stability, through an "equity" lens. From this perspective, we can see how different forms of inequality affect food and nutrition security and how they contribute to other inequalities, perpetuating a vicious circle.

Food and nutrition insecurity is not only related to food scarcity, but also to unequal or unfair access to land and territories, culture, health, education, employment, environment and other basic rights. The structural determinants of these rights violations or, in other words, the main drivers of food insecurity, require an understanding of the drivers as any natural or human-induced factor that directly or indirectly causes a change in a system. These include the concentration of wealth and power and unequal structural discrimination, including gender-based discrimination and global warming (HLPE, 2014).

One of the main roots of inequitable diets and food systems is the power structures that define the rules by which society is organised, and decisions and priorities are established (Prato, 2014). Power structures and political relations shape numerous aspects of society, including a country's agricultural and trading systems. They set the course of food distribution and production, influencing the accessibility of various foods for different sectors of the population (Mora & Muro, 2018). The concentration of wealth has increased in recent times. According to Oxfam (Pimentel & Lawson, 2018), billionaire wealth has risen by an annual average of 13 per cent since 2010, six times faster than the wages of ordinary workers, which have risen by a yearly average of just 2 per cent. The number of billionaires rose at an unprecedented rate of one every two days between March 2016 and March 2017. Furthermore, 82 per cent of the wealth generated in 2017 went to the richest 1 per cent of the global population, while the 3.7 billion people who make up the poorest half of the world saw no increase in their wealth (Willoughby & Gore, 2018). These numbers reveal that the global economy enables the wealthy elite to accumulate vast fortunes while hundreds of millions of people are struggling to survive on poverty wages. This same phenomenon can be found in different stages of the food supply chain. Available data show that 60 per cent of the market for seeds and chemical inputs are controlled by only three conglomerates. Although most farmers in the world are small-scale, 1 per cent of rural properties occupy 65 per cent of the world's agricultural land; four companies account for 70 per cent of trade in agricultural commodities globally by revenue; 50 food manufacturers account for half of all global food sales and just ten supermarkets account for over half of all food retail sales (Willoughby & Gore, 2018). The Global North is also incorporating technology into the processes of food production and consumption that, by its nature, is often not equally accessible to different population groups and countries. Both the adoption of certain technologies and the lack of access to them, can intensify inequities and inequalities.

This concentration of wealth and power has created production patterns that disadvantage small-scale farmers, a system which results in massive inequities. Production increased after the Second World War, in conjunction with regional specialisations, into a relatively narrow range of products, a process encouraged by the growth of international trade in agriculture. The benefits were concentrated in the hands of large production units and land-holders at the expense of small-scale producers and landless workers. Monocultures not only reward economies of scale, they also give a premium to the largest land-holders who are better positioned to achieve efficiency gains in this model. This process was strongly biased in favour of the Global North; over-production in the highly subsidised farming sectors of rich countries put downward pressure on agricultural prices, relegating many small farmers to subsistence agriculture for their own consumption (as they were not competitive in the markets), and accelerating rural-to-urban migration (de Schutter, 2018).

Some authors consider that we are now in an era of: (1) dematerialisation (a process that promotes the decrease of the physical substance of food and the increase of the market value of its immaterial dimensions); (2) digitalisation (increasingly automated, delocalised and informatised processes of production and commercialisation of food); and (3) financialisation (increasing the role played by financial markets within food systems). The consequences of these processes can be observed throughout the entire food system, from production to consumption. These processes contribute to the dispossession of small local farmers' knowledge and access to resources, by widening the gap between producers and consumers, and also facilitate the concentration of economic and political power in the hands of a new set of remote actors that master information and financial means (Filardi & Prato, 2018). We can see this corporate control play out across global food supply chains (including production; storage and distribution; processing and packaging; retail and markets) (Hawkes & Ruel, 2012). The concentration of resources, knowledge and power by large agri-food businesses at each stage of the food supply chain is illustrated by the large mergers of seed companies, biotechnology and agrochemicals. Farmers and society are increasingly dependent on these corporations. The same occurs in the food processing stage where ten companies account for the bulk of the food market, employing millions of workers worldwide. This results not only in the concentration of economic power but also in decisions on working conditions and the remuneration of these workers, as well as the parameters of negotiations of inputs for production and conditions of distribution and retail, leading to various imbalances and impacts (IPES-Food, 2017; Willoughby & Gore, 2018).

Another relevant driver of inequities in the food system is the structural discriminations that can be defined as a set of practices, cultural norms and institutional arrangements that are both reflective of and simultaneously help to create and maintain exclusion processes in societies. In this sense, food insecurity predominantly affects indigenous people, traditional communities, immigrants, refugees, among other marginalised groups of the global population. These groups usually are found in the poorest segments of society. Their food insecurity is a consequence of a multi-dimensional discrimination, resulting from the combination of a set of oppressions: poverty, violence, and cultural, religious and class exclusion among others (Knuth, 2009; Elsheikh & Barhoum, 2013).

The situation is even worse for women, who are affected by the aforementioned discrimination in a multi-burden situation associated with societal patriarchy. The exclusion process happens through two main channels. One is the limits on their access to education and employment opportunities, which curtails their economic autonomy and weakens their bargaining position within the family. Their weakened bargaining position translates into little or no voice in household decisions, differential feeding and caregiving practices favouring boys and men, food and nutrition insecurity, and lower health and nutrition outcomes. Second, the discrimination they face not only exposes women to material deprivation, it also makes it more difficult for them to fulfil their vital roles in food production, preparation, processing, distribution and marketing activities. These societal and institutional mechanisms of exclusion make women particularly vulnerable to climate variability and extremes, and their vulnerability derives from restricted access to the social and environmental resources required for adaptation (de Schutter, 2012; ADB, 2013; FAO et al., 2018).

The nutrition, health and environmental consequences of inequitable food systems

The dominant food system threatens people, the environment and the planet in a vicious circle. Ultimately it consistently violates the human rights of the majority of the world's population. The absolute number of undernourished people (those facing chronic food deprivations) was nearly 821 million in 2017. These levels are similar to those almost a decade ago (FAO et al., 2018). Many of these extremely poor people are smallholder farmers and landless people who are struggling to produce food, and to live and feed their families (World Bank, 2018). Small farmers have poor access to land, natural resources, technical assistance, credit and access to markets.

Inequities in food systems affect health consequences in different ways: (1) people work in unhealthy conditions; (2) people are affected by contaminants in water, soil or air; (3) people eat foods that are unsafe for consumption; (4) people have unhealthy diets; or (5) people are food-insecure and cannot access adequate and acceptable foods at all times (IPES-Food, 2017).

According to the World Health Organization (WHO, 2017), the double burden of malnutrition is characterised by the coexistence across the life course of undernutrition along with overweight and obesity, or diet-related non-communicable diseases (NCDs), within individuals, households and populations. In the context of a changing global nutrition landscape, influenced by unbalanced power relations, structural discrimination and climate change, diet-related epidemiology has seen a significant shift in recent decades. Worldwide in 2014, more than 1.9 billion adults (aged 18 years and older) were overweight, while 462 million adults were underweight. More than 600 million adults were obese. In the same year, 41 million children under the age of 5 were overweight or obese but 155 million children were affected by stunting (low height-for-age), while 52 million children were affected by wasting (low weight-for-height). Poor nutrition continues to cause nearly half of deaths in children under 5, while low- and middle-income countries are now witnessing a simultaneous rise in childhood overweight and obesity – increasing at a rate 30 per cent faster than in richer nations. These data reveal that almost 40 per cent of the global population are affected by inadequate diets. Moreover, the relationship between undernutrition and overweight and obesity is more than coexistence. Undernutrition in early ages may predispose to overweight and non-communicable diseases, such as diabetes and heart disease, later in life. Overweight in mothers is also associated with overweight and obesity in their offspring. Rapid weight gain early in life may predispose to long-term weight excess. These are just some of the examples of biological mechanisms, which along with environmental and social influences, are increasingly understood as important challenges for the global burden of malnutrition across the life course and for the food and nutrition system.

Another consequence of the agribusiness-dominant food system is its harmful impacts on environment. The spread of monocultures has resulted in a significant loss of agrobiodiversity; native and small farmers are gradually disappearing as they are displaced by the production of rice, maize, soy bean, sugar cane, wheat, planted forests and livestock, among others. Largely as a result of unsustainable farming practices, an estimated 33 per cent of soils worldwide are moderately to highly degraded, due to erosion, nutrient depletion and loss of organic matter, acidification, salinisation, compaction and chemical pollution. The resulting loss of natural soil fertility has forced an ever greater reliance on chemical fertilisers to increase yields, but this in turn has polluted water systems.

The loss of agrobiodiversity is huge: 75 per cent of plant genetic diversity has been lost as a consequence of the abandonment of locally adapted crop varieties for the genetically uniform and high-yielding varieties. Of the 250,000–300,000 known edible plant species, humans use only 150–200 (FAO, 2004). This process reinforces the concentration of resources for production, generating economic and technological dependence. It also impoverishes healthy food sources: 75 per cent of the world's food is derived from a mere 12 plants and 5 animal species. The apparent variety and diversity of products available in supermarkets are actually based on only a few staple crops and livestock. The food industry constantly re-engineers and recombines them into a variety of highly processed products (HLPE, 2017). Populations from low socio-economic groups tend to consume these products in high quantities (HLPE 2017). The low price of ingredients, the long shelf-life, high palatability, and clever marketing strategies, among other elements, make the accessibility and affordability of these products very high. Thus, consumption of these products illustrates another consequence of inequitable food systems.

Climate change is also a consequence of the global food system, while at the same time a major challenge for food and nutrition security. The dominant industrial food system is contributing to climate change. Considering the whole food chain, 20–30 per cent of greenhouse gases from human activity are linked to how food systems function (FAO, 2016a; 2016b; de Schutter, 2018). And global warming is in turn affecting people's access to adequate food and nutrition, especially the most vulnerable (FAO et al., 2018). Global warming is worsening the living conditions of farmers, fishermen, forest-dependent people, indigenous people, women living in developing countries, poor people, refugees and migrants who are already vulnerable and food-insecure. Hunger and malnutrition are increasing. Rural communities, particularly those living in already fragile environments, face an immediate and ever-growing risk of increased crop failure, loss of livestock, and reduced availability of marine, aquaculture and forest products. More frequent and more intense extreme weather events will have adverse impacts on food availability, accessibility, stability and utilisation, as well as on livelihood assets and opportunities in both rural and urban areas. Vulnerable people will be at risk of food and nutrition insecurity due to loss of assets and lack of adequate insurance cover. Rural people's ability to cope with the impact of climate change depends on the existing cultural and policy context, as well as on socio-economic factors, such as gender, household composition, age, and the distribution of household assets. Humans, plants, livestock and fish will be exposed to new pests and diseases that flourish only at specific temperatures and humidity. This will pose new risks for food security, food safety and human health (FAO, 2016a).

Priority actions going forward

Addressing the structural inequities in food and nutrition systems requires structural changes in the development model:

- the adoption of people-centred strategies of inclusion and sustainability;
- the articulation of a broader set of policies in different sectors;

- the establishment of accountability mechanisms;
- stronger governance with civil society participation to guarantee that food as a human right and a common good will be respected, protected and promoted (Prato, 2014).

The identification of characteristics that generate inequities throughout the food system points to strategies that will help reduce these inequities, as summarised in Table 3.1.

Another dimension of the food system is the *food environment*. This is defined as the physical, economic, political and socio-cultural context in which consumers engage with the food system to make their decisions about acquiring, preparing and consuming food. The key elements of the food environment that influence consumer food choices, food acceptability and diets are: (1) physical and economic access to food (proximity and affordability); (2) food promotion, advertising and information; and (3) food quality and safety (Caspi, Sorensen, Subramanian, & Kawachi, 2012; Hawkes et al., 2015; HLPE, 2017). Improved food environments would enable all consumers to purchase and consume more nutritious and healthy foods (Table 3.2).

TABLE 3.1 Examples of strategies that will enable more equitable food systems

Rights violations	Strategies
Land-grabbing	Promote access to land and natural resources for small producers, indigenous peoples and traditional communities
Intensive production of commercial crops	Protect the food heritage, protect and promote socio-biodiversity: ways of living and producing, protect and promote access to genetic diversity, health standards appropriate to the modes of production, control the use of pesticides and transgenic seeds, expansion of agro-ecological transition and organic production
Women's rights violations	Promote gender equity, recognition of the economic role of women's work, access to credit, resources for production, social equipment for childcare, division of domestic work, implement affirmative actions
Violations of the rights of vulnerable groups (indigenous people, traditional communities, migrants, etc.)	Implement affirmative actions, recognition of the values of different cultures, guarantee equitable access to education, transportation, housing, employment, and health care to all citizens, address the institutional discrimination in order to eliminate structural barriers to exclusion
Food supply oligopolisation	Access to markets for small farmers, short production and consumption circuits

Source: Based on HLPE (2017).

TABLE 3.2 Examples of strategies to influence consumers' more equitable food choices

Factors that influence consumers' food choice	Strategies
Accessibility and affordability	Short circuits, local markets to eliminate food deserts; food policies to guarantee access to healthy food (school feeding programmes, for example), public procurements, taxes, subsidies, trade policies
Knowledge, values and practices	Food and nutrition education to generate critical capacity and autonomy, labelling, control of marketing

Source: Based on HLPE (2017).

Brazil: an example of what can be achieved and reflections on the sustainability of the results

Although the agro-industrial model generates, on the one hand, sectors of great economic and political power, on the other, the environmental, social and economic consequences are undeniable, which increases opportunities for transformation. There is now a greater understanding of the interconnection of different aspects. This set of consequences in different aspects of human life generates potential for articulating agendas within different sectors of civil society and intersectoral actions within the public sector.

Until recently, Brazil was a good example. The Brazilian trajectory for guaranteeing food and nutritional security is connected to the process of understanding the roots of inequalities and hunger in the country, exemplified in a memorable way in the book, *Geography of Hunger*, by Josué de Castro in the 1950s (de Castro, 1952). The findings demonstrated the consequences in life, health and nutritional status related to the existing economic model that had generated public policies, such as the parameters for minimum wage definition, the composition of a basic food basket, and school feeding programmes, among others (Batista Filho & Soares, 2017).

More recently, in the process of democratisation following the military dictatorship, between the 1980s and the 1990s, hunger, food prices and access to land and territories were issues that mobilised civil society organisations. The Brazilian Forum on Food and Nutrition Security and Sovereignty (FBSSAN) was created by bringing together non-governmental organisations (NGOs), social movements and academics. The federal government implemented several intersectoral strategies to fight hunger, misery and poverty (President Itamar Franco's Plan to Fight Hunger, 1993 and 1994, and the Solidarity Community Program of President Fernando Henrique Cardoso, 1995–2002).

In 2003, with the election of President Lula, the theme of hunger gained a new central position with the elaboration and adoption of the Zero Hunger Programme. The programme proposed a series of actions in different sectors throughout the food system. At the same time, the National Council for Food and Nutrition Security (CONSEA) was established, which brought together representatives from civil society (two-thirds of the members). On the government side were represented all the sectors involved in actions to realise the human right to adequate food of the population in general, and of the most vulnerable, in particular. Agriculture, family farming, agro-ecology, environment, education, health, human rights, racial and ethnic equality, among others, were all members of the Council. CONSEA's civil society representatives were characterised by the diversity and representativeness of the different segments of Brazilian society: indigenous peoples, traditional communities, family farmers, urban movements and researchers. CONSEA reported directly to the president of the Republic, presenting analyses and proposals and was in direct dialogue with the Inter-ministerial Chamber of Food and Nutritional Security (CAISAN). Among its responsibilities were the proposal and monitoring of the guidelines and priorities of the Policy and the National Plan for Food and Nutrition (Caspi, Sorensen, Subramanian, & Kawachi, 2012).

The participation of the most diverse sectors of Brazilian society in the process of analysis, definition of priorities and proposal of actions contributed to the important results that Brazil achieved, in little more than a decade, to reduce hunger and poverty, especially among the most vulnerable. Between 2001 and 2015, Brazil saw a reduction in poverty from 26.6 per cent to 6.6 per cent, and a reduction in extreme poverty from 10.6 per cent to 2.7 per cent. By giving visibility to the demands of these groups and, moreover, by opening the dialogue for the proposals from different stakeholders, it was possible to do the following:

- implement actions that not only reduced inequalities but also protected the socio-biodiversity;
- defend the genetic and intangible heritage of these groups;
- regulate territories for traditional communities;
- open up markets to small-scale farmers;
- expand funding and technical assistance for organic and agro-ecological production.

The articulation of programmes directly related to food and nutrition security with macroeconomic measures increased the level of income and access to food of the Brazilian population to the point that in 2014, Brazil was no longer cited among the FAO Hunger Map countries (FAO, 2014; Silva et al., 2018; Vasconcelos et al., 2019).

In 2019, with the election of an extreme right-wing government, averse to social participation and critical of the idea of human rights, this experience came to an end. President Jair Bolsonaro's first measures included CONSEA's removal as well as the reorganisation of several sectors of the federal public administration that negatively affected the access of poor families to health, education, social assistance and pensions. In addition, measures have been implemented that threaten the rights of indigenous peoples, the protection of the environment and socio-biodiversity, and access to land for family farmers, among others.

Conclusion

Healthy and sustainable food systems are directly linked to equity. The degree of inequity indicates the parameters by which a society is structured and the model of development adopted. Today's global food system is neither equitable nor sustainable. It constantly violates the human rights of the majority of the world's population. The ways in which the food system contributes to inequity is through the dispossession of peasants' knowledge and access to resources; widening the gap between producers and consumers, and facilitating the concentration of economic and political power in the hands of a new set of remote corporate actors who control information and financial means.

The determinants of inequalities in outcomes of food and nutrition insecurity are therefore the concentration of wealth and power, the structural discrimination that excludes billions of people, including poor women, and increasing environmental degradation. In other words, the dominant food system threatens people, the environment and the planet in a vicious circle.

To overcome this situation, it is necessary to implement structural changes in the development model with the adoption of people-centred strategies of inclusion and sustainability; the articulation of a broader set of policies in different sectors; the establishment of accountability mechanisms; stronger governance with civil society participation to guarantee that food as a human right and a common good will be respected, protected and promoted.

Note

1 That is based on the production side, on monoculture, mechanisation, consumption of GMO seeds, fertilisers and pesticides. And on the supply side, on the massive expansion of supermarkets and similar facilities offering industrially produced food.

References

ADB (Asian Development Bank). (2013). Gender equality and food security: Women's empowerment as a tool against hunger. Mandaluyong City, the Philippines: Asian Development Bank. Available at: www.fao.org/wairdocs/ar259e/ar259e.pdf (accessed 16 March 2019).

Batista Filho, M., & Arlindo Soares, J. (2017). The "Geography of Hunger" legacy. *Revista Brasileira Saúde Materna Infantil*, 17, 213–214.

Brazil Ministry of Health. (2012). *Dietary guidelines for the Brazilian population*. Brasília: Ministry of Health, p. 150.

Caspi, C., Sorensen, G., Subramanian, S. & Kawachi, I. (2012). The local food environment and diet: A systematic review. *Health & Place*, 18(5), 1172–1187.

CESCR (Committee on Economic, Social and Cultural Rights). (1999). General comment 12: The right to adequate food. Geneva: United Nations. Available at: www.fao.org/fileadmin/templates/right tofood/documents/RTF_publications/EN/General_Comment_12_EN.pdf (accessed 16 March 2019).

de Castro, J. (1952). *Geography of hunger*. 1st edn. Boston: Little, Brown & Company.

de Schutter, O. (2012). Women's rights and the right to food. New York: United Nations General Assembly. Available at: www.srfood.org/images/stories/pdf/officialreports/20130304_gender_en.pdf (accessed 16 March 2019).

de Schutter, O. (2018). The political economy of food systems reform. *European Review of Agricultural Economics*, 44, 705–731. doi:10.1093/erae/jbx009

Elsheikh, E., & Barhoum, N. (2013). *Structural racialization and food insecurity in the United States*. Berkeley, CA: University of California. Available at: https://haasinstitute.berkeley.edu/sites/default/files/Structural%20Racialization%20%20%26%20Food%20Insecurity%20in%20the%20US-%28Final%29.pdf (accessed 16 March 2019).

FAO (Food and Agriculture Organization). (2004). What is agrobiodiversity? Fact sheet. Rome: Food and Agriculture Organization. Available at: www.fao.org/3/a- y5609e.pdf (accessed 16 March 2019).

FAO. (2012). Sustainable diets and biodiversity: Directions and solutions for policy, research and action. Rome: Food and Agriculture Organization. Available at: www.fao.org/docrep/016/i3004e/i3004e.pdf (accessed 16 March 2019).

FAO. (2014). The state of food insecurity in the world: Strengthening the enabling environment for food security and nutrition. Rome: Food and Agriculture Organization. Available at: www.fao.org/3/a-i4030e.pdf (accessed 16 March 2019).

FAO. (2016a). Climate change and food security: Risks and responses. Rome: Food and Agricultural Organization. Available at: www.fao.org/3/a-i5188e.pdf (accessed 16 March 2019).

FAO. (2016b). Energy, agriculture and climate change: Towards energy-smart agriculture. Rome: Food and Agriculture Organization. Available at: www.fao.org/3/a-i6382e.pdf (accessed 16 March 2019).

FAO, IFAD, UNICEF, WFP, & WHO. (2018). The state of food security and nutrition in the world 2018. Building climate resilience for food security and nutrition. Rome: Food and Agriculture Organization. Available at: www.fao.org/3/I9553EN/i9553en (accessed 16 March 2019).

Filardi, M., & Prato, S. (2018). Reclaiming the future of food: Challenging the dematerialization of food systems. when food becomes immaterial: confronting the digital age. Buenos Aires: Global Network for the Right to Food and Nutrition. Available at: www.righttofoodandnutrition.org/files/rtfn-watch-2018_eng.pdf (accessed 16 March 2019).

Hawkes, C., & Ruel, M. (2012). Value chains for nutrition: Reshaping agriculture for nutrition and health. International Food Policy Research Institute. Available at: http://ebrary.ifpri.org/utils/getfile/collection/p15738coll2/id/124831/filename/124832.pdf (accessed 16 March 2019).

Hawkes, C., Smith, T., Jewell, J., Wardle, J., Hammond, R., … Kain, J. (2015). Smart food policies for obesity prevention. *The Lancet*, 385(9985), 2410–2421.HLPE (High Level Panel of Experts). (2014). Food losses and waste in the context of sustainable food systems. A report by the High Level Panel of Experts on Food Security and Nutrition of the Committee on World Food Security. Rome: High Level Panel of Experts. Available at: www.fao.org/3/a-i3901e.pdf (accessed 16 March 2019).

HLPE. (2017). Nutrition and food systems. A report by the High Level Panel of Experts on Food Security and Nutrition of the Committee on World Food Security. Rome: High Level Panel of Experts. Available at: www.fao.org/3/a-i7846e.pdf (accessed 16 March 2019).

IPES-Food (International Panel of Experts on Sustainable Food Systems). (2017). Too big to feed: Exploring the impacts of mega-mergers, consolidation and concentration of power in the agri-food sector. Brussels: International Panel of Experts on Sustainable Food Systems. Available at: www.ip es-food.org/images/Reports/Concentration_FullReport.pdf (accessed 16 March 2019).

Knuth, L. (2009). The right to adequate food and indigenous peoples. How can the right to food benefit indigenous peoples?Rome: FAO. Available at: www.fao.org/3/a-ap552e.pdf (accessed 16 March 2019).

Mora, A., & Muro, P. (2018). Inequality and malnutrition. Advancing equity, equality and non-discrimination in food systems: Pathways to reform. *United Nations System Standing Committee on Nutrition*, 43, 15–24. Available at: www.unscn.org/uploads/web/news/UNSCN-News43-WEB.pdf (accessed 16 March 2019).

Norheim, O., & Asada, Y. (2009). The ideal of equal health revisited: Definitions and measures of inequity in health should be better integrated with theories of distributed justice. *International Journal for Equity in Health*, 8(40), 1–9.

Pimentel, D., & Lawson, M. (2018). Reward work, not wealth to end the inequality crisis, we must build an economy for ordinary working people, not the rich and powerful. Oxford: Oxfam. Available at: https://www.oxfam.org/en/research/reward-work-not-wealth (accessed 16 March 2019).

Prato, S. (2014). The struggle for equity: Rights, food sovereignty and the rethinking of modernity. *Development*, 57(3 4), 311–319.

Silva, A., Recine, E., Johns, P., Gomes, F., Ferraz, M., & Faerstein, E. (2018). History and challenges of Brazilian social movements for the achievement of the right to adequate food. *Global Public Health*. https://doi.org/10.1080/17441692.2018.1439516.

Vasconcelos, F., Machado, M., Medeiros, M., Neves, J., Recine, E., & Pasquim, E. (2019). Public policies of food and nutrition in Brazil: From Lula to Temer. *Revista de Nutrição*, 32, 1–13.

WHO (World Health Organization). (2017). The double burden of malnutrition. Policy brief. Geneva: World Health Organization. Available at: http://apps.who.int/iris/bitstream/handle/10665/255413/WHO-NMH-NHD-17.3-eng.pdf?ua=1 (accessed 16 March 2019).

Willoughby, R., & Gore, T. (2018). Ripe for change: Ending human suffering in supermarket supply chains. Oxford: Oxfam. Available at: https://policy-practice.oxfam.org.uk/publications/ripe-for-cha nge-ending-human-suffering-in-supermarket-supply-chains-620418 (accessed 16 March 2019).

World Bank. (2018). Poverty and shared prosperity 2018: Piecing together the poverty puzzle. Washington, DC: International Bank for Reconstruction and Development. Available at: https://openknowledge. worldbank.org/bitstream/handle/10986/30418/9781464813306.pdf (accessed 16 March 2019).

PART II

The food system

4

FOOD SYSTEM MODELS

John Ingram

Introduction

A food system comprises all the processes involved in keeping a population fed (Global Panel, 2016). The term "food system" is now frequently used in discussions about nutrition, health, development, environment and in the food industry. However, depending on the purpose for which it is used, it is variously taken to include some or all of the processes and infrastructure involved in feeding a population. A number of definitions therefore emphasise that food systems produce food, that they are made up of a broad set of activities from production to consumption and that they are influenced by external social, political and other drivers (Herforth & Ahmed, 2015).

Building on early agricultural economics literature, the food system concept has emerged over several decades. Writing in 1970, Padberg discussed the need for greater consumer protection for the "modern industrialized food system", noting how the food system was "vastly different" to that of only a generation earlier (Padberg, 1970). Shaffer goes on to explore some ideas and problems concerning a conceptual framework for organising knowledge of the relationship between political-economic organisation and performance (Shaffer, 1980). Driven by social and political concerns in 1990s, rural sociologists promoted a food systems approach (e.g. McMichael, 1994; Tovey, 1997), and several authors put forward frameworks for analysing food systems. Sobal et al. (1998), however, noted that few existing models broadly described the system and most focused on one disciplinary perspective or one segment of the system. They identified four major types of models: (1) food chains; (2) food cycles; (3) food webs; and (4) food contexts, and developed a more integrated approach, including nutrition. Dixon (1999) meanwhile proposed a cultural economy model to understand power in commodity systems, while Fraser et al. (2005) proposed a framework to assess the vulnerability of food systems to future shocks based on landscape ecology's 'Panarchy Framework'.

Despite these varied approaches, none were suitable for drawing attention to, let alone analysing the intricate interactions among, the wide range of aspects that are involved in achieving (or not) food security (Ingram, 2011). Driven by a heightened interest in the potential risks to food security due to climate change and other environmental and socio-economic stresses, researchers started to develop a more integrated approach that was more suitable for analysing the combined impacts of multiple, interacting stresses on food systems. As the adaptation agenda grew, an enhanced ability to analyse the consequences of different strategies on a range of other societal goals became increasingly important. Examples include income, rural development, employment, health, landscape, ecosystem services and animal welfare. This was particularly required for research in global environmental change which had hitherto largely focused on the impacts of climate change on agricultural yield and agro-ecology (Gregory et al., 1999).

Furthermore, while noting that the principal role of food systems is to deliver food security (i.e. stability of access to, and availability and utilisation of food, as distinct to just production), there was growing interest in their other socio-economic and environmental foods system drivers and outcomes (Ericksen, 2008; Ingram, 2011). A more integrated approach was hence developed (GECAFS, 2005; Ingram, Steffen, & Canadell, 2007) which recognised that the dynamics of change processes are particularly important in transforming food systems to deliver better social, economic and environmental outcomes (Geels, 2004). Food systems are, however, highly complex. They are classic examples of complex adaptive systems, with many interactive socio-economic and environmental drivers and feedbacks. They encompass a set of dynamic actors and activities with a wide range of power and vested interests operating under fragmented governance. There are, however, many policy, fiscal, social and technical options for change and many options for cooperation between actors. Understanding this and managing the change process require a systematic approach and conceptual models of the system are fundamental in disentangling the complexity.

A review of conceptual models of a food system

Food security is a primary societal goal, as noted in the widely cited definition stemming from the 1996 World Food Summit: "when all people, at all times, have physical, economic and social access to sufficient, safe, and nutritious food to meet their dietary needs and food preferences for an active and healthy life" (FAO, 1996; FAO, WFP, & IFAD, 2012) (Figure 4.1a). This goal is underpinned by food systems, and a number of conceptual models of varying complexity have been put forward to help provide a structured, analytical lens to research the highly complex food security agenda. They have built up from encompassing only the activities and outcomes to also include the drivers and feedbacks more representative of the complex adaptive, socio-ecological systems that are food systems. They often now also include the range of biophysical, socio-economic and political food system drivers across and along spatial, temporal and jurisdictional scales (Cash, 2006). Commonly used attributes therefore now include *activities, actors, drivers* and *outcomes*.

Activities include growing, harvesting or catching, packing, processing, transforming, transporting, marketing, consuming and disposing of food. This set is often termed the "food chain" or "value chain" (Gómez et al., 2011; Brown et al., 2015). *Actors* include all the people directly involved in the activities, e.g. the farmers, processors, retailers and consumers (Garnett, 2014). *Drivers* include the social, policy, technical, economics and environmental conditions that influence the behaviour of the actors and their decision-making (Swinburn, Egger, & Raza, 1999; Francis & Swoboda, 2016). *Outcomes* include the wide range of food security and other socio-economic and environmental factors resulting from the activities (Ericksen, 2008; Gustafson et al., 2016).

Perhaps the most fundamental approach is to link a number of activities with a number of outcomes as shown in Figure 4.1b. This diagrammatic representation has the advantage of simplicity, but several activities (comprising both many other actors and research communities) have

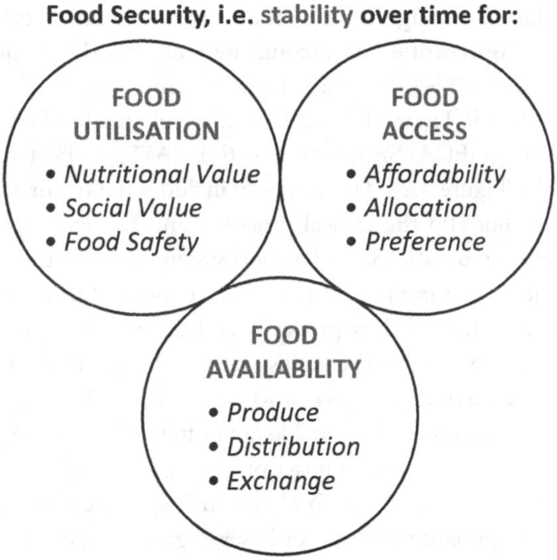

Food Security, i.e. stability over time for:
FOOD UTILISATION
• Nutritional Value
• Social Value
• Food Safety
FOOD ACCESS
• Affordability
• Allocation
• Preference
FOOD AVAILABILITY
• Produce
• Distribution
• Exchange

FIGURE 4.1a The three components, and their respective major elements, of food security, all of which need to be stable over time.
Source: Ingram (2011).

Food System ACTIVITIES
Storing
Transporting Trading
Producing
Processing/ Packaging
Wholesaling/ retailing
Consuming
Disposing/ Reusing
Food System OUTCOMES
Contributing to:
Social Welfare
• Income
• Employment
• Wealth
• Social capital
• Political capital
• Human capital
• ---
Food Security
Food Utilisation
Food Access
Food Availability
Environment
• Climate change
• water availability
• Water quality
• Biodiversity
• Biogeochemistry
• Soil degradation
• ---

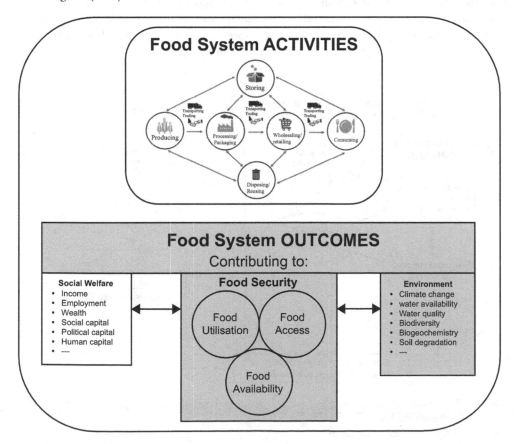

FIGURE 4.1b The combined notions of food system activities leading to a range of outcomes.
Source: Adapted from Ericksen (2008).

to be understood as included: fishing, hunting, food service, catering, cooking are all missing. Similarly, while high-level aspects of each outcome are included, the model gives no indication of scales or levels, drivers or feedbacks inherent in the system.

The basic model identified in Figure 4.1 was further developed by the Global Environmental Change and Food Systems (GECAFS) programme (GECAFS, 2005) to show the interaction with drivers and feedbacks (Figure 4.2). This not only includes the major activities and outcomes involved in food systems, but also the critical processes and factors influencing the social and environmental outcomes that are also part of a food system. It links these to help identify the nature of the outcomes at a point in time or space. This builds upon the idea that, within complex systems, it is possible to identify key processes and determinants that influence outcomes (Ericksen, 2008). A key development is the inclusion of both drivers and feedbacks to represent the dynamic nature of the system. It is important to note that, while much of the future of food security literature discusses the impact of a variable (and often this is a change in climate or water availability), it generally only discusses the impact on primary production. This model therefore serves as a reminder that, in reality: (1) the food system is subjected to the *interaction* of several variables, all of which are important to greater or lesser degrees depending on the circumstances; and (2) the determinants of food security are more than primary production. It also helps remind us that any intervention aimed at, e.g. improved nutrition or business goals will also have environmental consequences. Similarly, interventions aimed at reducing greenhouse gas emissions, or reducing pesticide usage through the use of genetically modified organisms will have socio-economic consequences, often these will be affordability or social acceptance. While this helps to identify potential synergies and trade-offs across societal goals, it does not include interactions across spatial, temporal and jurisdictional levels other than by inference.

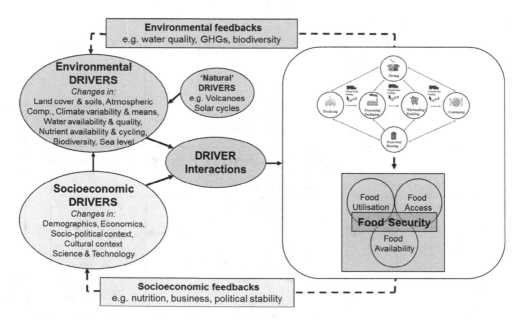

FIGURE 4.2 A food systems conceptual model developed specifically for global environmental change studies

Source: Adapted from Ericksen (2008).

Food systems are fundamentally underpinned by natural resources. A different food system conceptual model was developed by the United Nations Environment Programme's (UNEP) International Resources Panel specifically to analyse the impact of food system activities on such resources (UNEP, 2016). The model (Figure 4.3) was built on the premise that producing food in the form of agriculture or fisheries clearly depends on renewable resources, such as land, biodiversity, fresh water and marine resources, as well as on non-renewable resources, such as fossil fuels and minerals. However, it also notes that other food system activities (i.e. post-farm gate ones) also depend on natural resources. For instance, food processing on water; packaging on paper, card and aluminium; distributing and cooling on fossil fuels; cooking on fossil fuels and biomass.

Impacts on natural resources are clearer than in Figure 4.2, with clearer mechanisms of how food system activities draw on natural resources, and the consequent overall environmental effect. One advantage of this approach is to demonstrate the nature of impacts; the mechanism needs to be clear to be able to identify effective mitigation strategies. Feedback processes directly related to natural resources are included, but the wider feedbacks from food security outcomes to overarching socio-economic drivers are not.

Figure 4.4 shows a similar conceptual model to that of GECAFS, developed by the TransMango project (Brunori et al., 2015). Their approach made two contributions to Figure 4.2. First, they included an analytical distinction of natural and human-made assets, on which the food system activities draw. Second,

> [They] opened up the black box of regulative, normative and cognitive institutions by making the nature of institutional processes and their role in coordination of the dynamic interplay between food system activities, actors and assets an integral part of the analysis.
>
> *(Brunori et al., 2015)*

An improved understanding of how food systems operate will help food security planning by identifying where, when and how vulnerability arises, and hence what sorts of adaptation

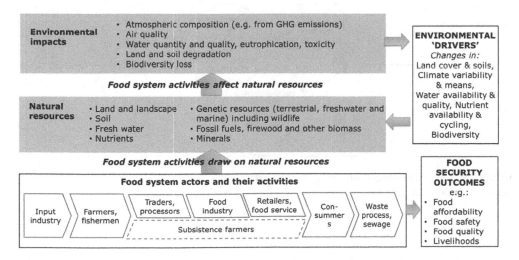

FIGURE 4.3 A food systems model developed to analyse impacts on natural resources
Source: Adapted from UNEP (2016).

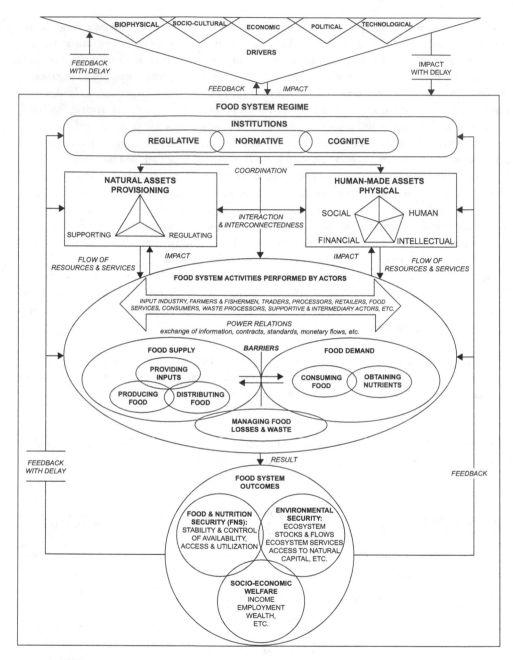

FIGURE 4.4 The TransMango conceptual framework
Source: Brunori et al. (2015).

interventions are needed, and where and when they would be most effective. The Trans-Mango conceptual framework aimed to assess the vulnerability of the food system to shocks and stresses in an integrated way by identifying outcomes to be avoided together with their root causes and dynamic pressures (vulnerability context) and pathways leading to them. The model therefore mapped these factors explicitly.

A further refined conceptual framework was developed by the EU project, "Metrics, Models and Foresight for European SUStainable Food And Nutrition" (SUSFANS; Figure 4.5). The overall SUSFANS objective is to build the conceptual framework, using the evidence base and analytical tools to underpin EU-wide food policies with respect to their impact on consumer diet and their implications for nutrition and public health in the EU, showing the impact on the environment, the competitiveness of the EU agri-food sectors, and global food and nutrition security. In this case, therefore, the aim was to develop a food system conceptual model specifically for EU policy goals (see bottom left of Figure 4.5). The basic food system activities and outcomes (cf. Figure 4.1b) are in the bottom right, and there is a first loop feedback via the direct drivers, making a sub-system. This sub-system leads to an estimation of performance (top right) against the stated policy goals, and this then leads to the goals themselves. The goals affect the work of the policy-makers and non-government organisations (NGOs) (the food system influencers), which in turn influences the first loop sub-system, thereby creating a second loop. The performance (top right in Figure 4.5) against the stated policy goals also affects higher-order indirect drivers (top left of Figure 4.5), thereby creating a third loop feedback. This nested set of feedbacks allows a range of direct and indirect actors and other interested parties to engage most effectively by *systematically* addressing what is a highly complex system.

Yet a different approach was taken by researchers working with the International Life Sciences Institute's Research Foundation "Center for Integrated Modeling of Sustainable Agriculture and Nutrition Security" (CIMSANS) project (Acharya, Fanzo, Gustafson, Ingram, & Schneeman, 2014) (Figure 4.6), again for a different purpose. This conceptual model was designed to identify the proximal causes of malnutrition, i.e. those consuming too few calories or nutrients, or those consuming too many calories for their physiological needs. Here the constraints on dietary choice and diversity, the post-farm gate activities, and the determinants of primary production were hierarchically linked, but also noting the wide-ranging feedbacks in the system as moderated by the social, political, business, science and technology and biophysical environments. Unlike the many models for addressing food insecurity based on the productionist paradigm, this model starts with the reasons for malnutrition and then works backwards through the food chain to the determinants of primary production. Given the major role access to food has in nutrition outcomes (Ingram, 2017), this model is better suited to discussions based on the World Food Summit definition above.

Akin to the CIMSANS conceptual model, the Global Panel on Agriculture and Food Systems for Nutrition (GLOPAN) developed a model aimed at explaining diet quality (Global Panel, 2016) (Figure 4.7). While the nested approach of this model illustrates well how diet is influenced by consumer attributes and food environment, there is no indication of feedback to the food supply system, which provides the overall context.

Finally, a different approach is to define the food system as a "dendritic cluster" of value chains (Reardon et al., 2018). They see these as linking: (1) input suppliers to farmers ("farm input value chains"); (2) farmers upstream to wholesalers and processors midstream, to retailers, then consumers downstream ("farm output value chains"); (3) "lateral service value

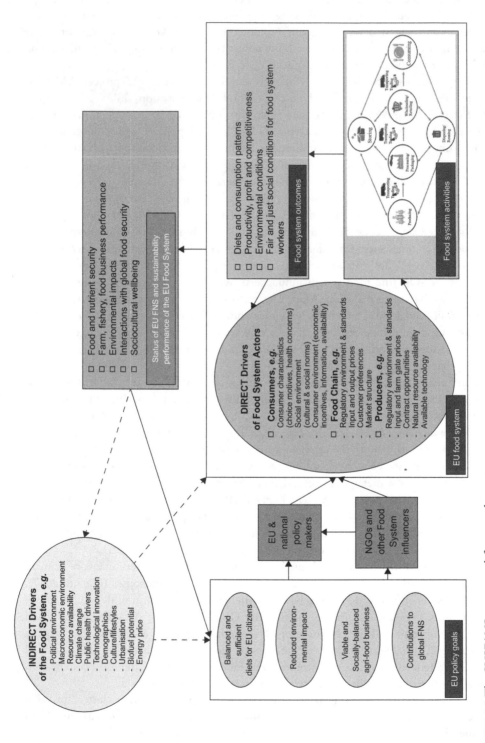

FIGURE 4.5 The SUSFANS conceptual framework

Source: From Zurek et al. (2016).

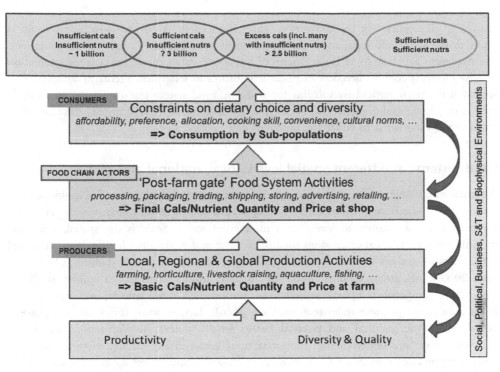

FIGURE 4.6 The CIMSANS framework
Source: Adapted from Acharya et al. (2014) and Ingram and Porter (2015).

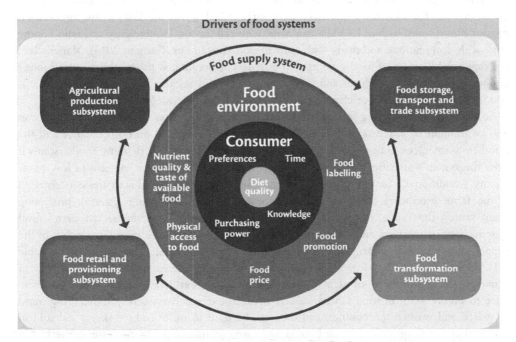

FIGURE 4.7 The GLOPAN conceptual framework for the links between diet quality and food systems
Source: Global Panel (2016).

chains" to all segments of the above two value chains (such as the transport supply chain as input to the wholesale segment of the output value chain); and (4) research, development, and extension suppliers to all the segments of the above value chains (such as the generation of new crop varieties by breeders in research institutes to extension agents to farmers). This approach has been particularly valuable for analysing food system transformation increasingly seen across the developing world, because, as Devaux et al. (2018) argue, standard value chain analysis has failed to tackle the problems in a holistic way.

Food systems at different spatial levels: local, national and global

A fundamental aspect of food systems is their inherent complexity due to the multiplicity of actors, feedforwards and feedbacks. A further reason for their complexity is the fact they function across a number of levels on a number of scales. Scale is the spatial, temporal, quantitative, or analytical dimensions used to measure and study any phenomenon, and level is the units of analysis that are located at different positions on a scale (Gibson, Ostrom, & Ahn, 2000; Cash, 2006). Depending on the situation, food systems span a number of different scales (e.g. spatial, temporal, jurisdictional, institutional, management) and a number of levels along each of these scales (e.g. national, global; days, seasons) (Ericksen et al., 2010). Social, economic, cultural and political factors largely determine interactions along and between scales, and understanding the interactions between and among them is critical to understanding the controls on food security; multi-scale, multi-level approaches are needed to complement the range of conceptual models discussed above.

There are still many cases where a major aspect of the food system is local, mostly in the developing world, where food chains are shorter and less complex. Some sections of society elsewhere aim for local food initiatives such as the Fife Diet in the UK, in overtly political peasant movements, such as La Via Campesina, who call for food sovereignty and who oppose large-scale corporations, and many within the organic movement (Garnett, 2014). Nonetheless, the rapid globalisation of food systems seen over recent decades, with greatly enhanced inter-connectivity between producer and consumer nations and regions, re-emphasises the spatial and social variability as major characteristics of globalisation (Marsden & Arce, 2017).

So, rather than classifying food systems only in terms of level on the spatial scale, they can also be thought of in terms of level along a complexity scale based on both distance and the number of interactions or nodes involved. Hence, a key element in defining food systems is how the system's activities and actors are linked to each other. Hence, systems of low complexity ("traditional") have a relatively short supply chain, with several activities concentrated at the farm: producing crops and animal products (in mixed farming systems), processing them within the home, and trading the raw and/or processed products. "Modern" food systems have many more areas of specialisation among activities and increase the length of the supply chain (UNEP, 2016) "Intermediate" food systems exhibit elements of each (Table 4.1). Irrespective of the degree of complexity, all food systems include the same set of activities, but the intensity of each varies according to context. For instance, and with reference to Figure 4.1b, in rural Ghana, cassava is cultivated and harvested (producing), ground or grated and washed (processing), and then can be fried to make *gari* (cooking) and sold in the market (retailing) before being bought and eaten (consuming). In contrast, in the UK, a simple modern food system dinner of cook-at-home pizza will have required all the same food system activities to have been completed, albeit at a more complex and intense manner.

TABLE 4.1 Main features of "Traditional", "Intermediate" and "Modern" food systems

Food system feature	'Traditional' food systems	Intermediate food systems	'Morden' food systems
Estimated number of people in system	-1 billion	-4 billion	-2 billion
Principal employment in food sector	In food production	In food production	In food processing, packaging and retail
Supply chain	Short, local; small-scale structures	Short to longer, supply chain has typically more actors than in 'modern' food systems	Long with many food miles and nodes; consolidation in input, processing and food retail segment; transnational companies and chains
Supply chain coordination system	Ad-hoc, spot exchange	Mainly ad-hoc, spot exchange	Contracts, standards, vertical integration
Food production system	Diverse, mixed production system (crops and animal production), varied productivity; low input farming systems. Food systems are the main source of energy	Combination of diverse, mixed production system and specialised operations with a certain degree of inputs, including fossil fuels	Few corps dominate (e.g. monoculture); specialisation and high productivity; high external input intensity, including fossil fuels. Food production consumes more energy than it delivers.
Typical farm	Family-based, small to moderate	Combination of small-holder farms and larger farms/fishery operations	Industrial, larger than in a traditional settings
Typical food consume	Basic locally-produce stables	Combination of basic products and processed food	Larger share of proceeds food with a brand name, more animal products
Food bough from	Small, local stop or market	Small local stop or market, share of supermarkets small but rapidly growing	Predominantly large supermarket chain, food service and catering (out of home)
Nutritional concern	Undernutrition	Both undernutrition and diet-related diseases	Diet-related diseases
Main source of national food shocks	Production shocks	International price and trade problems	International price and trade problems
Main source of household food shocks	Production shocks	International shocks leading to food poverty	International shocks leading to food poverty
Major environmental concern	Soil degradation, land clearing, water shortage	Combination of concerns in traditional modern systems	Emission of nutrients and pesticides, water demand, greenhouse gas emissions, and others due to fossil fuel use
Influential scale	Local to national	Local to global	National to global

Source: (UNEP, 2016).

Conclusion

Food system models help us to identify, map and analyse the interactions between the actors and their drivers, including each actor's activity, the outcomes of this activity, and the possibilities for, and consequences of, interventions. The models can be used in many applications. Governments can use them to help formulate food policy by assessing the probable efficacy and costs of e.g. regulation, taxes and subsidies. Food businesses can use models to instigate better practices to improve the nutrition and environmental impact of their products, while maintaining vibrant enterprises. Non-governmental organisations and civil society groups can use them to develop stronger arguments for advocacy and lobbying. And researchers can use them to identify areas for further work (Ingram, 2017).

The ability to develop food systems to enhance food security while meeting other societal goals, such as reducing the environmental footprint, would be increased if policy and technical options were considered more specifically in terms of complexity as well as spatially. This is, however, challenging, due to the diversity of stakeholder groups operating at the range of levels (e.g. government and NGOs; researchers and research funders; and business and civil society), all of whom have their own objectives (Liverman & Ingram, 2010). Furthermore, there are numerous interactions with higher and lower levels on these and other scales, such as temporal. Insufficient knowledge and awareness of actions taken at these other levels often lead to scale challenges (Cash, 2006), and food system conceptual models are an important tool in identifying how to capitalise on positive interventions and avoid unforeseen negative outcomes.

It is, however, important to use the most appropriate model for a given situation. This means being clear about the purpose (i.e. the objectives), the framing (e.g. which worldviews and/or type of user), the boundary (i.e. what is included and what is not); and their limitations (i.e. the major assumptions, omissions and/or uncertainties).

The chapters that follow in Part II will elaborate on the healthy and sustainable food systems components described in this chapter. In particular, each will focus on the prominent challenges being faced and the solutions available for the following system components to collectively achieve healthy and sustainable food systems: food production; food manufacturing; food retail and distribution; food service and restaurants; and food consumption.

References

Acharya, T., Fanzo, J., Gustafson, D., Ingram, J., & Schneeman, B. (2014). *Assessing sustainable nutrition security: The role of food systems.* Washington, DC: ILSI Research Foundation, Center for Integrated Modeling of Sustainable Agriculture and Nutrition Security.

Brown, M., Antle, J., Backlund, P., Carr, E., Easterling, W., Walsh, M., ... Tebaldi, C. (2015). *Climate change, global food security, and the U.S. food system.* Washington, DC: USDA.

Brunori, G., Bartolini, F., Avermaete, T., Brzezina, N., Mathijs, E., Marsden, T., ... Sonnino, R. (2015). Transmango Project: Assessment of the impact of global drivers of change on Europe's food and nutrition security (FNS), D2. Available at: transmango.wordpress.com/output

Cash, D. W., Adger, W. N., Berkes, F., Garden, P., Lebel, L., Olsson, P. ... Young, O. (2006). Scale and cross-scale dynamics: Governance and information in a multilevel world. *Ecology and Society*, 11(2), 8.

Devaux, A., Torero, M., Donovan, J., & Horton, D. (2018). Agricultural innovation and inclusive value-chain development: A review. *Journal of Agribusiness in Developing and Emerging Economies*, 8(1), 99–123.

Dixon, J. (1999). A cultural economy model for studying food systems. *Agriculture and Human Values*, 16(2): 151–160.

Ericksen, P. J. (2008). Conceptualizing food systems for global environmental change research. *Global Environmental Change*, 18, 234–245.

Ericksen, P. J., Stewart, B., Dixon, J., Barling, D., Loring, P. … & Ingram, J. (2010). The value of a food system approach. In J. Ingram, P. Ericksen, & D. Liverman (eds), *Food security and global environmental change*. London: Earthscan.

FAO (Food and Agriculture Organization). (1996). *Report of the World Food Summit*. Rome: FAO.

FAO, WFP, & IFAD. (2012). The state of food insecurity in the world: Economic growth is necessary but not sufficient to accelerate reduction of hunger and malnutrition. Rome: FAO.

Francis, C., & Swoboda, A. (2016). Evaluating the impacts of food systems. *Journal of Agriculture, Food Systems, and Community Development*, 6(2), 307–310.

Fraser, E., Mabee, W., & Figge, F. (2005). A framework for assessing the vulnerability of food systems to future shocks. *Futures*, 37(6): 465–479.

Garnett, T. (2014). Three perspectives on sustainable food security: efficiency, demand restraint, food system transformation. What role for life cycle assessment? *Journal of Cleaner Production*, 73, 10–18.

GECAFS. (2005). Science plan and implementation strategy. In J. S. I. Ingram, P. J. Gregory, & M. Brklacich (eds), *Earth system science partnership (IGBP, IHDP, WCRP, DIVERSITAS) Report No. 2*. Wallingford: CAB.

Geels, F. W. (2004). From sectoral systems of innovation to socio-technical systems: Insights about dynamics and change from sociology and institutional theory. *Research Policy*, 33(6–7), 897–920.

Gibson, C. C., Ostrom, E., & Ahn, T. K. (2000). The concept of scale and the human dimensions of global change: A survey. *Ecological Economics, 32*(2), 217–239.

Global Panel. (2016). Food systems and diets: Facing the challenges of the 21st century. Available at: www.glopan.org

Gómez, M., Barrett, C., Buck, L., De Groote, H., Ferris, S., Gao, H., … Pell, A. (2011). Research principles for developing country food value chains. *Science*, 332(6034), 1154–1155.

Gregory, P. J., Ingram, J. S. I., Goudriaan, J., Hunt, T., Landsberg, J., Linder, S. … Valentin, C. (1999). Managed production systems. In B. H. Walker, W. L. Steffen, J. Canadell, & J. S. I. Ingram (eds), *The terrestrial biosphere and global change: Implications for natural and managed ecosystems*. Cambridge: Cambridge University Press, pp. 229–270.

Gustafson, D., Gutman, A., Leet, W., Drewnowski, A., Fanzo, J., & Ingram, J. (2016). Seven food system metrics of sustainable nutrition security. *Sustainability*, 8(3), 196.

Herforth, A., & Ahmed, S. (2015). The food environment, its effects on dietary consumption, and potential for measurement within agriculture-nutrition interventions. *Food Security*, 7(3), 505–520. doi:10.1007/s12571–12015–0455–0458.

Ingram, J. (2011). A food systems approach to researching food security and its interactions with global environmental change. *Food Security*, 3(4), 417–431.

Ingram, J. (2017). Perspective: Look beyond production. *Nature*, 544(7651), S17.

Ingram, J. S. I. (2011). From food production to food security: Developing interdisciplinary, regional-level research. PhD thesis, Wageningen University.

Ingram, J. S. I., & Porter, J. R. (2015). Plant science and the food security agenda. *Nature Plants*, 1, 15173. doi:10.1038/nplants.2015.173.

Ingram, J. S. I., Steffen, W. L., & Canadell. J. (2007). Envisioning Earth system science for societal needs: The development of joint projects and the Earth System Science Partnership (ESSP). GECAFS Working Paper 6. Oxford: GECAFS.

Liverman, D., & Ingram, J. (2010). Why regions? In J. Ingram, P. Ericksen, & D. Liverman (eds), *Food security and global environmental change*. London: Earthscan.

Marsden, T., & Arce, A. (2017). The social construction of international food: A new research agenda. *The rural*. London: Routledge, pp. 87–106.

McMichael, P. (ed.) (1994). *The global restructuring of agro-food systems*. Ithaca, NY: Cornell University Press.

Padberg, D. I. (1970). Consumer protection for a modern industrialized food system. *American Journal of Agricultural Economics*, 52(5), 821–828. doi:10.2307/1237717.

Reardon, T., Echeverria, R., Berdegué, J., Minten, B., Liverpool-Tasie, S., Tschirley, D., & Zilberman, D. (2018). Rapid transformation of food systems in developing regions: Highlighting the role of agricultural research and innovations. *Agricultural Systems*. Available at: www.gldc.cgiar.org/wp-con tent/uploads/2018/05/Carberry-IFLRC18.pdf

Shaffer, J. D. (1980). Food system organization and performance: Toward a conceptual framework. *American Journal of Agricultural Economics, 62*(2), 310–318. doi:10.2307/1239706.

Sobal, J., Khan, L. K., & Bisogni, C. (1998). A conceptual model of the food and nutrition system. *Social Science & Medicine*, 47, 853–863.

Swinburn, B., Egger, G., & Raza, F. (1999). Dissecting obesogenic environments: The development and application of a framework for identifying and prioritizing environmental interventions for obesity. *Preventive Medicine*, 29(6), 563–570.

Tovey, H. (1997). Food, environmentalism and rural sociology: On the organic farming movement in Ireland. *Sociologia Ruralis*, 37(1), 21–37. doi:10.1111/1467–9523.00034.

UNEP. (2016). *Food systems and natural resources. A report of the Working Group on Food Systems of the International Resource Panel*. New York: UN.

Zurek, M., Ingram, J., Zimmermann, A., Garrone, M., Rutten, M., Tetens, I., … Deppermann, A. (2016). A framework for assessing and devising policy for sustainable food and nutrition security in the EU: The SUSFANS conceptual framework. *Sustainability*, 10(11), 4271.

5

FOOD PRODUCTION

*Mario Herrero, Daniel Mason-D'Croz, Jessica Bogard and
Mark Howden*

Introduction

Over the past 50–60 years, the global food system has seen significant changes, transforming
to meet growing and shifting demands from a global population that has grown from around
3 billion in 1960 to 7.3 billion in 2015 (UN, 2018), and a global economy that expanded
from US$11 trillion to more than US$75 trillion in 2010 (World Bank, 2018).

The transformation of food production during this time period was driven in part by the
Green Revolution, a package of technological innovations that increased agricultural productivity through the expansion of irrigation and the increasing application of mechanisation,
chemical inputs and improved breeding and farm management. This increase in productivity,
for example, by a factor between fourfold and sevenfold for the major crops since 1961
(FAO, 2019a), has reduced the demand for agricultural area expansion that would otherwise
have been needed (Ramankutty et al., 2018). Despite the productivity gains, total agricultural
land still increased by more than 4.1 million km^2 globally (about 9 per cent compared to
1961 levels), with the increase split about evenly between additional cropland and pasture
(FAO, 2018). Figure 5.1, from Ramankutty and colleagues, using FAOSTAT data, highlights
the historical drivers of increased global agricultural production by commodity, 1961–2014.
Figure 5.2 and Figure 5.3, also from Ramankutty and colleagues, show the trends in agricultural land-use by region.

Broad economic development has seen increasing productivity economy-wide leading to
urbanisation and industrialisation. The shifting allocation of resources across sectors has led to
increasing complexity and diversity of national economies (Reardon et al., 2018), with the
share of total economic activity accounted for by agriculture declining, even as agricultural
GDP has grown significantly. For example, at the start of the Green Revolution (the early
1970s), agriculture, forestry and fishing accounted for 37 and 42 per cent of GDP for South
Asia, and East Asia and Pacific respectively. By 1990, this had declined to 27 and 25 per cent,
even as agricultural GDP had increased by 61 and 114 per cent for South Asia and East Asia
and Pacific respectively (World Bank, 2018). Globally, agriculture now contributes between
3 and 4 per cent of global GDP, even as it still is a major source of employment (more than

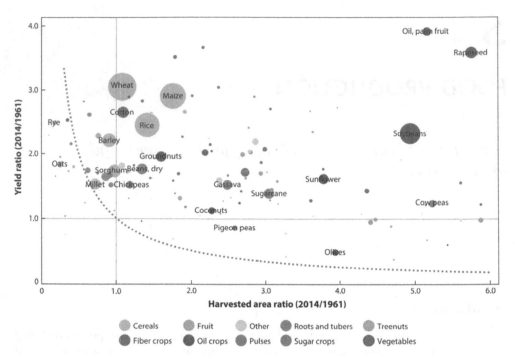

FIGURE 5.1 Trends in global harvested area and yields, 1961–2014
Source: (Ramankutty et al., 2018).

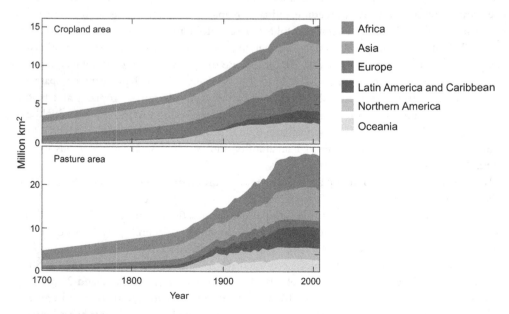

FIGURE 5.2 Summary of historical changes in cropland and pasture area, 1700–2014
Source: (Ramankutty et al., 2018).

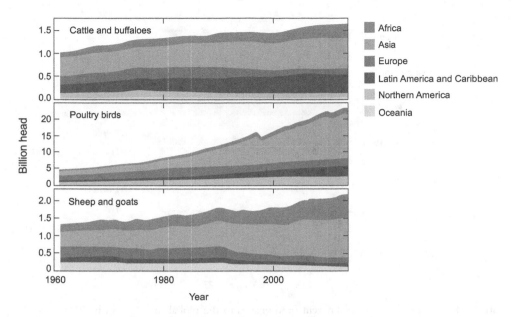

FIGURE 5.3 Summary of historical changes in livestock numbers, 1961–2014
Source: (Ramankutty et al., 2018).

25 per cent of all jobs are in the agriculture sector), particularly in the Global South, where employment in agriculture in 2015 in Sub-Saharan Africa, South Asia, and East Asia and Pacific was 57, 45, and 25 per cent respectively.[1]

Global economic development has raised living standards, impacting dietary patterns as wealthier consumers increasingly demand higher value and more resource-intensive agricultural commodities, such as animal source foods (meat, eggs, and dairy) and fruits and vegetables (Pingali, 2007; Clements & Si, 2017; Reardon et al., 2018). Economic development has also led to increasing demand for highly processed and discretionary foods, with growing demand for sugar and vegetable oils. Advances in other sectors have expanded the range of agricultural markets, as agricultural products increasingly are used as inputs for non-food purposes, such as industrial starches, biofuels, cosmetics and bioplastics. Figure 5.4 shows the increasing complexity of the global food system, and the contributions of key food system outcomes by food group.

The Livestock Revolution – as termed by Delgado and colleagues (Delgado, Rosegrant, Steinfeld, Ehui, & Courbois, 2001) – has for the most part been realised, as the growing demand for animal source foods (ASFs) has been a major driver of changes in agricultural production. In response to the growing demand for ASFs, particularly since 1990 as Chinese economic development began to take off, global production of ASFs has increased by more than 60 per cent (FAO, 2018). This increase in production has restructured and realigned much of agricultural production to provide key cereals and oil meals as inputs to the livestock sector, rather than for direct consumption by humans.

The increasing complexity of agricultural value chains, such as for the production of ASFs, is hinted at by global averages, where increasingly additional cereal demand is being driven by livestock feed and other demands. Between 1961 and 2015, globally 56 per cent of the

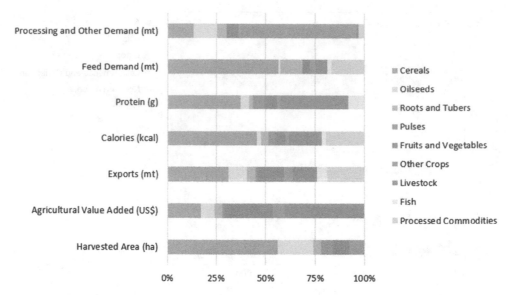

FIGURE 5.4 The contributions of different food groups to the global food system in 2015
Notes: Fish and processed commodity data were not available in the FAO's agricultural added value data set.
Source: Based on data from FAOSTAT Commodity Balance Sheets and Agriculture Added Value (FAO, 2018).

additional cereal demand came from non-direct food demand. In developed countries, over this time period, 80 per cent of increased cereal demand was from non-food demand, whereas direct food demand was still the main driver in increased cereal demand in developing regions like Africa (66 per cent) and Southern Asia (78 per cent). Faster-growing economies in the Global South have already begun to transition towards more complex food systems similar to developed countries (Reardon et al., 2018), and with economic projections suggesting continued economic development in Africa and Asia (Riahi et al., 2017), we can expect this transition to be consolidated in the coming decades.

The growing complexity of agricultural value chains has also seen increasing integration of regional and global agricultural markets with agricultural trade flows growing dramatically. This increasing integration is occurring while or even as most agricultural production is being consumed or processed first domestically. International agricultural trade is characterised primarily as regional, with trade taking place between nearby neighbours and with only a few major agricultural producers dominating global trade flows. Table 5.1 summarises some of the trends by region since 1960.

This transformation has not been without cost. The expansion has contributed to global greenhouse gas emissions through both land-use change (e.g. deforestation), increasing numbers of animals in the livestock sector (in particular, cattle) and increasing resource intensity (i.e. fertilisers). While the food system is not the largest contributor, it is a significant source of greenhouse gases and may contribute between 11–32 per cent of emissions, depending on estimation methodology and whether land-use is included (Tilman et al., 2014; Wollenberg et al., 2016). Area expansion and intensification put many additional pressures on the environment beyond greenhouse gas emissions, including increasing pressure

TABLE 5.1 Summary of trade trends for selected regions

Region	1960–1990	1990–present
World	Agricultural production (crop and livestock) more than tripled. With crop and ASF exports increasing fourfold and threefold respectively. In raw terms, these increases were driven mostly by cereal exports, which accounted for more than half of the increase of global agricultural exports. The fastest growth in exports globally during this period was seen for vegetable oils, which increased from 3 million tons to 23 million tons over the time period.	Agricultural production growth slows compared to the previous 30 years, although is still robust. Trade continues to increase at a faster rate than production, doubling between 1990 and 2010. Cereals continue to dominate in raw terms, but the rise of oil crops and vegetable oils hinted at in the previous time period become more prevalent. Trade in ASFs becomes a bigger part of the equation with meat exports nearly tripling from 14 to 42 million tons.
East and Southeast Asia	The region sees significant increases in agricultural production. However, population growth and demand grew faster as the region saw net agricultural imports increase across the region, with net imports as a share of agricultural production increasing from around 1–3 per cent. The region sees significant increases in cereal imports, but also see sees large increases in exports of vegetable oils, and starchy roots and tubers.	The rise of China dominates the region. Rapid economic growth in China spurs on demand for agricultural commodities, with net imports increasing from 3 per cent to close to 5 per cent of production, even as agricultural production in the region more than doubled. The region bifurcates, as China becomes a major importer, even as Southeast Asia increasingly becomes a major exporter of agricultural produce for Chinese markets. Agricultural value chains deepen and become more complex. Southeast Asia becomes a major producer of key crops for industrial biofuels (palm) and starches (cassava for tapioca) demanded in China and Europe. East Asia, while being a net importer of agricultural commodities, still sees significant increases in exports of fruits and vegetables.
Southern Asia	Southern Asia begins and ends the period as a net importer of agricultural commodities. Significant gains in agricultural productivity (cereal production more than doubles) are not sufficient to match growing demand. The region sees net imports of agricultural commodities increase.	South Asia continues being a net importer of agricultural commodities, but as a share of production imports they stay steady from 1990 and 2010. The region becomes a net exporter of animal source foods, driven in large part from increased exports of milk and meat from India, which saw a significant increase in dairy production, and a muted increase in meat demand.
Africa	Africa begins the period as a small net exporter of agricultural commodities. It sees smaller productivity gains from the Green Revolution as compared to Asia and Latin America and, by 1990, Africa has become a net importer of agricultural commodities, particularly of cereals.	Agricultural production nearly doubles between 1990 and 2010. However, this continued to be insufficient to meet growing demand, which exceeded production by around 13 per cent. The region is a net exporter of many cash crops, including fruits and vegetables to Europe, and coffee, tea and cacao to global markets.

Region	1960–1990	1990–present
Latin America and the Caribbean	Started the period as a small net export of agricultural commodities. Exports of oil crops increased dramatically, due to large increases in soybean production in Brazil and Argentina. The region also saw rapid increase in exports of fruits and vegetables to supply growing demand in North America and, to a lesser extent, Europe.	Latin America consolidates its position as a major source of global exports, led by the expansion of agricultural production in Brazil and Argentina. Exports grew at a faster pace than agricultural production, in part to satisfy the dramatic increase in demand for agricultural commodities from China. Cereals, oil crops, and fruits continue being key exports. Sugar and vegetable oils also increasingly become important, particularly as Brazil becomes a major player in biofuels.
Europe and North America	Contributed two-thirds of the global increase in crop and ASF exports. Meat exports increased significantly from around 2 million tons to 9.5 million tons. Oilseed, vegetable oil, and sugar exports grew significantly, reflecting shifts towards more processed foods, and more intensive livestock production processes in developed countries. High incomes in the region also lead to increasing imports of fruits and vegetables.	The region continues being an important source of agricultural trade. However, the share of global trade originating in the region declines significantly with the rise of Latin America, and China. The region continues to be a major exporter of cereals and oil crops, as well as ASFs. The region also increases its imports of fruits and vegetables, at the same time as the region also increased imports of sugar and vegetable oils.

Source: Authors' analysis based on detailed trade statistics from FAOSTAT (FAO, 2018).

on ground and surface water supplies, water pollution from agricultural runoff, air pollution from over-application of fertilisers, degrading ecosystems leading to biodiversity loss, to name a few examples. The food system threatens the environmental safe operating space in which human society has evolved (Rockström et al., 2009), putting at risk the gains realised over the past 50 or more years.

Local, national and regional variations in food production

The nature of agriculture and food production varies widely throughout the world and is shaped by environmental factors (such as climate, topography and soil quality), as well as economic factors (such as access to technology and inputs), and sociocultural factors related to dietary patterns. All of these factors affect not only what is produced but also productivity, quality, variability, the scale of farm enterprises and the economics of production (Figure 5.5). Large farms (>50 hectares) dominate production systems in North and South America, Australia and New Zealand, while small and medium farms produce the majority of major food groups globally, and very small farms (<2 hectares) contribute about 30 per cent of agricultural production in parts of Asia and Sub-Saharan Africa (Herrero et al., 2017).

Despite this diversity across regions, there is, however, a global trend towards increasing homogeneity in production systems over time, whereby national food supplies are becoming more similar (Khoury et al., 2014). This reduction in diversity is being driven by a number of factors related to both food supply and demand, including trade liberalisation, the globalising nature of food industries, transitions towards more Western diets and the standardisation and

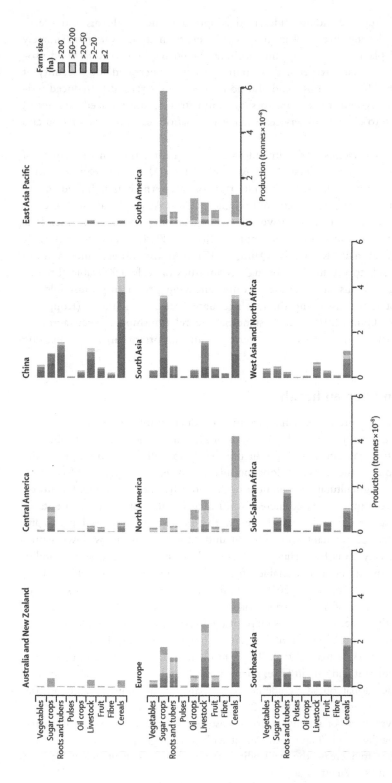

FIGURE 5.5 Distribution of production of key commodity groups by region and farm size
Source: (Herrero et al., 2017).

modernisation of agriculture, including widespread adoption of new cultivars and breeds often at the expense of locally diverse plant and animal genetic material. Of approximately 6,000 edible cultivated plant species, only nine account for 66 per cent of total food production (FAO, 2019b). In many respects, these transitions have increased food security at local and national levels. However, this trend also poses several risks related to reduced resilience within production systems to respond to shocks and stresses, and reduced capacity of agriculture to contribute to ecosystems services, such as pollination, carbon sequestration and pest control (FAO, 2019b) .

Diversity of production systems is also linked to dietary quality, though the nature of this relationship is highly context-dependent. At a global scale, the increasing homogeneity of production systems related to the adoption of Western diets is linked to the growing prevalence of overweight, obesity and related NCDs. At the local level, greater on-farm production diversity can improve dietary quality of household members who rely on their own produce for consumption (Jones, 2014; Jones, Shrinivas, & Bezner-Kerr, 2014; Koppmair, Kassie, & Qaim, 2017). On the other hand, a more market-oriented approach to production through economies of scale achievable through less diverse production systems can increase income, allowing producing households to purchase a diversity of foods (assuming there is adequate access to markets) (Koppmair et al., 2017; Sibhatu & Qaim, 2018). Understanding the relationship between agrobiodiversity and human nutrition across scales remains an important area for ongoing research.

Food production and human health

There are multiple pathways through which agricultural production influences human health. Most directly, through the nutritional quality of foods produced and how they contribute to dietary patterns and nutritional status. Food production has historically focused on producing sufficient and cheap food for the growing global population in terms of quantity (Swinburn et al., 2019). To this end, agricultural development in the latter half of the twentieth century, through the Green Revolution, saw rapid increases in the availability of energy-dense staple foods, particularly wheat, maize and rice. However, the benefits of increased per capita energy consumption and the resultant reductions in undernourishment across low-income countries have been partially offset by declines in nutritional quality, with reduced availability and affordability of micronutrient-rich vegetables, fruit, pulses, nuts and seeds (IFPRI, 2002; Gómez et al., 2013; Mason D'Croz et al., 2019). This focus on staple foods at the expense of dietary diversity is a key driver of micronutrient malnutrition globally.

At the other end of the scale, global oversupply of energy-rich staple cereal and oil crops has also contributed to the proliferation of low-cost, energy-dense, nutrient-poor, ultra-processed foods (Headey & Alderman, 2019). These foods tend to be high in saturated fat, sodium and free sugar content and low in fibre, micronutrients and phytochemicals, and are a significant driver of the global obesity epidemic and related non-communicable diseases (Monteiro, Moubarac, Cannon, Ng, & Popkin, 2013).

This imbalance in oversupply of starchy, energy-dense staples and undersupply of micronutrient-rich foods is highlighted in Figure 5.6. Albeit with some regional variation, there is a clear need for agriculture to increase the availability of nuts, legumes, fruit, vegetables and fish to support healthy diets (Willett et al., 2019).

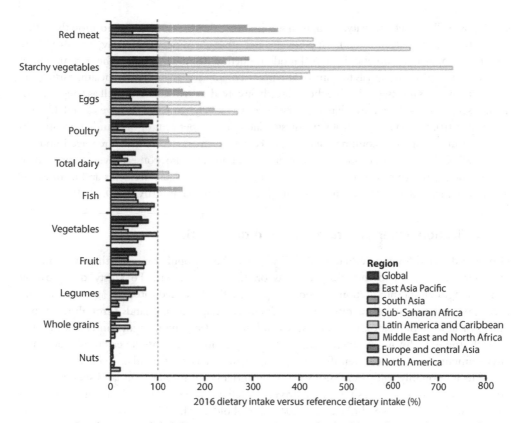

FIGURE 5.6 Gap between global dietary patterns in 2016 and a healthy reference dietary intake
Source: (Willett et al., 2019).

Analysis indicates that the nutritional inadequacies of the food supply will likely continue into the future, with the consequences disproportionately affecting some regions more than others (Nelson et al., 2018). Under a "business-as-usual" scenario of moderate socio-economic growth, availability of carbohydrates and protein remain in more than adequate supply globally to 2050, however, key micronutrients such as iron, calcium, vitamin A and vitamin B12 are lacking in low- and middle-income countries. On the other hand, oversupply of saturated fat and sugar, which are harmful to health when consumed in excess, also persist, particularly in high-income regions, though with relatively greater increases in lower-income countries. Even under a scenario of rapid and equitable economic growth in the poorest regions with concomitant diversification of diets (and supply-side responses from agriculture), food production will continue to fail to provide the basis for healthy diets into the future, if current trends continue.

Agricultural production also influences human health through food safety, and environmental and occupational health of those directly involved in agricultural production. Food safety hazards include biological, chemical or physical contaminants and can be introduced at any stage of the food supply chain, including agricultural production. Under warm and humid conditions, mycotoxins can proliferate on crops (both pre- and post-harvest), posing a significant risk to humans both directly and indirectly through consumption of animal products following feed contamination (Wu, Groopman, & Pestka, 2014). Exposure to these mycotoxins is linked to various forms of cancer, as well as acute toxicity, compromised immune function and impaired growth. Other concerns relate to contamination from pesticides and other chemical agents, heavy metals and the use of hormones and antibiotics in animal food production (IAASTD, 2009). The transmission of infectious diseases from animals to humans also poses a significant risk to human health, particularly as farming systems intensify, both for those directly involved in production as well as consumers of animal-source foods. Foodborne illness has been conservatively estimated to have caused 420,000 deaths in 2010, and 33 million disability adjusted life years; 98 per cent of this burden occurred in low- and middle-income countries, and 40 per cent was experienced by children aged under 5 years (WHO, 2015). Occupational deaths in agriculture are also conservatively estimated at 170,000 deaths per year, related to machinery- and equipment-related accidents and from exposure to chemicals, animal diseases, toxic agents and ergonomic hazards (IAASTD, 2009).

Intensification, extensification and land degradation

Growing demand for agricultural production, due to both population growth and economic development, has led to increasing impacts on the environment. To satisfy this growing demand, agricultural production has both expanded the land dedicated to agricultural purposes (extensification) and increased the productivity of agricultural lands through the application of new technologies, including seeds and increased chemical inputs (intensification).

Both these pathways to increasing agricultural production, however, have had their environmental impacts. Extensification is a major driver of land-use change, which accounts for roughly half of emissions from the agriculture, forestry and land sectors (FAO, 2019c). Extensification is also a major driver of deforestation, habitat degradation and loss and biodiversity loss (Newbold et al., 2015; Newbold et al., 2016; Griscom et al., 2017; Tilman et al., 2017). The expansion of agriculture additionally has had significant impacts on biodiversity, both by decreasing the size of the ecosystems that species occupy, and increasingly fragmenting these ecosystems into smaller and more isolated areas. Land-use change is not uniform globally. Some high-income regions, such as Europe, are in the process of reversing agricultural land expansion (Mather, 2002). However, significant deforestation, driven by agricultural extensification, continues in many tropical and sub-tropical regions of South America, Africa, Southeast Asia and Australia (Laurance, Sayer & Cassman, 2014; WWF, 2015; Griscom et al., 2017).

While agricultural extensification has played a role in increased agricultural production, since 1960, the majority of additional agricultural production is due to increased agricultural productivity (Byerlee, Stevenson, & Villoria, 2014). Unlike agricultural extensification, which is generally seen as having negative environmental impacts, the impacts of agricultural intensification are more mixed. Increased productivity of land and labour over time has been considered one of the major drivers of industrialisation, urbanisation and economic development, leading to significant changes to economies and societies, with both positive and negative impacts. Intensification has helped to reduce food prices and ultimately reduce food insecurity globally. Increased agricultural productivity has also likely eased pressures on agricultural land expansion on average, even though it may have encouraged deforestation and expansion on the agricultural frontier (Stevenson, Villoria, Byerlee, Kelley, & Maredia, 2013). Increasingly intense use of agricultural areas, however, have also added additional environmental burdens. Agriculture is the primary user of freshwater, globally accounting for 70 per cent of freshwater withdrawals, and 90 per cent of consumptive uses

(Siebert et al., 2010). Irrigated agriculture contributed significantly to unsustainable groundwater withdrawal, which not only threatens to deplete groundwater resources in many regions (Gleeson, Wada, Bierkens, & van Beek, 2012; Wada, van Beek, & Bierkens, 2012), but may contribute directly to sea-level rise (Wada et al., 2010). Agriculture is also a significant source of water pollution, with runoff of nitrogen and phosphorus negatively impacting aquatic ecosystems (Diaz & Rosenberg, 2008), and leaching reducing the quality of groundwater resources that are key sources of drinking water (Hansen, Thorling, Schullehner, Termansen, & Dalgaard, 2017). Nitrogen fertiliser use is also a significant source of GHG emissions, specifically nitrous oxide, as well as ammonia, which is the main driver of acid rain. Nitrogen fertilisers, additionally, are significant sources of local air pollution (PM2.5) in intensive agricultural areas of Europe, the USA, and China (Bauer, Tsigaridis, & Miller, 2016). Still, evidence suggests, that in many places the sustainable intensification of agriculture and livestock systems is the lesser of the two evils for driving agricultural production growth (Garnett et al., 2013; Balmford et al., 2018), as long as environmental pollution, animal welfare, biodiversity, and social welfare are improved in the process.

Many agricultural systems are subject to some form of degradation which reduces the potential biological productivity of land or reduces the quality of production. These arise through the interaction of proximate and often highly contextual physical, chemical, biological and human factors which can themselves be a function of larger-scale drivers, such as climate change or economic or social systems. Specific processes can include *inter alia* soil erosion by water or wind, acidification, salinisation, compaction, surface sealing, nutrient and carbon depletion, waterlogging and deposition (e.g. shifting dunes). Degradation can also arise from pollution by heavy metals, pesticides and other chemicals, by woody thickening or through changes in biological composition (either loss of critical components or introduction of pest plants or animals). Degradation processes can occur in either intensive or extensive systems and they can operate over very short time-scales (e.g. storm-driven erosion) or long timescales (e.g. dryland salinisation).

The framing and definition of degradation have been contested over a significant period leading to very different estimates of the consequences of degradation on agricultural systems. One estimate using remote sensing indicated that biological productivity is declining on 22–24 per cent of global land area (Bai, Dent, Olsson, & Schaepman, 2008) with soil degradation potentially reducing crop yields by up to 25 per cent in some regions (Bindraban et al., 2012), thereby increasing yield gaps and reducing food security. In terms of soil erosion rates on agricultural fields, these are between 16 and 360 times greater than soil formation rates (Montgomery, 2007). Degradation also increases the variability of the food supply (particularly in response to climate events) requiring action and investment at other points in the food system (e.g. storage) to compensate so as to meet the stability dimension of food security.

Climatic changes affect degradation by influencing many of the processes listed above. For example, observed and projected increases in rainfall intensity (IPCC, 2014) and other climate changes are highly likely to increase the rates of water erosion (Li & Fang, 2016) and other degradation processes, resulting in yield reductions in addition to those caused directly by climate changes (Bindraban et al., 2012). In other cases, climate change may reduce the degradation risk, particularly in cool temperate regions where potential biomass production may increase. Degradation can also contribute to climate changes by emissions of CO_2 from soils and biomass, via albedo changes which raise the temperature and through changes in the hydrological cycle.

The degradation of agricultural systems is heavily influenced by both tactical and strategic risk management decisions in response to climate, financial, technological, policy and other factors. Best practice risk management can reduce the degradation risk but not remove it. Mismatches between expectations of system biomass production and other performance metrics and the actual risk profiles appear to be a contributing factor in some degradation events (McKeon, Hall, Henrey, Stone, & Watson, 2004). In other cases, degradation is driven by critical needs (e.g. food access during drought), illustrating the need for highly contextual responses so as to help provide healthy and sustainable food systems.

Climate change: impacts, adaptation and mitigation

Climate variability has historically been the major factor driving variability in the availability of most foodstuffs and in relation to the degradation of the natural resource base on which a sustainable food system depends. Climate variability affects several aspects of food production at different scales. For example, at the plant level, phenological stages such as flowering are sensitive to changes in mean temperatures, as well as night-time temperatures or degree days. At the plot level, yields are partly determined by inter-annual and intra-seasonal rainfall variability. At more aggregated levels, it has been shown that in countries largely dependent on agriculture, GDP fluctuates in similar cyclical cycles to those of rainfall. Climate variability is, however, harder to project than mean climate, and there is significant uncertainty on how it might evolve in the future. Table 5.2, from Thornton and colleagues (Thornton, Ericksen, Herrero, & Challinor, 2014), shows the observed and projected changes of key climate variability indicators.

There is increasing evidence that climate change is already affecting crop yields at both global (Challinor et al., 2014) and national scales, e.g. Hughes, Lawson, & Valle (2017). Broadly, these impacts are negative, particularly so for wheat and maize and for the tropical and Mediterranean zones. Projections of crop yields for the forthcoming decades have considerable uncertainty arising from both the climate and crop modelling capacities and their combination. Nevertheless, our understanding of the interactions of the underlying crop physiology and management would suggest a high degree of confidence that in the absence of adaptation, crop yields will be reduced via: (1) higher temperatures that will shorten the growth periods of most annual crops; (2) supra-optimal temperatures for growth and reproduction, especially in the tropics and mid-latitudes which will damage pollination and seed set; and (3) decreased water use efficiency due to increased vapour pressure deficit, which will reduce crop yield per unit water used (Porter et al., 2014). Additionally, projections of decreased rainfall in the sub-tropics and mid-latitudes will tend to reduce productivity of both dryland and irrigated agricultural systems (the latter because of issues with availability) and likely increased rainfall variability and increase in the frequency and magnitude of climate extremes will reduce the stability dimension of food security. In contrast, there are some prospects for increased production in cold-climate agriculture due to lessening of climate constraints, although these gains are likely to be limited by soil and land-use constraints. Broadly, these reductions in yields tend to increase over time to the end of this century and they are particularly problematic for many developing nations (Porter et al., 2014). Similar patterns of response arise for livestock systems although they are less studied than cropping systems (Rivera-Ferre et al., 2016). Climate change is also likely to act as a threat multiplier in relation to many of the issues of land degradation raised above (e.g. rainfall intensity and

TABLE 5.2 Summary of observed and projected changes of five climate extremes at a global scale

Variable/phenomenon	Observed changes since 1950	Attribution of observed changes	Projected changes up to 2100
Temperature	Very likely* decrease in number of unusually cold days and nights. Very likely increase in number of unusually warm days and nights. Medium confidence in increase in length or number of warm spells or heatwaves in many regions. Low or medium confidence in trends in temperature extremes in some sub-regions due either to lack of observations or varying signal within sub-regions.	Likely anthropogenic influence on trends in warm/cold days/nights globally. No attribution of trends at a regional scale with a few exceptions.	Virtually certain decrease in frequency and magnitude of unusually cold days and nights. Virtually certain increase in frequency and magnitude of unusually warm days and nights. Very likely increase in length, frequency, and/or intensity of warm spells or heatwaves over most land areas.
Precipitation	Likely statistically significant increases in the number of heavy precipitation events in more regions than those with statistically significant decreases, but strong regional and sub-regional variations in the trends	Medium confidence that anthropogenic influences have contributed to intensification of extreme precipitation at the global scale	Likely increase in frequency of heavy precipitation events or increase in proportion of total rainfall from heavy falls over many areas of the globe, in particular, in the high latitudes and tropical regions, and in winter in the northern mid-latitudes
El Niño and other modes of variability	Medium confidence in past trends towards more frequent central equatorial Pacific El Niño-Southern Oscillation (ENSO) events. Insufficient evidence for more specific statements on ENSO trends.	Anthropogenic influence on trends in North Atlantic Oscillation (NAO) is about as likely as not. No attribution of changes in ENSO.	Low confidence in projections of changes in behaviour of ENSO and other modes of variability because of insufficient agreement of model projections
Droughts	Medium confidence that some regions of the world have experienced more intense and longer droughts, in particular, in southern Europe and West Africa, but opposite trends also exist	Medium confidence that anthropogenic influence has contributed to some observed changes in drought patterns. Low confidence in attribution of changes in drought at the level of single regions due to inconsistent or insufficient evidence.	Medium confidence in projected increase in duration and intensity of droughts in some regions of the world, including southern Europe and the Mediterranean region, central Europe, central North America, Central America and Mexico, northeast Brazil, and southern Africa. Overall low confidence elsewhere because of insufficient agreement of projections.

Variable/phenomenon	Observed changes since 1950	Attribution of observed changes	Projected changes up to 2100
Floods	Limited to medium evidence available to assess climate-driven observed changes in the magnitude and frequency of floods at the regional scale. There is low agreement on this evidence, and so low confidence at the global scale regarding even the sign of these changes. High confidence in trend towards earlier occurrence of spring peak river flows in snowmelt- and glacier-fed rivers.	Low confidence that anthropogenic warming has affected the magnitude or frequency of floods. Medium to high confidence in anthropogenic influence on changes in some components of the water cycle (precipitation, snowmelt) affecting floods.	Low confidence in global projections of changes in flood magnitude and frequency because of insufficient evidence. Medium confidence that projected increases in heavy precipitation would contribute to rain-generated local flooding in some catchments or regions. Very likely earlier spring peak flows in snowmelt- and glacier-fed rivers.

Source: Thornton et al. (2014).

* Likelihood assessment: virtually certain, 99–100%; very likely, 90–100%; likely, 66–100%; more likely than not, 50–100%; about as likely as not, 33–66%; unlikely, 0–33%; very unlikely, 0–10%; and exceptionally unlikely, 0–1%.

soil erosion). However, for some degradation processes, such as dryland salinity (which is driven by water percolating past the root zone and then re-surfacing downslope), reductions in rainfall may reduce this hazard.

There are many potential adaptations to respond to the above impacts. For example, selecting crop varieties with greater thermal time requirements so as to delay progression through developmental stages with higher temperatures. Additionally, changing planting times and methods to adjust for changing rainfall and temperature regimes. For example, instead of dryland crop sowing following rainfall events, there is an emerging practice of dry sowing so that seeds germinate with the first substantial rains. This can increase production risk but it also expands the effective growing season and reduces soil moisture loss, increasing yields. In livestock systems, there are options to manage the feedbase, provide effective shade and shelter and breed more heat-tolerant animals among many other adaptations (Stokes & Howden, 2010).

While tending to increase plant production, particularly in dry conditions and for C3 crops, elevated atmospheric CO_2 concentrations also reduce nutritional quality in a variety of crops (Myers, Wessells, Kloog, Zanobetti, & Schartz, 2015; Beach et al., 2019), and even increased toxicity in others (Gleadow, Evans, McCaffery, & Cavagnaro, 2009). Carbon fertilisation, however, is unlikely to fully mitigate the yield reductions caused by temperature increases and changes in precipitation (Ruane et al., 2018). Adaptation responses include breeding crops which maintain or increase the concentrations of these nutrients, management through fertiliser applications during growth or addition to the foodstuffs or diet during processing (Ziska et al., 2012).

Agriculture and associated activities are also a major source of greenhouse gas emissions, with these contributing close to 10 $GTCO_2eq/yr$, and representing 18–22 per cent of global emissions (Smith et al., 2014). The primary source of agricultural greenhouse gas emissions is land-use change (about 5 Gt CO_2eq/yr), enteric fermentation from livestock, and from the application of nitrogen fertilisers. Mitigation efforts to reduce emissions following global accords such as the Paris Agreements could enable emissions pathways that would be compatible with some of the less severe climate scenarios used by the IPCC (IPCC, 2013; van Vuuren et al., 2013). As a major source of emissions, the agriculture, forestry and other land use (AFOLU) sector will need to play a significant role to produce more food with a smaller carbon footprint (Smith et al., 2014; Wollenberg et al., 2016; Willett et al., 2019). However, the policies needed to bring down agricultural emissions may be costly, and, if poorly designed and targeted, could have negative unintended consequences and slow progress towards the eradication of hunger and malnutrition in all its forms (Springmann et al., 2016; Hasegawa et al., 2018).

Conclusion

In an era of healthy and sustainable food systems, agriculture must be recognised as a key driver of multiple outcomes relevant to human and planetary health. Global, regional and national policies must reflect these priorities. Conceptually, this requires adjustment to the key indicators used to measure agricultural success; yield or calorie production alone will no longer suffice. Practically, this will require a multitude of actions, including increased efficiencies and improvements in production practices of both crop and livestock systems, reduced waste and greater alignment of production with the needs of human health. Yields will need to increase, particularly of nutrient-rich, non-staple food crops, including vegetables, fruit, legumes and nuts. This will require significant investment in research and development for these foods, along with incentives for producers to transition towards more diverse and nutritious systems. Increases in yields will need to be obtained within closely monitored environmental bounds. Greenhouse gas emissions will need to be reduced to curb the impacts of climate change, land use change will need to be reduced to the minimum, biodiversity and watersheds protected, and nutrient run-off reduced. These aspects will need to be highlighted accordingly, depending on the region and their main constraints. Achieving agricultural production to feed the growing population will require embracing a variety of production systems. In some cases, these will be highly diverse crop and livestock systems, agroecology and regenerative systems, pastoral production in low opportunity cost lands, all the way to highly intensive production. New, transformational technologies and ways to produce food will need to be seriously embraced to meet food demand shortfalls and/or improve environmental or social aspects. Circular food systems, for example, have a broader role to play. Novel products, such as meat substitutes or digital agriculture, will also be key to spur the next food revolution. One that is ethical, environmental and promotes human and planetary well-being.

Note

1 For comparison, agriculture contributed less than 5 per cent of total GDP and employment in OECD countries.

References

Bai, Z. G., Dent, D. L., Olsson, L., & Schaepman, M. E. (2008). Proxy global assessment of land degradation. *Soil Use Management*, 24(3), 223–234.

Balmford, A., Amano, T., Bartlett, H., Chadwick, D., Collins, A. ... Eisner, R. (2018). The environmental costs and benefits of high-yield farming. *Nature Sustainability*, 1(9), 477–485.

Bauer, S. E., Tsigaridis, K., & Miller, R . (2016). Significant atmospheric aerosol pollution caused by world food cultivation. *Geophysical Research Letters*, 43(10), 5394–5400.

Beach, R. H., Sulser, T. B., Crimmins, A., Cenachi, N., Cole, J., Fukagawa, N. K. ... Ziska, L. H. (2019). Combining the effects of increased atmospheric carbon dioxide on protein, iron, and zinc availability and projected climate change on global diets: A modelling study. *The Lancet Planetary Health*, 3(7): e307–e317, doi:10.1016/S2542-5196(19)30094-4.

Bindraban, P. S., van der Velde, M., Ye, L., van den Berg, M., Materechera, S. ... van Lynden, G. (2012). Assessing the impact of soil degradation on food production. *Current Opinion in Environmental Sustainability*, 4(5), 478–488.

Byerlee, D., StevensonJ., & Villoria, N. (2014). Does intensification slow crop land expansion or encourage deforestation? *Global Food Security*, 3(2), 92–98.

Challinor, A. J., Watson, J., Lobell, D. B., Howden, S. M., Smith, D. R., & Chhetri, N. (2014). A meta-analysis of crop yield under climate change and adaptation. *Nature Climate Change*, 4, 287.

Clements, K. W., & Si, J. (2017). Engel's Law, diet diversity, and the quality of food consumption. *American Journal of Agricultural Economics*, 100(1), 1–22.

Delgado, C., Rosegrant, M., Steinfeld, H., Ehui, S., & Courbois, C. (2001). Livestock to 2020: The next food revolution. *Outlook on Agriculture*, 30(1),27–29.

Diaz, R. J., & Rosenberg, R. (2008). Spreading dead zones and consequences for marine ecosystems. *Science*, 321(5891), 926–929.

FAO (Food and Agriculture Organization). (2018). FAOSTAT: Commodity balances. Available at: www.fao.org/faostat/en/#data/BC (accessed 4 September 2018).

FAO. (2019a). *Food and agricultural data*. Rome: FAO.

FAO. (2019b). *The state of the world's biodiversity for food and agriculture*, J. Bélanger & D. Pilling (eds). Rome:FAO Commission on Genetic Resources for Food and Agriculture Assessments.

FAO. (2019c). FAOSTAT: Emissions by sector. Available at: www.fao.org/faostat (accessed 25 March 2019).

Garnett, T., Appleby, M. C., Balmford, A., Bateman, I. J., Benton, T. G. ... Godfrey, H. C. J. (2013). Sustainable intensification in agriculture: Premises and policies. *Science*, 341(6141), 33–34.

Gleadow, R. M., Evans, J. R., McCaffery, S., & Cavagnaro, T. R. (2009). Growth and nutritive value of cassava (Manihot esculenta Cranz.) are reduced when grown in elevated CO_2. *Plant Biology*, 11 (Suppl. 1), 76–82.

Gleeson, T., Wada, Y., Bierkens, M. F. P., & van Beek, L. P. H. (2012). Water balance of global aquifers revealed by groundwater footprint. *Nature*, 488, 197.

Gómez, M. I., Barrett, C. B., Raney, T., Pinstrup-Andersen, P., Meerman, J. ... Thompson, B. (2013). Post-Green Revolution food systems and the triple burden of malnutrition. *Food Policy*, 42, 129–138.

Griscom, B. W., Adams, J., Ellis, P. W., Houghton, R. A., Lomax, G. ... Fargione, J. (2017). Natural climate solutions. *Proceedings of the National Academy of Sciences*, 114(44), 11645–11650.

Hansen, B., Thorling, L., Schullehner, J., Termansen, M., & Dalgaard, T. (2017). Groundwater nitrate response to sustainable nitrogen management. *Scientific Reports*, 7(1), 8566.

Hasegawa, T., Fujimori, S., Mason-D'Croz, D., Wiebe, K. D., Sulser, T. B., ... Witzke, P. (2018). Risk of increased food insecurity under stringent global climate change mitigation policy. *Nature Climate Change*, 8(8), 699–703.

Headey, D., & Alderman, H. (2019). The relative caloric prices of healthy and unhealthy foods differ systematically across income levels and continents. *The Journal of Nutrition*, doi:10.1093/jn/nxz158.

Herrero, M., Thornton, P. K., Power, B., Bogard, J. R., Remans, R. ... Havlík, P. (2017). Farming and the geography of nutrient production for human use: A transdisciplinary analysis. *The Lancet Planetary Health*, 1(1), 33–42.

Hughes, N., Lawson, K., Lawson, & Valle, H. (2017). *Farm performance and climate: Climate adjusted productivity for broadacre cropping farms*. Canberra, Australia: Australian Bureau of Agricultural and Resource Economics.

IAASTD. (2009). Agriculture at a crossroads: Synthesis report, B. D. McIntyre, *et al.* (eds). New York: UN.

IFPRI. (2002). Green Revolution: Blessing or curse?Washington, DC: International Food Policy Research Institute.

IPCC. (2013). *Climate change 2013: The physical science basis. Contribution of Working Group I to the Fifth Assessment Report of the Intergovernmental Panel on Climate Change*, T. F. Stocker, et al. (eds). Cambridge: Cambridge University Press.

IPCC. (2014). *Climate change 2014: synthesis report. Contribution of Working Groups I, II and III to the Fifth Assessment Report of the Intergovernmental Panel on Climate Change*, Core Writing Team, R. K. Pachauri, & L. A. Meyer (eds). Geneva, Switzerland: IPCC.

Jones, A. D. (2014). The production diversity of subsistence farms in the Bolivian Andes is associated with the quality of child feeding practices as measured by a validated summary feeding index. *Public Health Nutrition*, 18(2), 329–342.

Jones, A. D., ShrinivasA., & Bezner-Kerr, R. (2014). Farm production diversity is associated with greater household dietary diversity in Malawi: Findings from nationally representative data. *Food Policy*, 46, 1–12.

Khoury, C. K., Bjorkman, A. D., Dempewolf, H., Ramirez-Villegas, J., Guarino, L. … Struik, P. C. (2014). Increasing homogeneity in global food supplies and the implications for food security. *Proceedings of the National Academy of Sciences*, 111(11), 4001–4006.

Koppmair, S., Kassie, M., & Qaim, M. (2017). Farm production, market access and dietary diversity in Malawi. *Public Health Nutrition*, 20(2), 325–335.

Laurance, W. F., Sayer, J., & Cassman, K. G. (2014). Agricultural expansion and its impacts on tropical nature. *Trends in Ecology & Evolution*, 29(2), 107–116.

Li, Z. & Fang, H. (2016). Impacts of climate change on water erosion: A review. *Earth-Science Reviews*, 163, 94–117.

Mason-D'Croz, D., Bogard, J. R., Sulser, T. B., Cenacchi, N., Dunston, S., Herrero, M., Wiebe, K.*et al.* (2019). Gaps between fruit and vegetable production, demand, and recommended consumption at global and national levels: An integrated modelling study. *The Lancet Planetary Health*, 3(7), e318–329, doi:10.1016/S2542-5196(19)30095-6.

Mather, A,. (2002). The reversal of land-use trends: The beginning of the reforestation of Europe. In I. Bicik, et al. (eds), *Land use/land cover changes in the period of globalization*. Prague: Charles University and IGU-LUCC, pp.23–30.

McKeon, G., Hall, W., Henrey, B., Stone, G., & Watson, I . (2004). *Pasture degradation and recovery in Australia's rangelands: Learning from history*. Queensland:Department of Natural Resources, Mines and Energy.

Monteiro, C. A., Moubarac, J. C., Cannon, G., Ng, S. W., & Popkin, B. (2013). Ultra-processed products are becoming dominant in the global food system. *Obesity Reviews*, 14, 21–28.

Montgomery, D. R. (2007). Soil erosion and agricultural sustainability. *Proceedings of the National Academy of Sciences*, 104(33), 13268–13272.

Myers, S. S., Wessells, K. R., Kloog, I., Zanobetti, A., & Schartz, J. (2015). Effect of increased concentrations of atmospheric carbon dioxide on the global threat of zinc deficiency: A modelling study. *The Lancet Global Health*, 3(10), e639–e645.

Nelson, G., Bogard, J., Lividini, K., Arsenault, J., Riley, M. … Rosegrant, M. (2018). Income growth and climate change effects on global nutrition security to mid-century. *Nature Sustainability*, 1(12), 773–781.

Newbold, T., Hudson, L. N., Arnell, A. P., Contu, S., De Palma, A. … Purvis, A. (2016). Has land use pushed terrestrial biodiversity beyond the planetary boundary? A global assessment. *Science*, 353 (6296), 288–291.

Newbold, T., Hudson, L. N., Hill, S. L. L., Contu, S., Lysenko, I. … Purvis, A. (2015). Global effects of land use on local terrestrial biodiversity. *Nature*, 520, 45.

Pingali, P. (2007). Westernization of Asian diets and the transformation of food systems: Implications for research and policy. *Food Policy*, 32(3), 281–298.

Porter, J. R., Challinor, A. J., Cochrane, K., Howden, S. M., Iqbal, M. M., ... Ziska, L. (,2014). Food security and food production systems. In C. B. Field, et al. (eds), *Climate change 2014: Impacts, adaptation, and vulnerability. part a: global and sectoral aspects. Contribution of Working Group II to the Fifth Assessment Report of the Intergovernmental Panel on Climate Change*. Cambridge: Cambridge University Press.

Ramankutty, N., Mehrabi, Z., Waha, K., Jarvis, L., Kremen, C., Herrero, M., & Rieseberg, L. H. (2018). Trends in global agricultural land use: Implications for environmental health and food securit y. *Annual Review of Plant Biology*, 69, 789–815.

Reardon, T., Ruben, E. G., Berdegué, J. A., Minten, B., Liverpool-Tasie, L. S., Tschirley, D., & Zilberman, D. (2018). Rapid transformation of food systems in developing regions: Highlighting the role of agricultural research & innovations. *Agricultural Systems*, 142, 47–59.

Riahi, K., van Vuuren, D. P., Elmar, K., Edmonds, J., O'Neill, B. C. ... Tavoni, M. (2017). The shared socioeconomic pathways and their energy, land use, and greenhouse gas emissions implications: An overview. *Global Environmental Change*, 42, 153–168.

Rivera-Ferre, M. G., López-i-Gelats, F., Howden, M., Smith. P., Morton, J. F., & Herrero, M. (2016). Re-framing the climate change debate in the livestock sector: Mitigation and adaptation options. *Climate Change*, 7(6), 869–892.

Rockström, J., Steffen, W., Noone, K., Persson, A., ChaplinIII, S. ... Foley, J. A. (2009). A safe operating space for humanity. *Nature*, 461, 472.

Ruane, A. C., Antle, J., Elliott, C., Folberth, G., Hoogenboom, D. ... Rosenzweig, C. (2018). Biophysical and economic implications for agriculture of +1.5° and +2.0°C global warming using AgMIP Coordinated Global and Regional Assessments. *Climate Research*, 76(1), 17–39.

Sibhatu, K. T., & Qaim, M. (2018). Review: Meta-analysis of the association between production diversity, diets, and nutrition in smallholder farm households. *Food Policy*, 77, 1–18.

Siebert, S., Burke, J., Faures, J. M., Frenken, K., Hoogeveen, J., Döll, P., & Portmann, P. T. (2010). Groundwater use for irrigation: A global inventory. *Hydrology and Earth System Sciences*, 14(10), 1863–1880.

Smith, P., Ahammad, H., Clark, H., Dong, H., Elsiddig, E. A. ... van Minnen, J. (2014). Agriculture, Forestry and Other Land Use (AFOLU). In O. Edenhofer, et al. (eds), *Climate change 2014: Mitigation of climate change. Contribution of Working Group III to the Fifth Assessment Report of the Intergovernmental Panel on Climate Change*. Cambridge: Cambridge University Press.

Springmann, M., Mason-D'Croz, D., Robinson, S., Wiebe, K., Godfrey, C. J., Rayer, M., & Scarborough, P. (2016). Mitigation potential and global health impacts from emissions pricing of food commodities. *Nature Climate Change*, 7, 69.

Stevenson, J. R., Villoria, N., Byerlee, D., Kelley, T., & Maredia, M. (2013). Green Revolution research saved an estimated 18 to 27 million hectares from being brought into agricultural production. *Proceedings of the National Academy of Sciences*, 110(21), 8363–8368.

Stokes, C., & Howden, M. (2010). *Adapting agriculture to climate change: Preparing Australian agriculture, forestry and fisheries for the future*. Canberra: CSIRO Publishing.

Swinburn, B. A., Kraak, V. I., Allender, S., Atkins, V. J., Baker, P. I., Bogard, J. R. ... Devarajan, R. (2019). The global syndemic of obesity, undernutrition, and climate change: The Lancet Commission report. *Lancet*, doi:10.1016/S0140–6736(18)32822–32828.

Thornton, P. K., Ericksen, P. J., Herrero, M., & Challinor, A. J. (2014). Climate variability and vulnerability to climate change: A review. *Global Change Biology*, 20(11), 3313–3328.

Tilman, D., Clark, M., Williams. D. R., Kimmel, K., Polasky, S., & Packer, C. (2017). Future threats to biodiversity and pathways to their prevention. *Nature*, 546, 73.

UN (United Nations). (2018). World population prospects: Revision 2017. Available at: https://population.un.org/wpp/ (accessed 10 February 2019).

van Vuuren, D. P., Stehfest, E., den Elzen, M. G. J., Kram, T., van Vliet, J. ... van Ruijven, B. (2011). RCP2.6: Exploring the possibility to keep global mean temperature increase below 2°C. *Climate Change*, 109(1), 95.

Wada, Y., van Beek, L. P. H., & Bierkens, M. F. P. (2012). Nonsustainable groundwater sustaining irrigation: A global assessment. *Water Resources Research*, 48(6).

Wada, Y., van Beek, L. P. H., van Kempen, C. M., Reckman, J. W. T. M., Vasak, S., & Bierkens, M. F. P. (2010). Global depletion of groundwater resources. *Geophysical Research Letters*, 37(20).

WHO. (2015). WHO estimates of the global burden of foodborne diseases: Foodborne disease burden, Epidemiology Reference Group 2007–2015. Geneva: World Health Organization.

Willett, W., Rockström, J., Loken, B., Springmann, M., Lang, T., Vermeulen, S., … Murray, C. J. L. (2019). Food in the Anthropocene: The EAT–Lancet Commission on healthy diets from sustainable food systems. *Lancet*. doi:10.1016/S0140-6736(18)31788–31784.

Wollenberg, E., Richards, M., Smith, P., Havlik, P., Obersteiner, M. … Campbell, B. M. (2016). Reducing emissions from agriculture to meet the 2 °C target. *Global Change Biology*, 22(12), 3859–3864.

World Bank. (2018).World development indicators. Available at: https://datacatalog.worldbank.org/dataset/world-development-indicators (accessed 10 February 2019).

Wu, F., Groopman, J. D., & PestkaJ. J. (2014). Public health impacts of foodborne mycotoxins. *Annual Review of Food Science and Technology*, 5(1), 351–372.

WWF (World Wildlife Fund). (2015). Saving forests at risk. In R. Taylor (ed.), *WWF living forests report*. Gland, Switzerland:World Wildlife Fund.

Ziska, L. H., Bunce, J. A., Shimono, H., Gealy, D. R., Baker, J. T. … Wilson, L. T. (2012). Food security and climate change: On the potential to adapt global crop production by active selection to rising atmospheric carbon dioxide. *Proceedings. Biological Sciences*, 279(1745), 4097–4105.

6

FOOD MANUFACTURING

Processed foods and big food corporations

Gyorgy Scrinis

Introduction

The food manufacturing industry has played an important role in the industrialisation and globalisation of food systems. Food manufacturers transform raw agricultural commodities into processed and packaged food and beverage products. As large-scale purchasers of agricultural produce, they have a significant influence on the social and ecological relations of primary food production. Food manufacturers also have a profound effect on the nutritional quality of the food supply, population dietary patterns and diet quality. Transnational food manufacturing corporations – Big Food – in particular have come under increased scrutiny for the nutritional quality of their products and the environmental sustainability of their practices. This chapter examines the health and environmental impacts of manufactured foods and beverages, the power and practices of transnational food manufacturing corporations, and some policy initiatives that aim to create more nutritious and environmentally sustainable manufactured foods.

The production and distribution of processed and packaged foods and beverages

The food manufacturing sector produces a diverse range of relatively affordable, palatable, safe, durable and convenient foods and beverages. They include minimally-processed foods and ingredients that can be used in home cooking, such as canned tomatoes, dried pasta, bread, fruit juices, and unflavoured fermented yoghurts. Since the 1970s, there has been a proliferation of industrially-produced, ready-to-eat, ready-to-heat and novel meals, snacks and beverages. The bulk of the sales of packaged foods and beverages include products such as sugar-sweetened beverages, ready-to-eat breakfast cereals, infant formula, flavoured yoghurt, canned soups, frozen pizza, ice cream and salty snacks.

Food manufacturers are able to mass-produce foods similar to those that can be produced in the home or in artisanal restaurants. But manufacturers also use a range of industrial food processing technologies, techniques, and additives in order to create certain types of products with particular characteristics, such as enhanced flavours, reduced costs and greater durability and longevity of products. These techniques and technologies include various forms of freezing and heating, high pressure processing, extraction, pasteurisation, smoking, fractionation, grinding, extrusion, advanced meat recovery, hydrogenation and packaging. Manufacturers also use a range of industrially-produced additives, such as colour and flavour enhancers, emulsifiers, sweeteners and preservatives. A key characteristic of highly processed foods is that they are made up of ingredients that have been broken down into their components, further processed, and then reconstituted and recombined into the final food products. Such formulated or fabricated products are referred to as *processed-reconstituted foods*, as these foods typically have few intact or whole ingredients (Scrinis, 2013).

To produce cheap yet tasty and desirable products, food manufacturers have tended to rely heavily on a small range of ingredients, such as grains (particularly wheat and corn), soya beans, vegetable oils (such as palm and soy oils), and sugars (such as sugar beet and corn-based sweeteners), as well as milk and meat, each of which may be processed in various ways before being added to the final formulated products. These ingredients are typically cheap and generic grain crops and animal products produced on a large scale and often sourced globally. While food manufacturers profit from the ability to add value to raw ingredients, keeping the price-point low is a key selling point of many processed foods. This is typically achieved through a number of strategies, such as the use of cheap raw ingredients; mass production and technological innovation; low pay and poor conditions for workers; and an industry-friendly regulatory environment.

While the production of cheap, tasty and convenient products has been important in the growth of sales, so too are the distribution and marketing strategies developed by these manufacturers. A key strategy has been to ensure the products are ubiquitous, and available anywhere and any time. Supermarkets have been an important vector for the distribution of manufactured foods. Anthony Winson has referred to the *spatial colonisation* of industrial foods as the "power of food processors to place product in the most visible and effective selling spaces in a food environment" (Winson, 2013). We can also observe what I will refer to here as the *temporal colonisation* of processed foods, whereby processed food products are available to be purchased and consumed at any time of the day or night, and consumers are confronted with around-the-clock advertising.

With sales of packaged foods in the Global North starting to plateau in recent years, much of the growth in food product sales has occurred in low- and middle-income countries. Trade liberalisation policies and the deregulation of foreign direct investments since the 1980s have paved the way for the penetration of foreign transnational corporations into these countries, allowing supermarket and food manufacturing corporations to establish local subsidiaries (Friel et al., 2013). The lowering of trade barriers has also facilitated the increased global trade in final food products and of the commodities that make up the bulk ingredients in packaged foods and beverages (Hawkes, 2010). The rise of supermarkets in the Global South since the 1990s has been important in the spread of packaged foods in low- and middle-income countries. But the distribution of these foods has not only relied on supermarkets and food stores, but also involved the development of local distributional channels in places where retail infrastructure is not well established, such as door-to-door sales (Gómez & Ricketts, 2013).

Industry structure and corporate power: Big Food and Big Soda

The food manufacturing sector is enormous in terms of global sales and encompasses a diverse range of small, medium and large enterprises. This includes small-scale producers servicing local markets, medium-scale nationally-based companies that own nationally-recognised brands, and large transnational corporations that have manufacturing facilities in multiple countries. The trend in industry structure has been the growth and concentration of transnational corporations, which has been achieved through organic growth; the buy-out of small and medium companies and their proprietary brands and products; their expansion into other countries and regions; and mergers with other transnational corporations. These corporations are also developing financial investment arms to seed-fund or acquire small start-up companies that produce innovative products and brands, and that tap into new consumer and health trends (Clapp & Isakson, 2018).

The top 10 global food and beverage manufacturing corporations include Nestlé, Pepsico, Coca-Cola, Unilever, Mondelez, Kelloggs, Kraft and Mars. The level of corporate concentration in the food manufacturing sector is not as pronounced as in other sectors of the food system, such as agricultural inputs and retailing, due to the many small and medium-sized firms in operation in particular countries and regions. Nevertheless the 50 largest food manufacturers account for around half of all global sales (Heinrich Böll Foundation, 2017). The concentration of market share is higher within particular countries and product sectors. In Latin America, for example, the top four firms selling carbonated soft drinks control over 80 per cent of the market, and over 75 per cent of the breakfast cereal market (PAHO, 2015).

Big Food and Big Soda corporations use their market power to grow the sales of their products, to gain advantages over smaller competitors, and to leverage their power over other actors. This includes being able to invest in product innovation, consumer research and testing, and scientific research and technological innovation. Large food corporations are able to devote enormous budgets to the marketing of their products and brands through multiple media platforms and other means, such as through sponsorship of sporting and community groups. The buying power of corporations also allows them to dictate prices paid to farmers for agricultural produce, and to shape the product quality and environmental standards of agricultural production.

Big Food's market power also translates into more direct political power, and their ability to shape national and local government policies and regulations. The range of *corporate political activities* these companies pursue – a term first used by researchers to identify the political activities of tobacco companies – include:

- the direct lobbying of policy-makers;
- the creation of industry front groups;
- the sponsorship of expert groups and civil society organisations;
- the funding of scientific research to deliver favourable scientific evidence;
- public campaigns against regulatory initiatives (Mialon, Swinburn, Allender, & Sacks, 2016).

Nutritional quality and health impacts of manufactured foods and beverages

Processed and packaged foods and beverages have had a range of impacts – beneficial and detrimental – on the nutritional quality of the food supply and on the health of the population. Food processing technologies, practices, ingredients and additives can enhance or detract from the nutritional quality of a food. Traditional and some modern food processing techniques not only can help to retain and preserve the nutritional qualities of foods, but can potentially enhance their nutritional quality or make their nutritional components more available and digestible. Traditional fermentation practices, for example, such as turning milk into yoghurt, can make milk more digestible and add beneficial micro-organisms to the end product. The primary processing and preservation of basic foods and ingredients ensure these foods are convenient, affordable and available all year round, and assist in the home preparation of meals. The production of final-food products can provide convenient and relatively healthy meals, particularly in the context of time-poor working households where the burden of cooking continues to fall on women (Jackson, Brembeck, Everts, & Fuentes, 2018). Processed final-food products also facilitate the diversification of diets and cuisines, allowing ready access to less familiar foods or time-consuming preparation.

Processing techniques and practices can, however, also diminish the nutritional quality of whole foods in various ways. Primary processing techniques that refine or extract components from whole foods remove valuable parts of the food, and concentrate components, such as sugar and refined grain. More advanced processing techniques that involve subjecting foods to high pressure, high temperature heating, or chemical transformation, such as deep frying and hydrogenation, have in some cases been found to be harmful (Fardet, 2018). Many processed and packaged foods and beverages are heavily adulterated with refined and processed ingredients, such as added sugars, refined starches, added fats, and salt, each of which may be sourced from a number of interchangeable bulk ingredients. These foods also tend to have little if any intact or whole ingredients, but instead rely on a range of additives to compensate for their lack of taste and texture.

The rise in consumption of poor quality processed foods and beverages is now linked to a range of non-communicable diseases, such as diabetes, cancer and cardiovascular disease; and the rise in levels of overweight and obesity (Fardet, 2018). The conventional way in which processed foods are evaluated and their disease pathways are understood by nutrition experts is primarily in terms of their nutrient composition, which is a characteristic of what is referred to as the dominant ideology or paradigm of "nutritionism", or nutritional reductionism (Scrinis, 2013). In particular, the concern is over the high levels of nutrients-to-limit – sodium, sugars, saturated fats, trans-fats and energy – and the relative absence of beneficial nutrients. Over the past two decades nutrition experts have also begun to study the health effects of particular processed food products, though usually on the grounds that they have high levels of particular nutrients-to-limit. A primary focus has been on sugar-sweetened beverages (SSB), with studies demonstrating a link between SSB consumption and poor health outcomes, such as obesity incidence and diabetes (Singh et al., 2015). The rapid rise in processed food consumption in low- and middle-income countries over the past two decades is of particular concern, particularly where poor quality processed foods displace the consumption of traditional and minimally processed foods and meals, and reduce dietary diversity (Stuckler & Nestle, 2012).

A systematic approach to studying the nutritional quality and health impacts of processed foods has been pioneered by Monteiro and colleagues, who have developed a classification system for foods based on levels of processing, rather than nutrient composition (Monteiro et al., 2018). They distinguish four categories of foods: (1) minimally processed foods; (2) processed culinary ingredients; (3) processed foods; and (4) ultra-processed foods. *Ultra-processed foods* are defined as "formulations made mostly or entirely from substances derived from foods and additives", and include both packaged foods and beverages and fast-foods (Monteiro et al., 2018). A key aspect of the definition of ultra-processed foods is the presence of industrial additives, such as colours, flavour enhancers and processing aids. The category of ultra-processed foods essentially identifies the class of foods manufactured by the food industry that cannot be or are not typically produced in the home or artisanal food businesses. Beyond their composition, Monteiro and colleagues define the overall *purpose* of ultra-processing as being "to create branded, convenient (durable, ready-to-consume), attractive (hyper-palatable) and highly profitable (low-cost ingredients) food products designed to displace all other food groups" (Monteiro et al., 2018). A number of country-based studies have demonstrated that – as a class of food – ultra-processed foods have considerably higher concentrations of nutrients-to-limit, and that higher levels of consumption of these foods are associated with higher rates of obesity and the incidence of a number of non-communicable diseases (Monteiro et al., 2018).

Food manufacturers often market packaged foods and beverages with nutritional and health claims. In contrast to mandatory micronutrient fortification of staple foods regulated by government agencies, food manufacturers voluntarily and arbitrarily fortify many of their products with micronutrients, often accompanied by the front-of-pack marketing of these micronutrients. Big Food corporations are now actively distributing and marketing micronutrient-fortified foods to people in low- and middle-income countries who are at risk of micronutrient deficiencies, and this is a key strategy being used to target and grow sales to people at the bottom of the economic pyramid (Kimura, 2013; Scrinis, 2016). Food manufacturers also produce foods that contain ingredients which they market with direct or implied health claims for optimal or targeted health benefits. These so-called "functional foods", or what can more accurately be described as *functionally-marketed foods*, may be minimally processed or ultra-processed (Scrinis, 2008). Whether individual fortified and functionalised foods are able to replicate – much less improve upon – the diverse and complex combination of nutrients and food components delivered by wholefoods, and whether they deliver their claimed enhanced health benefits in the context of people's overall dietary patterns, are the subject of intense expert debates (Nestle, 2013). Nutrient and health claims may also create a "health halo" and a nutritional façade around otherwise poor-quality products. Some studies have demonstrated that poorer quality foods are more likely to be marketed with nutrient and health claims (Christoforou, Dachner, Mendelson, & Tarasuk, 2018).

With rising public and government concerns over the quality and health impacts of processed foods, food manufacturers face both regulatory and market threats to their products and practices. The sales of some types of products – such as SSB and heavily processed and sweetened breakfast cereals – have started to decline in some markets as many consumers look for healthier options, and follow the trend towards minimally processed, additive-free and "natural" packaged foods and beverages (Popkin & Hawkes, 2016; Asioli et al., 2017). Food manufacturers have responded by voluntarily and systematically reformulating their products to reduce the levels of nutrients-to-limit, as well as reducing some artificial additives and adding beneficial nutrients and "whole" ingredients. Food corporations have for many decades offered "reduced" or "lesser evil" versions of their products (Nestle, 2013). Sugar-sweetened beverages, for example, have had their sugar content reduced or replaced with artificial sweeteners.

Many food corporations have now developed policies for systematically reformulating their entire product portfolios. Nestlé and Unilever, for example, have developed their own nutrient profiling systems that they pledge all their products will eventually meet. Yet the nutrient standards and limits they set for their products are often much more lenient than those set by independent experts and organisations. Aside from the specific nutrient standards, an inherent limitation of nutrients-to-limit reformulation is that, while these relatively modest reductions may reduce the harmfulness of high sugar/salt/fat products, they do not necessarily result in the production of *nutritious* foods (Scrinis & Monteiro, 2018).

Until recently, most government initiatives have taken the form of voluntary measures intended either to encourage manufacturers to improve the quality of their products, or to encourage consumers to change their consumption choices. But with mounting evidence of harm, and the weakness of industry initiatives, many governments have begun to implement stronger, mandatory and innovative policies and regulations, such as front-of-pack labelling schemes, mandatory nutrient limits, sugar taxes, restrictions of marketing to children, school-food policies, and new forms of dietary guidelines (Hawkes, Hawkes, Jewell, & Allen, 2013). Importantly, however, several low- and middle-income countries are taking the lead with these initiatives (Pérez-Escamilla et al., 2017).

In terms of reformulation policies, governments have so far been reluctant to set mandated nutrient limits. Exceptions are limits on trans-fat content in some countries, beginning with Denmark in 2004 (Hyseni et al., 2017). Limits on sodium content are also starting to be introduced, with South Africa introducing limits on a range of processed food categories in 2016 (Peters et al., 2017). Front-of-pack labelling initiatives include: the Multiple Traffic Light labelling system first introduced in the UK in 2013, and since introduced to Uruguay; the Health Star Rating system used in Australia since 2014; and the black "stop" sign label, introduced in Chile in 2017. Chile's black stop label is the strongest of these initiatives, for it is underpinned by stricter nutrient standards, and does not include a promotional dimension that can be perceived as a positive endorsement for a product (such as a green traffic light or a high-star rating). The Chilean labelling laws also prohibit products that carry a warning sign from being marketed to children or sold in schools (Corvalán, Reyes, Garmendia, & Uauy, 2013). Many governments are now also turning to the use of food taxes as a pricing mechanism to reduce consumption as well as production of poor quality foods (Baker, Jones, & Thow, 2018). Studies of the Mexican tax on SSB introduced in 2014 suggest that it has been effective in reducing the consumption of SSBs (Colchero, Rivera-Dommarco, Popkin, & Ng, 2017).

Ecological impacts and sustainability initiatives of food manufacturers

Much of the evidence on the environmental impacts and sustainability of food systems focuses on agricultural produce, such as meat and dairy, rather than manufactured foods. Yet a large portion of agricultural produce is typically processed to some degree by the food manufacturing or food service industries before they are consumed. There are multiple ways in which the products and practices of the food manufacturing sector are contributing to energy and resource consumption and pollution emissions, and more generally to structures and cultures of production, distribution and consumption that are environmentally unsustainable. These include:

- the production and sourcing of key ingredients in manufactured foods;
- the process of manufacturing, packaging and distributing packaged foods and beverages;
- food waste and packaging;
- the unnecessary production and consumption of ultra-processed foods that are of little or no nutritional value.

The large-scale production and sourcing of some of the key ingredients that serve as inputs into the manufacture of packaged foods – wheat, corn, soy, palm oil, milk and even water – have considerable environmental as well as social impacts. The manufacturing sector has been a key driver of the global expansion of production of soy and vegetable oil crops such as palm. Palm oil is used both as an ingredient and as frying oil for packaged foods, as well as by the food service sector, and these sectors have driven the expansion of palm production. Much of the world's palm tree production is concentrated in Indonesia and Malaysia, and has involved the burning and deforestation of forests on an immense scale. Soy bean crops, on the other hand, have more varied uses, but include soy oil for frying and soy fractions as ingredients in packaged foods. The continued growth in demand for soy has contributed to the large-scale deforestation of the Amazon in South America (Sage, 2012).

Many global food manufacturing corporations have developed sustainable sourcing policies for some of the agricultural commodities that they rely so heavily upon. Sustainable sourcing can incorporate not only environmental considerations but also animal welfare and farmer livelihoods, such as ensuring fairer prices for farmers and better working conditions for agricultural workers. This may involve signing up to third party certification and auditing schemes, such as Fair Trade accredited products, or developing company-own, self-regulated certification schemes, such as Nestlé's "Cocoa Plan". Food corporations are also active players in multi-stakeholder "roundtable" governance mechanisms, such as the Responsible Soy Roundtable and the Roundtable on Sustainable Palm Oil (RSPO). Nestlé and Unilever, for example, have supported RSPO, though this scheme has been criticised for its weak standards and ineffectiveness in halting deforestation. Food manufacturing corporations have until recently demonstrated little concern for animal welfare issues, but some corporations have begun acting more proactively in this area, e.g. adopting cage-free egg policies (Amos & Sullivan, 2017). Sustainable sourcing policies can be understood not only as being driven by sustainability concerns, as they also enable food corporations to better manage and discipline agricultural producers, and to ensure an ongoing supply of high quality ingredients for their products (Elder & Dauvergne, 2015). These sustainability policies also provide legitimation for the continued growth in the production and consumption of packaged foods and beverages, rather than questioning the need for the production, distribution and consumption of these products (Scott, 2018).

Food and beverage manufacturers are also heavy water users, both for the manufacturing process and as an ingredient in bottled water and carbonated beverages. Enormous quantities of water are required for every stage of the processing and manufacturing of foods, such as for washing raw produce, for cleaning equipment, and for heating and cooling processes (Baldwin, 2015). Manufacturing plants typically produce large quantities of contaminated liquid waste that requires treatment, though the strength of laws regulating these discharges varies greatly between countries. For the production of bottled water and soft drinks, food manufacturers typically draw freshwater from rivers and underground sources. The large-scale extraction and use of potable water by food corporations have involved the privatisation of public water supplies, and often directly compete with the availability of water for household use, and have led to conflicts between food corporations and local communities (Jaffee & Newman, 2013)

There are considerable energy demands in the manufacture of foods, as well as packaging, refrigeration and transportation. Food processing is estimated to account for around 20 per cent of total energy use within the US food system, with a large portion used to provide heating and cooling technologies (Lau, Tang, & Swanson, 2000; Canning et al., 2010; Baldwin, 2015). A UK study estimated that the food manufacturing sector accounts for 12 per cent of the energy used in the UK food system (Garnett, 2011). There have been ongoing technological innovations in the food manufacturing sector that have enabled the more efficient use of energy per unit produced as well as higher outputs, though these innovations have primarily been driven by the need to reduce costs rather than to achieve environmental benefits (Misra et al., 2017).

The food manufacturing sector directly contributes to food waste in the food manufacturing process itself, with some estimates of 10 per cent of the total food waste generated along the supply chain (Gustavsson, Cederberg, & Sonesson, 2011). A portion of packaged foods and beverages also become food waste at the retail and household level when they pass their expiry dates (Stuart, 2009). The relatively new category of supermarket ready-meals is likely to produce higher rates of wastage than tinned and other more durable convenience foods (Sage, 2012). There are initiatives in some countries to reform the standards for use-by and best-before dates.

A major environmental impact associated with packaged foods and beverages is in the production and disposal of the packaging itself, as well as the distribution and cold storage of packaged foods and beverages. The production of packaging can be energy- and greenhouse-gas intensive, particularly for various types of plastics manufactured from oil (Garnett, 2011). In the European Union, food and beverage packaging accounts for around two-thirds of all packaging waste by weight. Much of this packaging waste is destined either for landfill or pollutes rivers and oceans. Packaging materials can also release harmful chemicals into the foods and into environment, such as colorants, flame retardants, and bisphenol A (BPA) (Worldwatch Institute, 2015). Only around 10 per cent of all packaging is recycled in some way (Mason & Lang, 2017), though even the recycling and the production of biodegradable packaging are energy-intensive processes.

A common argument put forward by the food and packaging industries is that food packaging is not simply an environmental liability, but provides environmental benefits through their role in protecting foods, preventing spoilage, maintaining food quality and thereby preventing food waste along the supply chain (Williams & Wikström, 2011; Nestlé, 2018). Proponents of food packaging even argue that – based on lifecycle assessment studies – packaging actually delivers a net environmental benefit, given the relative environmental impacts of food waste, despite the resources consumed and waste produced by food packaging. However, such narrowly-framed environmental accounting ignores the fact that it is often unnecessary to manufacture processed foods that require such environmentally-destructive and non-reusable packaging, and also ignores the various ways that packaging actually contributes to the generation of food waste by enabling the increased production and long-distance transportation of perishable foods.

The questions of the nutritional quality and environmental sustainability more clearly intersect in the production and consumption of ultra-processed foods which have little or no nutritional value to offer (Hadjikakou, 2017). The significant level of consumption of foods that are at best not nutritious, and, at worst, directly or indirectly cause harm, suggests that there would be both health and environmental benefits from reductions in the production and consumption of these types of packaged foods and beverages. An obvious case in point is the health impacts and packaging waste created by sugar-sweetened soft drinks.

Conclusion

Food manufacturing corporations have started to develop comprehensive sustainability policies to address the resource use, sustainable sourcing, and pollution and waste generated by their manufacturing processes, products and packaging. These corporate sustainability policies are in the first instance driven by their need to maintain their access to the raw ingredients they require into the future. But food manufacturing corporations are yet to face serious government and public scrutiny or regulatory pressure over their sustainability initiatives. A more immediate challenge for these corporations is to negotiate concerns over the health impacts of their "junk food" products; the market trends towards minimally processed and "natural" convenience foods; and the inevitable growth of government regulation of their products and marketing practices. These health concerns represent both threats and opportunities for the packaged food sector, as they aim to reduce the harmfulness of their products while also marketing the benefits of their fortified and functionalised foods. But any improvements in the nutritional quality or ecological sustainability of manufactured foods must be evaluated in the context of the continued growth in production and consumption of these foods globally, and particularly in low- and middle-income countries. This growth in production and consumption threatens to exacerbate the current health and environmental impacts of ultra-processed foods. Most government and industry policies currently favour relatively minor modifications of these products – such as nutritional reformulation to reduce sugar/salt/fats, and creating greater production and packaging efficiencies – rather than more substantive changes or reductions in production and consumption. By contrast, the revised Brazilian Dietary Guidelines, released in 2014, proposed limiting or reducing current levels of consumption of ultra-processed and packaged foods as a means of creating food systems that "nourish humanity and the planet".

References

Amos, N., & Sullivan, R. (eds) (2017). *The business of farm animal welfare*. London: Routledge.

Asioli, D., Aschemann-Witzel, J., Caputo, V., Vecchio, R., Annunziata, A. … & Varela, P. (2017). Making sense of the "clean label" trends: A review of consumer food choice behavior and discussion of industry implications. *Food Research International*, 99, 58–71.

Baker, P., Jones, A., & Thow, A. M. (2018). Accelerating the worldwide adoption of sugar-sweetened beverage taxes: Strengthening commitment and capacity: comment on "the untapped power of soda taxes: incentivizing consumers, generating revenue, and altering corporate behavior". *International Journal of Health Policy and Management*, 7(5), 474.

Baldwin, C. (2015). *The 10 principles of food industry sustainability*. Chichester: John Wiley & Sons.

Canning, P. N., Charles, A., Huang, S., Polenske, K. R., & Waters, A. (2010). *Energy use in the US food system*. Washington, DC: USDA.

Christoforou, A., Dachner, N., Mendelson, R., & Tarasuk, V. (2018). Substitute foods are more likely than their traditional food counterparts to display front-of-package references. *FACETS*, 3(1), 455–468. doi:10.1139/facets-2017-0094.

Clapp, J., & Isakson, S. R. (2018). *Speculative harvests: Financialization, food and agriculture*. Winnipeg: Fernwood.

Colchero, M. A., Rivera-Dommarco, J., Popkin, B. M., & Ng, S. W. (2017). In Mexico, evidence of sustained consumer response two years after implementing a sugar-sweetened beverage tax. *Health Affairs*, 36(3), 564–571.

Corvalán, C., Reyes, M., Garmendia, M. L., & Uauy, R. (2013). Structural responses to the obesity and non-communicable diseases epidemic: The Chilean Law of Food Labeling and Advertising. *Obesity Reviews*, 14(S2), 79–87.

Elder, S. D., & Dauvergne, P. (2015). Farming for Walmart: The politics of corporate control and responsibility in the Global South. *The Journal of Peasant Studies*, 42(5), 1029–1046.

Fardet, A. (2018). Characterization of the degree of food processing in relation with its health potential and effects. *Advances in Food and Nutrition Research*, 85, 79–129. doi:10.1016/bs.afnr.2018.02.002.

Friel, S., Hattersley, L., Snowdon, W., Thow, A. M., Lobstein, T., Sanders, D., ... Kelly, B. (2013). Monitoring the impacts of trade agreements on food environments. *Obesity Reviews*, 14(S1), 120–134.

Garnett, T. (2011). Where are the best opportunities for reducing greenhouse gas emissions in the food system (including the food chain)? *Food Policy*, 36, S23–S32.

Gómez, M. I., & Ricketts, K. D. (2013). Food value chain transformations in developing countries: Selected hypotheses on nutritional implications. *Food Policy*, 42, 139–150.

Gustavsson, J., Cederberg, C., & Sonesson, U. (2011). *Global food losses and food waste*. Rome: FAO.

Hadjikakou, M. (2017). Trimming the excess: Environmental impacts of discretionary food consumption in Australia. *Ecological Economics*, 131, 119–128.

Hawkes, C. (2010). The influence of trade liberalisation and global dietary change: The case of vegetable oils, meat and highly processed foods. In C. Hawkes, C. Blouin, S. Henson, N. Drager, & L. Dubé (eds), *Trade, food, diet and health: Perspectives and policy options*. Chichester: John Wiley & Sons Ltd.

Hawkes, C., Hawkes, J., Jewell, K., & Allen. (2013). A food policy package for healthy diets and the prevention of obesity and diet-related non-communicable diseases: The NOURISHING framework. *Obesity Reviews*, 14(S2), 159–168.

Heinrich Böll Foundation. (2017). *Agrifood atlas: Facts and figures about the corporations that control what we eat*. Berlin: Heinrich Böll Foundation.

Hyseni, L., Bromley, H., Kypridemos, C., O'Flaherty, M., Lloyd-Williams, F., Guzman-Castillo, M., ... Capewella, S. (2017). Systematic review of dietary trans-fat reduction interventions. *Policy*, 95(12).

Jackson, P., Brembeck, H., Everts, J., & Fuentes, M. (2018). *Reframing convenience food*. Cham: Palgrave Macmillan.

Jaffee, D., & Newman, S. (2013). A more perfect commodity: Bottled water, global accumulation, and local contestation. *Rural Sociology*, 78(1), 1–28.

Kimura, A. (2013). *Hidden hunger: Gender and the politics of smart foods*. Ithaca, NY: Cornell University Press.

Lau, M., Tang, J., & Swanson, B. (2000). Kinetics of textural and color changes in green asparagus during thermal treatments. *Journal of Food Engineering*, 45(4), 231–236.

Mason, P., & Lang, T. (2017). *Sustainable diets: How ecological nutrition can transform consumption and the food system*. London: Routledge.

Mialon, M., Swinburn, B., Allender, S., & Sacks, G. (2016). Systematic examination of publicly-available information reveals the diverse and extensive corporate political activity of the food industry in Australia. *BMC Public Health*, 16(1), 1.

Misra, N. N., Koubaa, M., Roohinejad, S., Juliano, P., Alpas, H., Inacio, R. S., ... Barba, F. J. (2017). Landmarks in the historical development of twenty-first-century food processing technologies. *Food Research International*, 97, 318–339. doi:10.1016/j.foodres.2017.05.001.

Monteiro, C. A., Cannon, G., Moubarac, J. C., Levy, R. B., Louzada, M. L. C., & Jaime, P. C. (2018). The UN Decade of Nutrition, the NOVA food classification and the trouble with ultra-processing. *Public Health Nutrition*, 21(1), 5–17. doi:10.1017/S1368980017000234.

Nestlé. (2018). Nestlé in society: Creating shared value and meeting our commitments 2017. Vevey: Nestlé.

Nestle, M. (2013). *Food politics: How the food industry influences nutrition and health*, 10th ed. Berkeley, CA: University of California Press.

PAHO. (2015). *Ultra-processed food and drink products in Latin America: Trends, impact on obesity, policy implications*. Washington, DC: Pan American Health Organization.

Pérez-Escamilla, R., Lutter, C., Rabadan-Diehl, C., Rubinstein, A., Calvillo, A., Corvalán, C., ... Kline, L. (2017). Prevention of childhood obesity and food policies in Latin America: From research to practice. *Obesity Reviews*, 18, 28–38.

Peters, S. A. E., Peters, S., Dunford, E., Ware, L., Harris, T., Walker, A., ... Neal, B. (2017). The sodium content of processed foods in South Africa during the introduction of mandatory sodium limits. *Nutrients*, 9(4), 404.

Popkin, B., & Hawkes, C. (2016). Sweetening of the global diet, particularly beverages: Patterns, trends, and policy responses. *The Lancet Diabetes & Endocrinology*, 4(2), 174–186.

Sage, C. (2012). *Environment and food*. London: Routledge.

Scott, C. (2018). Sustainably sourced junk food? Big Food and the challenge of sustainable diets. *Global Environmental Politics*, 18(2), 93–113.

Scrinis, G. (2008). Functional foods or functionally-marketed foods: A critique of, and alternatives to, the category of functional foods. *Public Health Nutrition*, 11, 541–545. doi:10.1017/S1368980008001869.

Scrinis, G. (2013). *Nutritionism: The science and politics of dietary advice*. New York: Columbia University Press.

Scrinis, G. (2016). Reformulation, fortification and functionalization: Big Food corporations' nutritional engineering and marketing strategies. *The Journal of Peasant Studies,* 43(1), 17–37. doi:10.1080/03066150.2015.1101455.

Scrinis, G., & Monteiro, C. A. (2018). Ultra-processed foods and the limits of product reformulation. *Public Health Nutrition*, 21(1), 247–252. doi:10.1017/S1368980017001392.

Singh, G. M., Micha, R., Khatibzadeh, S., Lim, S., Ezzati, M., Mozaffarian, D.*et al.* (2015). Estimated global, regional, and national disease burdens related to sugar-sweetened beverage consumption in 2010. *Circulation*, 132(8), 639–666. doi:10.1161/CIRCULATIONAHA.114.010636.

Stuart, T. (2009). *Waste: Uncovering the global food scandal*. New York: W.W. Norton & Co.

Stuckler, D., & Nestle, M. (2012). Big food, food systems, and global health. *PLoS Medicine*, 9(6), e1001242.

Williams, H., & Wikström, F. (2011). Environmental impact of packaging and food losses in a life cycle perspective: A comparative analysis of five food items. *Journal of Cleaner Production*, 19(1), 43–48.

Winson, A. (2013). *The industrial diet: The degradation of food and the struggle for healthy eating*. Vancouver: UBC Press.

Worldwatch Institute. (2015). Global plastic production rises, recycling lags. Washington, DC: Worldwatch Institute.

7

FOOD RETAIL AND DISTRIBUTION

A focus on supermarkets

Sandra Murray and Martin Caraher

Introduction

The food retail, particularly supermarkets, and distribution sectors are key drivers of the global food-related health and sustainability challenges. The food retail sector generally includes any business where food is sold to customers, and retail food is defined as "food, other than restaurant food, that is purchased by consumers and consumed off-premises" (Seth & Randall, 1999). Food distribution, often known as post-farmgate activities, refers to a combination of activities and functions including production, handling, storage, transport, processing, packaging, wholesale and retail (Estrada-Florez & Larsen, 2010).

Food retailers, and in particular supermarkets, are key paths via which food is channelled from growers to consumers. They are embedded in the food distribution system and are also closely connected to pre-farmgate activities, with significant impacts on small-scale farmers, agricultural workforces and women's inequalities (Oxfam, 2018). Given that supermarkets are powerful gatekeepers of the supply chain, they can play a key role in enabling provision and consumption of healthy and environmentally sustainable foods as everyday practices (Mason & Lang, 2017).

The chapter begins by describing the contribution of supermarkets as key players in the current unsustainable food system and looks at ways to transform them to be positive components of healthy and sustainable food systems. Using the UK and Australia as two case studies, the chapter then goes on to explore opportunities and barriers to changes in food provisioning in relation to health and sustainability considerations. The UK has a system dominated by five or six key retailers. Australia shares similarities with a duopoly of retail control, however, this is being challenged with new competition from what are called the "hard discounters" with their emphasis on own-brand labels, smaller store size and a focus on operations management. Retailer dominance through supermarkets results in dominance of all parts of the food chain from farmers to consumption. From the perspective of health and sustainable food systems, there are lessons that emerge from the analysis of the UK and Australia that are global and broadly relevant to many other middle- and high-income countries, as well as emerging economies.

Overview of the current status of global food retail and distribution

The profile of the global food retail environment is changing dramatically, with an influx of large supermarkets and fast-food outlets. This is creating an increasing tension between the big supermarket giants versus smaller food stores, food social enterprises, farmers markets, bartering and food hubs (Estrada-Florez & Larsen, 2010). These changes in the food retail environment have contributed to a nutrition transition towards greater consumption of highly processed nutrient-poor foods, resulting, ultimately, in high levels of malnutrition and diet-related disease. The rate of transition has been accelerating, with food systems and environments in emerging economies being transformed within a 3–5-year period (das Nair, 2018; Popkin & Reardon, 2018).

At the same time, the distribution of food from producers, via food retailers, to customers plays a significant role in the environmental performance of the food supply chain. One of the major environmental concerns is the amount of greenhouse gas (GHG) emissions resulting from the transportation of food products (Estrada-Florez & Larsen, 2010). The World Economic Forum (Schwab, 2009) estimated that the global footprint of logistics and transport is 5.5 per cent of the total annual GHG emissions generated by human activity. In absolute terms, road freight makes the highest contribution to GHG emissions at around 57 per cent of the total, followed by ocean freight at 17 per cent.

Globally, supermarkets are at the centre of the many changes in the food system and therefore offer opportunities and barriers to health and environmental concerns. There is great penetration by transnational food retail corporations (TNFRCs) into high-, middle- and low-income countries, accompanied by increasing concentration and control of the market by a very small number of TNCs. Table 7.1 shows the top ten global retailers (by sales) and the corporate headquarters of each company. These are global trends with regional variations – Tesco in some areas, Carrefour in others, and through mergers and acquisitions in other territories, Walmart. The concentration of power among retailers also demonstrates a north/south divide, with major TNCs being based or originating in the rich Global North and expansion and growth taking place in developing markets in the Global South (Reardon, Timmer, & Berdegué, 2005).

Figure 7.1 shows how supermarkets in Europe exert control across the food supply chain. Note this funnel model is not exclusive to Europe (Howard, 2016). Not only do they control what is available for purchase by consumers but the supermarkets' buying desks also control the volume and type of food that is grown and produced. This gives supermarkets significant power along the whole supply chain (Monteiro et al., 2018; Popkin & Reardon, 2018), and affects the relative availability, affordability and acceptability of healthy to unhealthy foods, as well as the environmental sustainability practices used across the system.

Weatherspoon and Reardon (2003) identified that supplying supermarkets presented "both potentially large opportunities and big challenges for producers", often resulting in many producers being dependent on supermarkets. Being part of the supermarkets' supply chain results in amalgamations to meet bulk contracts, and investment in phytosanitary procedures and equipment to gain contracts. Through contracts and contract specification, supermarkets encourage producers to focus on growing monocultures. Howard (2016) shows that the growth of supermarkets has followed a path from regional to global dominance with health and sustainability issues beginning to emerge. The impacts on livelihoods are also enormous

TABLE 7.1 Top ten global retailers by sales, 2015

Name	Country of origin	Sales per year 2015 (billions UK pounds)**	Comments
Walmart	US	267	3 million employees worldwide. Largest global food retailer with annual sales equal to Carrefour, Tesco, Metro and Aeon combined. In the UK, they operate as ASDA.
Carrefour	France	89	Recently expanded into Middle Eastern countries, including Iraq, Iran and Syria
Tesco	UK	62	Major operations and financial success in the UK. Failed expansion to the US. Currently withdrawing from countries such as Poland and facing problems in Thailand.
Metro	Germany	61	Focus on wholesale and food service
Aeon	Japan	56	Corporate mantra is "Act global, think local"
7-11 Holdings	Japan	55	Also own hospitality enterprises, including the Denny's restaurant chain
Kroger	US	51	US-based, no expansion outside the US. In 2009, they donated 10.9 per cent of their pre-tax profits (US$64 million) to charity.
Lidl	Germany	50	Known as a "hard discounter", now in 30+ countries, expansion plans continue. Not successful in Norway and exited that market.
Costco	US	47	Pay for membership, then benefit from wholesale prices
Auchban	France	46	Innovative and not afraid to try new markets. In the US, they shut down their outlets after not making a profit. Current expansion is focused on Eastern European countries, especially Russia.

Note: **Estimated using data from Forbes and Kantar World Panel data, 2014–2016, authors' own calculations.

as farms consolidate and people move off the land (Oxfam, 2018), and as the retail food sector has grown, it has become a major employer, often with poor employment practices, including a lack of security and low wages.

A consequence of this vertical control by the retailers is that alternative sources of supply, such as wholesalers, are "written out" of the supply chain. The nature of the scale of these TNCs and the size of their operations mean that they rely on global food supply chains going where prices are low and building in added value via processing. Processing of foods has two advantages for the retailers. First, processed foods store and travel better than fresh foods and, second, they develop consumer dependence and deskilling (Lang, Barling, & Caraher, 2009). However, these advantages come at a cost to the health and sustainability of the global food system. This has driven consumption towards highly-processed foods, resulting in longer food chains and issues for sustainability (Monteiro et al., 2018; Popkin & Reardon, 2018). Major retailers claim that the scale of operation results in economies of scale, including less damage to the

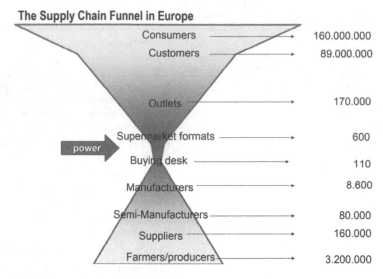

FIGURE 7.1 The food supply chain "funnel", Europe
Source: Grievink (2003).

environment (Desrochers & Shimizu, 2012). Multiple small shops are more wasteful, according to this premise, relying on many lines of supply and repeating processing at the local level (Seth & Randall, 2005). However, the counter-argument is that the global nature of the food chain operated by supermarkets allows costs and damage to the environment and health to be hidden along the way; so low wages in growing countries, degradation of local environments, pollution along the food distribution chain can more easily be concealed (Mason & Lang, 2017). In terms of economics, raw goods are often produced and then exported for processing in importing countries, meaning that the added value does not remain in the country of origin. Coffee offers an example, where the coffee grower in Africa receives AUS$0.30 per kilo for a product that eventually sells for AUS$35 in the Australian supermarket (Oxfam, 2018). There is a need to leave more money at the farm gate – cheap food can often be an illusion especially when the costs to health and sustainability, such as damage to livelihoods and the environment, are factored in.

National and regional variation in food retail and distribution

The UK and the changing supermarket situation

The UK underwent a recession (2007–12) that led to changes in shopping behaviours driven by the twin influences of increases in food prices (30 per cent increases) and greater awareness of sustainability and food waste issues. The monthly shop has been replaced by top-up shopping and the return of the supermarkets back to town centres, after abandoning them in the 1990s and early 2000s. The "food deserts" have now been filled with smaller size supermarket stores offering a limited range of essential goods at prices often up to 15 per cent higher than they sell for at their "big bins" or online.

The growth in small supermarket format on the high street is being led by the major supermarkets and does not reflect a growth in independent ownership. All this is possible because of technology and changes in supply chains. Supermarkets do not keep stocks of food on site, new systems such as just-in-time retailing allow goods to be shipped as they are bought and move off the shelves. From a health and sustainability perspective, there are moves to use electric vehicles and carbon-neutral approaches for transport, with some major supermarkets and their suppliers now using the rail (rather than road) networks to transport food from the European continent to central hubs in the UK (Behrends, 2012).

Tesco, the dominant supermarket chain in the UK, has set up a cheap new discount chain (Jack's) to combat the loss of sales to what are called the "hard discounters", namely, Aldi and Lidl. It is important to remember that these "hard discounters" are not new models of operation but variants on a dominant model; they offer a smaller range of goods at cheaper prices. In the early stages of their incursion into the UK and Irish markets, the model was based on large warehouse provision with goods being imported from the European main-land. Recent developments have shown them offering more and more goods produced in the UK or Ireland. This is especially true for fresh meat and vegetables, while large amounts of processed goods continue to be imported.

The hard discounters have grown at the expense of the major chains; there is no new or growing consumer base, the supermarket wars for customers are based on cannibalising cus-tomers from competitors. Some of the supermarkets with smaller market shares (Waitrose, Iceland, Marks & Spencer) have positioned themselves as offering sustainable food as part of their core offer but this comes at a price. The offer is aimed at a core customer base that is older, with higher income levels and concerned with sustainability. The supermarket, Ice-land, is a notable exception to this with low-income consumers and a produce range of mainly frozen goods (see their commitment to the environment at www.iceland.co.uk). This changing supermarket situation is prefaced by tensions in the food system with the consumer demanding local and sustainable goods but at the same time driven by price reductions and the lure of a bargain (Mason & Lang, 2017).

In the UK, between 2000 and 2008, a few supermarkets set up and experimented with local buying offices attempting to develop local supply lines. This coincided with increased consumer awareness and demand for local food, organic food and increases in oil prices. The recession from 2007 to 2012 resulted in consumers becoming more price-conscious and a decline in demand for locally produced foods, resulting in UK supermarkets shutting down their local buying offices. The decline in oil prices made it again more competitive to source goods from abroad.

Since the official end of the recession from 2012, there is a mixed economy of provision with local food offered at a premium and specifically around some key product categories. Many of the supermarkets now promote fresh beef from the UK and Ireland as this is a product category that consumers are concerned about, especially fraud and contamination (due perhaps to the horsegate and BSE scandals). The retail sector in the UK is heavily dependent on imports and the intention of the UK to leave the European Union will have major impacts on food supply chains. For sustainability, the border-free transfer of goods within the European Union will cease, resulting in increases in delivery times and transports being held up at border crossing (Millstone, Lang, & Marsden, 2017). This will result in longer temporal food supply chains leading to increased nuisance and pollution on the seas and roads.

A new emerging entrant to the UK food distribution systems is Amazon with the infra-structure for home delivery. Currently online retail shopping remains small as opposed to online ordering of take-away foods such as the like of Ubereats and Deliveroo. Online-only grocery retailers are benefiting from what is called "sofa surfing", with UK sales increasing from £1.1 billion in 2010, to an estimated £2.3 billion in 2015 out of a total retail spend of £120 billion+ (MINTEL, 2016). This trend is set to increase with the major supermarkets in the UK heavily investing in infrastructure to deliver food to the home. This issue is picked up later in the discussion along with the opportunities and threats this poses for healthy and sustainable food supply systems.

Australia and the changing supermarket situation

Australia by-passed the development of its own system of agriculture and imported a Eur-opean model with two key periods of change in the Australian foodscape: the industrialisa-tion of the garden, the pantry and then the kitchen (Symons, 1998), followed by the domination of the Australian plate and palate by supermarkets (Santich, 2012). This has had impacts on retail and food systems, with the model of operation reflecting production methods and now the move to highly-processed foods (Pulker, Scott, & Pollard, 2018).

The demands of the global food economy and the pressure to grow crops for cash have had implications for local communities in Australia. It effectively made the market less amicable to farmers (through oversupply) and encouraged the environmental degradation of the land through unsustainable farming. The effects have been devastating for the health and welfare of the rural sector with fewer family farms and the growth of corporate forms of agricultural production (Lawrence, Share, & Campbell, 1992). This has led to the death of many small rural towns with local shops being driven out by supermarkets (Knox, 2014).

Similar to the present situation in the UK, power within the Australian food retail sector is unequally concentrated with two main supermarket chains, Coles and Woolworths, holding a combined 61 per cent share of the total grocery market (Figure 7.2). Of the total grocery market in the 12 months to December 2017, Woolworths had a market share of 32.2 per cent and Coles 28.8 per cent. Hard discounter Aldi has also emerged in Australia, challenging the dominant supermarket players with a market share of 12.1 per cent (Figure 7.2). Aldi's approximately 1,350 or so products pale in comparison to Coles and Woolworths' broad and deep product ranges. Yet this provides them with lower supply chain costs and greater effi-ciencies. The market share of other supermarkets such as Independent Grocers Australia (IGA) has dropped to 7.4 per cent market share, as seen in Figure 7.2.

Fresh food has become a highly competitive segment for the major supermarkets with Figure 7.2 indicating that all the major supermarkets have a lower market share of the fresh food market than their overall grocery market share. The best performer in this segment is the non-supermarket group with 30.2 per cent share. Roy Morgan (2018) notes that this is a result of the non-supermarket group – such as bread shops, fruit shops, butchers, seafood retailers – being able to compete in the fresh food segment. What this also suggests is that consumers are increasingly using their purchasing power to support smaller food retailers for reasons that may include the sustainability of how they source their food.

From the perspective of food distribution, the sheer geographical size of Australia makes the transport of food almost inevitable but there are inconsistencies in the production and transport of foods. Perth, sometimes referred to as the most isolated city in the southern

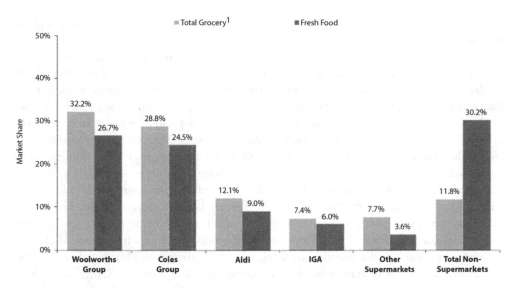

FIGURE 7.2 Share of Australian total grocery market versus share of fresh food market
Base: Grocery buyers aged 14+, 12 months ended December 2017, n = 12,313. [1]Includes fresh food.
Source: Roy Morgan (2018).

hemisphere, has one of the largest food storage and distribution centres in the world, yet this comes with an environmental cost. An improved understanding of the factors affecting GHG emissions, fuel use and potential vulnerabilities in the supply chain of food products will be important to their ongoing viability. What was once viewed as a miracle of logistics of food distribution, transporting food from one side of Australia to the other is now seen as an environmentally costly folly.

The challenges of food retail and distribution in contributing to healthy and sustainable food systems

Given the stranglehold that supermarkets have over both producers and consumers, they are key to changes in the delivery of sustainable and nutritious foods. Currently such moves seem to be driven not by concerns about these issues but by consumer demand, opportunity for niche products and issues of margins and profits.

The objective of supermarkets is to make a profit for their shareholders rather than deliver healthy and sustainable food. Debates over how to encourage supermarkets to engage with the ecologically integrated approach to health and environment set out above and develop more sustainable food supply systems have long raged. The irony with goods such as food, which carry both a private and public goods aspect to them, is that the public good is not factored in. Traditional cost accounting hides the true or full cost of goods. While there are moves to introduce full cost accounting procedures for foods, so far the work on this has come from industries, such as coal (Epstein et al., 2011). Short or local food chains or organics may be good for ecological and human health (Mason & Lang, 2017) but their place on the supermarket shelf is determined by price not cost. Food needs to be reconceived as a public good not just a consumer one and the power of supermarkets needs to be maximised in delivering the social good, which does not mean they cannot continue to make a profit but that the externalities are built into the equation.

The UK Sustainable Development Commission (2008) has argued for regulation by government to ensure that supermarkets meet their moral obligations. To date, little has occurred to advance this policy agenda, with the focus remaining on voluntary corporate social responsibility and fair-trade initiatives. This brings to mind the public health approach originally set out by Geoffrey Rose that small changes across a whole population achieve more than big changes in a small section of the population (Rose, Khaw, & Marmot, 2008). Similarly, for sustainable food chains, the problem facing us all in the future is to achieve changes across many food products and categories, not just a niche group sold at premium prices to affluent consumers. This is linked to debates that we do not need to grow more but should change existing food growing and production practices. Berners-Lee, Kennelly, Watson, and Hewitt (2018) say that the current production of crops is sufficient to provide enough food for the projected global population of 9.7 billion, but this must occur within a framework of changes to the dietary choices of the majority (replacing most meat/dairy with plant-based alternatives, and greater acceptance of human-edible crops currently fed to animals). Supermarkets with their powerful position in the food chain are well placed to deliver on such future sustainable development initiatives. But will they do so without government policy? The Berners-Lee hypothesis means that we may have to engage with a new concept of sustainability that is not just about sourcing, but also more closely aligned to human health and global rights.

Food transport, specifically freight, remains an ongoing challenge, with pressures of rising energy costs, potential carbon prices and increasing vulnerability in food supply chains challenging food producers and businesses, and they have important implications for food availability, access and utilisation – and hence food security (Estrada-Florez & Larsen, 2010). As observed in Australia, sustainability has become a concern as food is transported many thousands of kilometres, often criss-crossing the country in its moves from raw product to processed goods. The challenge of such logistics has become a concern to the major retailers who, when oil prices were low, saw this as an operational issue that could be absorbed as a "hidden cost", now the increased cost of oil has made this difficult to ignore. Yet we cannot leave food systems to the mercy of oil prices.

This chapter asserts that the future trends shaping grocery and supermarket expansion will come in the virtual world of internet ordering and delivery. Although currently small in overall financial terms, this is set to grow. The expansion of Amazon into home food delivery and its acquisition of Wholefoods are indicative of this trend. This offers opportunities as well as threats to sustainability. In the UK, the online grocer Ocado has just sold its services and expertise to Kroger supermarkets in the US, highlighting a new kind of merger and acquisition (Monaghan, 2018). It is likely that the Amazon expansion into food will herald similar models, maybe making links to local food producers at a price; this would enable it to promote local fresh sustainable food without much risk.

Conclusion

What is to be done about supermarkets and their stranglehold on the food retail sector? Drawing on Mason and Lang's (2017) notion of eco-nutrition, one way to rebalance the supermarkets' power is a move to a food system which is locally driven, and which pays attention to the issues of local "foodways" and ecological sustainability. The challenge for existing supermarket food distribution systems is to transport goods between producers and customers with the lowest possible impact on the environment, improving health, while rewarding growers and employees with fair wages and incomes. Farm and consumer-led initiatives offer great ways to do this. These types of systems, including farmers markets; marketing cooperatives; community-supported agriculture, direct and online sales hubs, will promote shorter distances between producers and consumers. All this can form the basis of a plan of action for policy to support local food provisioning. The benefits to supermarkets that engage in these forms of distribution systems are at both ends of the food chain; the production and processing element results in fewer costs in transport and processing, and at the retail end of the chain, it appeals to customers' concerns about health and the environment.

References

Behrends, S. Ö. (2012). The urban context of intermodal road-rail transport: Threat or opportunity for modal shift? *Procedia: Social and Behavioral Sciences*, 39, 463–475. doi:10.1016/j.sbspro.2012.03.122.

Berners-Lee, M., Kennelly, C., Watson, R., & Hewitt, C. (2018). Current global food production is sufficient to meet human nutritional needs in 2050 provided there is radical societal adaptation. *Elementa: Science of the Anthropocene*, 6(1), 52.

das Nair, R. (2018). The internationalisation of supermarkets and the nature of competitive rivalry in retailing in southern Africa. *Development Southern Africa*, 35(3), 315–333. doi:10.1080/0376835X.2017.1390440.

Desrochers, P., & Shimizu, H. (2012). *The locavore's dilemma: In praise of the 10,000-mile diet.* New York: Public Affairs.

Epstein, P., Buonocore, J., Eckerle, K., Hendryx, M., Stout III, B., Heinberg, R., … Glustrom, L. (2011). Full cost accounting for the life cycle of coal. *Annals of the New York Academy of Sciences*, 1219(1), 73–98.

Estrada-Florez, S., & Larsen, K. (2010). *Best practice food distribution systems.* Melbourne: Victorian Eco-Innovation Lab.

Grievink, J. W. (2003). The changing face of the global food industry. Paper presented at Changing dimensions of the food economy: Exploring the policy issues, The Hague, OECD.

Howard, P. (2016). *Concentration and power in the food system: Who controls what we eat?* London: Bloomsbury.

Knox, M. (2014). Supermarket monsters: Coles, Woolworths and the price we pay for their domination. *The Monthly*, August.

Lang, T., Barling, D., & Caraher, M. (2009). *Food policy: Integrating health, environment and society*Oxford: Oxford University Press.

Lawrence, G., Share, P., & Campbell, H. (1992). The restructuring of agriculture and rural society: Evidence from Australia and New Zealand. *Journal of Australian Political Economy*, 30, 1–23.

Mason, P., & Lang, T. (2017). *Sustainable diets: How ecological nutrition can transform consumption and the food system.* London: Routledge.

Millstone, E., Lang, T., & Marsden, T. (2017). Will the British public accept chlorine-washed turkey for Christmas dinner, after Brexit? In *Food research collaboration.* London: Centre for Food Policy.

MINTEL. (2016). Grocery retailing UK 2016 report. London: MINTEL.

Monaghan, A. (2018). Ocado shares soar 45% as US deal makes it worth more then M&S. *The Guardian*, 18 May, p. 35.

Monteiro, C. A., Cannon, G., Moubarac, J.-C., Levy, R. B., Louzada, M. L. C., & Jaime, P. C. (2018). The UN Decade of Nutrition, the NOVA food classification and the trouble with ultra-processing. *Public Health Nutrition*, 21(1), 5–17.

Oxfam. (2018). *Ripe for changes: Ending human suffering in supermarket supply chains.* Oxford: Oxfam International.

Popkin, B., & Reardon, T. (2018). Obesity and the food system transformation in Latin America. *Obesity Reviews*, 19, 1028–1064.

Pulker, C., Scott, J., & Pollard, C. (2018). Ultra-processed family foods in Australia: Nutrition claims, health claims and marketing techniques *Public Health Nutrition*, 21(1), 38–48.

Reardon, T., Timmer, P. C., & Berdegué, J. A. (2005). Supermarket expansion in Latin America and Asia: Implications for food marketing systems. In A. Regmi, & M. Gehlhar (eds), *New directions in global food markets*. Washington, DC: Economic Research Service/USDA.

Rose, G., Khaw, K., & Marmot, M. (2008). *Rose's strategy of preventive medicine*. Oxford: Oxford University Press.

Roy Morgan (2018). Woolworths increases lead in $100b+ grocery war, 2018. Available at: www.roymorgan.com/findings/7537-woolworths-increases-lead-in-$100b-plus-grocery-war-201803230113 (accessed 22 May 2018).

Santich, B. (2012). *Bold palates: Australia's gastronomic heritage*. Kent Town, South Australia: Wakefield Press.

Schwab, K. (2009). *The global competitiveness report 2009–2010*. Geneva: World Economic Forum.

Seth, A., & Randall, G. (1999). *The grocers: The rise and rise of the supermarket chains*. London: Kogan Page.

Seth, A., & Randall, G. (2005). *Supermarket wars: Global strategies for food retailers*. London: Palgrave.

Sustainable Development Commission. (2008). Green, healthy and fair: A review of government's role in supporting sustainable supermarket food. London: Sustainable Development Commission.

Symons, M. (1998). *The pudding that took a thousand cooks: The story of cooking in civilisation and daily life*. Ringwood, Vic: Viking.

Weatherspoon, D., & Reardon, T. (2003). The rise of supermarkets in Africa: Implications for agrifood systems and the rural poor. *Development Policy Review, 21*(3), 333–355. doi:10.1111/1467-7679.00214;03.

8

FOOD SERVICE AND RESTAURANT SECTORS

Vivica Kraak

Introduction

Food systems are a major driver of human-induced climate change, inefficient land and water use and loss of biodiversity – which affect the food security and health of people worldwide (Myers et al., 2017). Food production and consumption are responsible for 19–29 per cent of greenhouse gas (GHG) emissions, and the carbon footprint of businesses contribute to the health and environmental challenges associated with climate change (UNSCN, 2017). In 2015, 150 leaders from 193 Member States, the business and civil society sectors convened to support the implementation of the United Nations (UN) 17 Sustainable Development Goals (SDGs) by 2030 to end poverty, ensure economic prosperity, and protect the planet from the effects of climate change (Stockholm Resilience Centre, 2018).

The process of creating healthy and sustainable food systems is linked to all 17 SDGs (Johnston, Fanzo, & Cogill, 2014; Stockholm Resilience Centre, 2018). However, about 80 per cent of major transnational food and beverage firms' revenue aligns with only three goals: zero hunger (SDG 2); population health and well-being (SDG 3); and responsible production and consumption practices (SDG 12) (Wan, 2017). Businesses have many opportunities: to address poverty (SDG 1); ensure gender equality (SDG 5); create jobs (SDG 8); reduce workplace-related inequities and inequalities (SDG 10); and promote climate action (SDG 13) to mitigate their impact on people and the planet (Stockholm Resilience Centre, 2018).

Achieving healthy and food-secure populations, as outlined in the UN's SDG agenda, will require collaborations across sectors and settings to promote the co-benefits of healthy and sustainable food systems, and respond to the evolving challenges related to the poor stewardship of natural resources that contribute to poor health and climate change (Johnston et al., 2014; James, 2015; FAO, 2017).

The transnational chain and non-chain restaurants and food service industry sectors are important food system actors who feed millions of customers daily. These sectors offer a variety of inexpensive and convenient meals either consumed by customers on the premises, through takeaway, or delivered at home. As technology evolves, customers will demand greater convenience to order through global positioning system-enabled, mobile applications, self-serve kiosks, and delivery services. In many countries, restaurant, food service and hospitality businesses are partnering with delivery service businesses, such as Yum! Brands with Grubhub, McDonald's with UberEATS, and DoorDash with Postmates, which enable people to customise their orders and delivery locations (Mintel, 2018). Through these new partnerships, restaurants have the potential to influence upstream and midstream procurement practices and downstream eating and environmental stewardship behaviours of populations to support healthy and sustainable food systems (Goggins et al., 2018).

The extent to which transnational chain restaurants, independent restaurants and food service operations have adopted comprehensive healthy and sustainable food system policies and practices has not been described. Drawing principally on experiences in the USA, this chapter summarises evidence to inform the restaurant and food service industry sectors' efforts to use marketing mix and choice architecture (MMCA) strategies to promote business practices supportive of healthy and sustainable food systems that align with the one health vision and the UN SDG agenda by 2030.

History and expansion of the US restaurant industry

The US quick-service restaurant (QSR) industry emerged during the 1950s due to several factors, including the development of new food technology, rising disposable income, changing work and family lifestyles, a motorised travel infrastructure, and an increased market demand for convenient and inexpensive food and beverage products. During the 1970s, McDonald's Corporation, Subway, Yum! Brands, Domino's Pizza and Burger King expanded into international markets using a franchising business model that allowed these restaurant chains (franchisor) to contract with an individual (franchisee) who paid to use the company's trade name, branded products and services and operating standards (Daszkowski, 2017; Rush Wirth, 2017). Franchisees provide a location, train employees, adhere to the corporate brand standards, and develop a marketing plan (Daszkowski, 2017). Figure 8.1 sets out the US restaurant-sector structure including independent non-chain restaurants, limited-

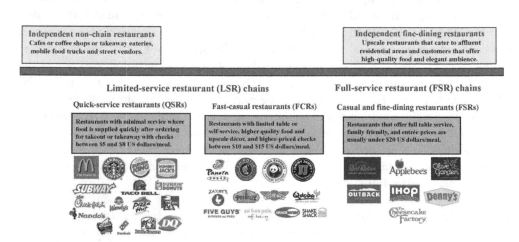

FIGURE 8.1 Structure of the chain and non-chain restaurant industry
Source: Based on Kraak et al. (2017a) and Statista (2018).

service restaurants (LSRs), such as QSR and fast-casual restaurant (FCR) chains, full-service restaurant (FSR) chains, and independent fine-dining restaurants (Kraak, Englund, Misyak, & Serrano, 2017a; Statista, 2018).

Principles, frameworks and strategies to create healthy and sustainable restaurants

Food system stakeholders and actors have several principles to guide the integration of health and sustainability into food system activities (Barilla Center for Food and Nutrition, 2018; Stockholm Resilience Centre, 2018). The Fair Food, Good Food, Slow Food, and Sustainable Food Movements have evolved over decades, in response to concerns about the harmful impacts of the fast-food culture and large-scale food and agricultural systems on the diet quality and health of populations (Morath, 2014). These movements have advocated for food to be healthy, green, humane, fair and equitable, affordable and profitable; they have supported local food cultures and traditions; raised awareness about how food is grown and processed; and educated citizens about how their choices support either sustainable or unsustainable food systems practices (Morath, 2014). The reality is that business leaders, policy-makers and the public make trade-offs that prioritise certain principles over others in current local, national and global food systems.

The restaurant, food service, hospitality and health care industries have many frameworks, guidelines, standards and metrics to promote heathy and sustainable food systems at upstream points (i.e. materials, supply chain and transportation); midstream points (i.e. green menu design, storage, cooking, service, packaging and marketing); and downstream points (i.e. customer service, recycling, and food waste and packaging management) (Wang, Chen, Lee, & Tsai, 2013). For example, businesses can incorporate sustainable goods and building materials into the design, construction and outdoor landscaping of physical structures. They can select sustainable or recycled furniture, fixtures and fittings; and use organic or eco-label-certified cleaning products. Restaurants can promote energy and water efficiency; use locally, regionally and seasonally sourced foods and goods; and adhere to best practices and laws to ensure that they serve healthy and safe foods (Wang et al., 2013; Green Restaurant Association, 2018).

Sustainable principles and practices are also available for food service management firms and operations such as cafeterias, concessions, caterers of professional meetings and vending machines (Figure 8.2) (The Sustainable Restaurant Association, 2015; World Obesity Federation, 2015; Sodexo, 2017; Culinary Institute of America & Harvard T.H. Chan School of Public Health and President and Fellows of Harvard College, 2018).

Restaurant businesses could also use MMCA strategies or "nudges" to cue healthy and sustainable behaviours (Kraak, Englund, Misyak, & Serrano, 2017b). Choice architecture or nudges represent how options are framed or presented to individuals in environments, deemed effective based on the assumptions that:

1. People choose options that require the least amount of mental or physical effort.
2. People value immediate rewards or avoid short-term costs versus long-term benefits or consequences of specific actions.
3. People align their behaviour with prevailing social norms.
4. People identify with peer groups that reinforce specific lifestyle behaviours

(Mols et al., 2015).

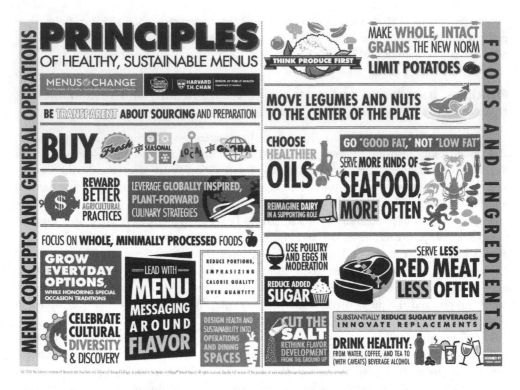

FIGURE 8.2 Menus of change: principles to support healthy and sustainable restaurant menus
Source: Culinary Institute of America, Harvard T.H. Chan School of Public Health, and President and Fellows of Harvard College (2018). Copyright permission has been granted.

By definition, choice architecture and nudges exclude pricing or fiscal strategies, such as subsidies and taxes, which are powerful interventions to influence consumers' behaviour and reduce health inequities. Therefore, MMCA strategies can be strategically combined to maximise their synergistic effects to promote population and environmental health (Kraak et al., 2017a; 2017b).

A MMCA framework is available to enable restaurants to promote healthy food environments that offer eight strategies, aligned with expert bodies' recommended targets and actions, to encourage healthy food environments (Figure 8.3). These strategies include:

- place (ambience and atmospherics),
- profile (nutrient composition),
- portion (serving size),
- pricing (strategic and proportionate),
- promotion (responsible marketing),
- healthy default picks (side dishes and beverages),
- priming or prompting (information and labelling),
- proximity (strategic positioning)

(Kraak et al., 2017a).

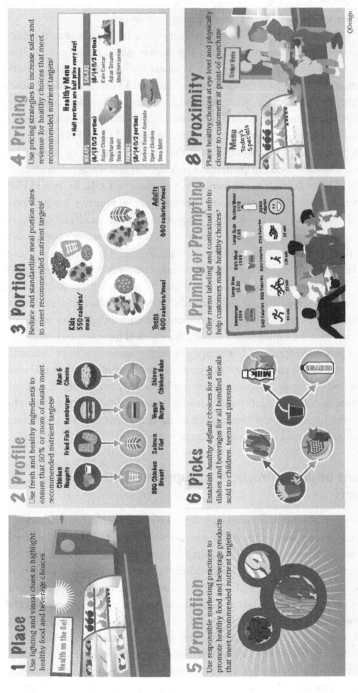

FIGURE 8.3 Marketing mix and choice architecture strategies to promote healthy restaurant environments

Source: Kraak et al. (2017b). Permission has been granted to reprint this image through a creative commons copyright.

[1] Quick-service, fast-casual and full-service chain restaurants and non-chain restaurants.

These voluntary strategies complement government-mandated standards, legislation, regulations and laws that require restaurants to meet food safety guidelines, food labelling requirements, nutrient composition targets, and responsible food and beverage marketing practices that influence the decisions of children, teens and their parents.

Starting in May 2018, the US menu labelling law required that calorie labelling be accompanied by contextual information to help Americans to make healthy choices when eating out at chain restaurants. The information states for children: 1,200–1,400 calories/day is used for general nutrition advice for ages 4–8 years and 1,400–2,000 calories/day for ages 9–13 years, but calorie needs vary. For adults: 2,000 calories/day is used for general nutrition advice, but calorie needs vary. Upon a customer's request, restaurants must provide written nutrition information for total calories, fat, saturated fat, trans-fats, sodium, protein, carbohydrates, added sugars and fibre (FDA, 2018).

An evaluation of US restaurant industry practices that used the MMCA framework assessed the sector's performance to promote healthy food environments for American customers between 2006 and 2017 (Kraak et al., 2017b). The evaluation found some progress made by QSR, FCR and FSR chains to reduce meal portions, but limited progress to use strategic pricing, improve product profiles, establish healthy default picks, and use responsible promotion, priming and prompting to promote healthy choices. No evidence was available to assess the US restaurant sector's use of place or proximity to promote healthy food environments (Kraak et al., 2017b). The evaluation found that most US restaurant offerings exceeded the expert-recommended nutrient targets for energy (≤ 600–700 calories or ~2,500–3,000 kJ/meal); fat (≤ 35% total energy); saturated fat (≤ 10% total energy); free or added sugars (≤ 35% total energy); and sodium (≤ 210–410 milligrams/meal item) (Kraak et al., 2017a; 2017b). The expert and US government-recommended nutrient targets included: energy (≤ 600 calories/meal for children and ≤ 700 calories/meal for teens and adults).

The consumption of ultra-processed foods and beverages in large portions at chain and non-chain restaurants is associated with poor diet quality and increased overweight and obesity rates among children, adolescents and adults in many countries worldwide (Kraak et al., 2019). An evaluation of progress by transnational restaurant chains found great variability in actions taken by chain restaurants across countries to reformulate menu items to meet nutrient targets, and reduce or standardise portion sizes to encourage a healthy diet (Kraak et al., 2019).

Transforming restaurant business practices to support healthy and sustainable food systems

People's views of the environmentally friendly business practices to produce "green restaurants" differ across countries. US consumers who visit green restaurants report that they value fresh ingredients, health, easy access, and environmentally sustainable food choices (Dewald, Bruin, & Jang, 2014). However, US restaurants and food service industries have encountered barriers to expanding healthy and sustainable meals that include: low customer demand for, satisfaction with, and acceptance of new options; a limited selection of products from upstream vendors; and increased time, cost, and workforce training to prepare and serve items that may not be financially sustainable (Jilcott Pitts et al., 2018). Restaurant owners in low- to middle-income countries can face other barriers to implementing environmentally sustainable "green restaurant" policies. A study in Malaysia identified several challenges faced by green restaurants, including weakly enforced national environmental laws and regulations, scarce or unreliable sustainable supply chains, low customer demand for sustainable choices, and domestic agricultural and international trade policies that do not support sustainable outcomes (Kasim & Ismail, 2012).

The US National Restaurant Association (NRA) has identified several sustainable practice trends for food systems, such as: increasing water efficiency; promoting recyclable, edible and biodegradable packaging (Strom, 2017); and reducing food production loss and consumer food waste (ReFED, 2018). Managing food waste is important to save money for businesses while also reducing GHG emissions to mitigate the adverse effects of climate change. The US economy wastes about 63 million tons of food annually, of which about 11 million tons is generated by the restaurant industry, costing US$25 billion (ReFED, 2016). Businesses that interact with consumers generate about 40 per cent of the food waste by weight (ReFED, 2018).

Restaurant businesses could save US$8 for every dollar invested in food-waste reduction actions (ReFED, 2016). Since 2011, members of the US Food Waste Reduction Alliance (i. e. NRA, McDonald's, Yum! Brands and Darden) have reported having reduced their food waste by increasing food donations to needy people, and diverting food waste from landfills through repurposing and recycling efforts (GMA, 2013). However, these seemingly sensible activities can themselves be more complex than first appears. For instance, activities involving the donation of unsold food to needy people have been criticised for being motivated primarily by a desire to reduce the cost of disposing of unwanted food, and while they may provide a short-term fix to food insecurity, this risks diverting attention away from the need to tackle the underlying causes of food insecurity (Riches & Silvasti, 2016).

Chain and non-chain restaurant businesses can contribute to food waste reduction through various policies and strategies, such as:

- providing customers with smaller plates in self-serve or buffet settings;
- promoting trayless dining and eliminating "all you can eat" promotions;
- replacing plastic food packaging containers with recyclable containers and edible wrapping;
- tracking food waste practices to inform changes;
- using diverted food waste in menus to reduce costs;
- supporting institutional composting

(NRA, 2018; ReFED, 2018).

The tracking and management of food waste diversion by QSR businesses are complicated because corporate headquarters often have limited control over franchised restaurant operations that engage with different actors for food donations, recycling and disposal at local or state levels (BSR, 2014).

Some transnational restaurant chains have committed to supply-chain sourcing policies and practices that support sustainable menus and products. Civil society organisation campaigns have used accountability scorecards and publicised the results through social media to accelerate industry action. Several restaurant chains have committed to providing customers with antibiotic-free meat and poultry through global food supply chain sourcing practices (Friends of the Earth et al., 2017).

By 2017, 14 of 25 transnational restaurant companies (i.e. Panera, Chipotle, Subway and Chick-fil-A) had adopted and disclosed a policy to reduce or eliminate antibiotics in chicken obtained through their supply chains, whereas Starbucks, Burger King, KFC and Domino's Pizza have not yet made meaningful public commitments (Friends of the Earth et al., 2017). Civil society groups pressured McDonald's Corporation to implement an antibiotic-free chicken policy that the firm committed to implement in all global markets by 2027 (Consumers International, 2017).

McDonald's Corporation and Darden's Red Lobster chains have also committed to "sea to plate" transparency and traceability for sustainably harvested fish and seafood (Aquaculture Stewardship Council, 2018). By 2018, 40 major US restaurant chains had made cage-free egg pledges (Cage Free Future, n.d.). Dunkin' Donuts and Subway have committed to eliminate palm oil in their products to protect rainforest biodiversity, animal habitats and communities. Yum! Brands, Wendy's, Domino's, Burger King and Starbucks have not yet made meaningful palm oil commitments (Union of Concerned Scientists, 2015).

MMCA strategies that can promote healthy and environmentally sustainable meals

The Menus of Change initiative examined progress achieved by US restaurants and food service operators across 16 health and sustainability issues from 2014 to 2018 (Culinary Institute of America & Harvard T.H. Chan School of Public Health and President and Fellows of Harvard College, 2018). The 2018 report documented that some progress has been made to support supply-chain resiliency and transparency, change food industry investment standards, support local and regional food systems, and reduce antibiotics in the food supply. However, limited or no progress was made: to promote water sustainability; to engage in sustainable practices for fish, seafood and oceans; or to support sustainable land use and farming practice (Culinary Institute of America & Harvard T.H. Chan School of Public Health and President and Fellows of Harvard College, 2018).

Businesses have many opportunities to promote healthy and sustainable food system choices that influence customers' preferences for a "plant-forward" Mediterranean or flexitarian diet that reduces but does not eliminate meat from menus, and to expand whole-grain choices (Dibb & de Llaguno, 2017; Culinary Institute of America & Harvard T.H. Chan School of Public Health and President and Fellows of Harvard College, 2018). Restaurant owners and managers can provide training for chefs and cooks to combine MMCA strategies that promote both healthy choices or "blue nudges" and environmentally sustainable choices or "green nudges". Examples of blue nudges are designing menus to feature high quality but smaller portions of red meat (i.e. lamb and beef) and larger portions of fruits, vegetables or salads to occupy half of the plate or to feature meat-alternative options at the top of menus. Restaurant managers could also use proximity as a strategy to highlight meat-free or meat-alterative options at the beginning of self-serve counters and buffets (Dibb & de Llaguno, 2017; Culinary Institute of America & Harvard T.H. Chan School of Public Health and President and Fellows of Harvard College, 2018).

Green nudges could include offering upstream food system strategies by selecting third party-certified fair trade coffee, tea and chocolate products; organic produce and meat; and sustainably harvested seafood (BSD Consulting, 2018). Chain restaurants could also use priming, prompting and promotion to emphasise carbon footprint labelling to raise awareness about how one's food choices contribute to GHG emissions and planetary health (Macdiarmid, Douglas, & Campbell, 2016).

In 2018, McDonald's announced major planetary health commitments to work with franchisees and suppliers globally to reduce the business-related, GHG emission carbon footprint by 36 per cent by 2030 (McDonald's Corporation, 2018). This commitment, and others adopted by other leading transnational restaurant and food service industry businesses, could substantially influence supply-chain practices, improve energy efficiency, adopt recyclable packaging, and reduce food waste through food recovery and food recycling activities.

Conclusion

Transnational chain restaurants and non-chain food service operations can use principles, guidelines, standards and metrics to support healthy and sustainable food systems. Few transnational restaurant chains are yet to use comprehensive MMCA strategies to encourage customers to make healthy and environmentally sustainable choices in countries where they operate franchise businesses. In the future, restaurant and food service industry businesses should harmonise universal nutrition and environmental sustainability guidelines and standards to support healthy and sustainable meals for customers across countries and regions. Government and civil society organisations and researchers should monitor the implementation of these commitments, and evaluate the impact on outcomes to hold restaurants accountable for promoting healthy and sustainable food systems that align with the one health vision and the SDG agenda by 2030.

References

Aquaculture Stewardship Council. (2018). Available at: www.fishchoice.com/seafood-program/aquaculture-stewardship-council (accessed 10 December 2018).

Barilla Center for Food and Nutrition. (2018). Double pyramid: Healthy food for people, sustainable food for the planet, 2018. Available at: www.barillacfn.com/m/publications/pp-double-pyramid-healthy-diet-for-people-sustainable-for-the-planet.pdf (accessed 10 December 2018).

BSD Consulting. (2018). Equitable food initiative: Driving change across agricultural systems. Available at: www.equitablefood.org/single-post/2018/02/27/EFI-is-Making-an-Impact (accessed 10 December 2018).

BSR. (2014). Analysis of U.S. food waste among food manufacturers, retailers, and restaurants. Prepared for the Food Waste Reduction Alliance. Food Marketing Institute, Grocery Manufacturers Association, National Restaurant Association. Available at: www.foodwastealliance.org/wp-content/uploads/2014/11/FWRA_BSR_Tier3_FINAL.pdf (accessed 10 December 2018).

Cage Free Future. (n.d.). Corporate commitments on farm animal confinement issues: Restaurant chains. Available at: http://cagefreefuture.com/wp/commitments/(accessed 10 December 2018).

Consumers International. (2017). Consumers International welcomes McDonald's improvement in global policy on antibiotics, 25 August 2017 (media release). Available at: www.consumersinternational.org/news-resources/news/releases/consumers-international-welcomes-mcdonald-s-improvement-in-global-policy-on-antibiotics/ (accessed 10 December 2018).

Culinary Institute of America, Harvard T.H. Chan School of Public Health, and President and Fellows of Harvard College. (2018). Menus of change. The business of healthy, sustainable, delicious food choices: 2018 annual report. Available at: www.menusofchange.org/images/uploads/pages/2018_Menus_of_Change_Annual_Report_FINAL.pdf (accessed 10 December 2018).

Daszkowski, D. (2017). The expansion of American fast food franchises, *The Balance*. Available at: www.thebalancesmb.com/how-american-fast-food-franchises-expanded-abroad-1350955 (accessed 10 December 2018).

Dewald, B., Bruin, B. J., & Jang, Y. J. (2014). US consumer attitudes towards "green" restaurants. *Anatolia*, 25(2), 171–180.

Dibb, S., & de Llaguno, E. (2017). The future of eating is flexitarian: Companies leading the way. Eating better for a fair, green, healthy future. Available at: www.eating-better.org/uploads/Documents/2017/Eating%20Better_The%20future%20of%20eating%20is%20flexitarian.pdf (accessed 10 December 2018).

FDA (Food and Drug Administration). (2018). Menu labeling requirements. September 14, 2018. Available at: www.fda.gov/food/food-labeling-nutrition/menu-labeling-requirements

FAO (Food and Agriculture Organization). (2017). Nutrition and food systems. A report by the High Level Panel of Experts on Food Security and Nutrition of the Committee on World Food Security. Rome: United Nations. Available at:www.fao.org/3/a-i7846e.pdf (accessed 10 December 2018).

Friends of the Earth, Natural Resources Defense Council, Consumers Union, Food Animal Concerns Trust, Keep Antibiotics Working, Center for Food Safety & Union. (2017). Chain reaction III: How top restaurants rate on reducing use of antibiotics in their meat supply. Available at: www.consumer.org.hk/ws_en/news/press/473/antibiotics.html (accessed 10 December 2018).

GMA (Grocery Manufacturers Association). (2013). Food waste reduction alliance. Available at: www.foodwastealliance.org/

Goggins, G. (2018). Developing a sustainable food strategy for large organizations: The importance of context in shaping procurement and consumption practices. *Business Strategy and the Environment*, 27, 838–848.

Green Restaurant Association. (2018). Green Restaurant Certification Standards. Available at: www.dinegreen.com/certification-standards (accessed 10 December 2018).

James, S. W., & Friel, S. (2015). An integrated approach to identifying and characterising resilient urban food systems to promote population health in a changing climate. *Public Health Nutrition*, 18(13). 2498–2508.

Jilcott Pitts, S., Schwartz, B., Graham, J., Warnock, A. L., Mojica, A.… Harris, D. (2018). Best practices for financial sustainability of healthy food service guidelines in hospital cafeterias. *Preventing Chronic Disease*, 15, E58.

Johnston, J. L., Fanzo, J. C., & Cogill, B. (2014). Understanding sustainable diets: A descriptive analysis of the determinants and processes that influence diets and their impact on health, food security, and environmental sustainability. *Advances in Nutrition*, 5(4), 418–429.

Kasim, A., & Ismail, A. (2012). Environmentally friendly practices among restaurants: Drivers and barriers to change. *Journal of Sustainable Tourism*, 20(4), 551–570.

Kraak, V., Englund, T., Misyak, S., & Serrano, E. L. (2017a). A novel marketing mix and choice architecture framework to nudge restaurant customers toward healthy food environments to reduce obesity in the United States. *Obesity Reviews*, 18(8), 852–868.

Kraak, V., Englund, T., Misyak, S., & Serrano, E. L. (2017b). Progress evaluation for the restaurant industry assessed by a voluntary marketing-mix and choice-architecture framework that offers strategies to nudge American customers toward healthy food environments, 2006–2017. *International Journal of Environmental Research and Public Health*, 14(7), 760.

Kraak, V., Rincón-Gallardo Patiño, S., Renukuntla, D., & Kim, E. (2019). Progress achieved by transnational restaurant chains to reformulate products and standardize portions to meet healthy dietary guidelines, 2000–2018: A scoping and systematic review to inform policy. *International Journal of Environmental Research and Public Health*, 16(15), 2732, doi:10.3390/ijerph16152732.

Macdiarmid, J. I., Douglas, F., & Campbell, J. (2016). Eating like there's no tomorrow: Public awareness of the environmental impact of food and reluctance to eat less meat as part of a sustainable diet. *Appetite*, 96, 487–493.

McDonald's Corporation. (2018). McDonald's announces global commitment to support families with increased focus on Happy Meals, February 15, 2018.

Mintel. (2018). Thought bubble: Fast food evolution. 15 February 2018. Available at: www.mintel.com/blog/foodservice-market-news/thought-bubble-fast-food-evolution (accessed 10 December 2018).

Mols, F., Haslam, S. A., Jetten, J., & Steffens, N. K. (2015). Why a nudge is not enough: A social identity critique of governance by stealth. *European Journal of Political Research*, 54(1), 81–98.

Morath, S. (2014). *From farm to fork: Perspectives on growing sustainable food systems in the twenty-first century.* Akron, OH: University of Akron Press.

Myers, S. S., Smith, M. R., Guth, S., Golden, C. D., Vaitla, B.… Huybers, P. (2017). Climate change and global food systems: Potential impacts on food security and undernutrition. *Annual Review of Public Health*, 38(1), 259–277.

NRA. (2018). The state of restaurant sustainability 2018. Available at: www.restaurant.org/getattachment/News-Research/Research/State-of-Restaurant-Sustainability/Sustainability_FINAL_pdf.pdf (accessed 10 December 2018).

ReFED (Rethinking Food Waste through Economics and Data). (2016). A roadmap to reduce U.S. food waste by 20%. Available at: https://assets.rockefellerfoundation.org/app/uploads/20160310153850/ReFED_Roadmap_to_Reduce_Food_Waste.pdf

ReFed (Rethinking Food Waste through Economics and Data). (2018). Restaurant food waste action guide. Available at: www.refed.com/downloads/Restaurant_Guide_Web.pdf#page=6 (accessed 1 August 2019).

Riches, G., & Silvasti, T. (2016). *First World hunger revisited: Food charity or the right to food?*Basingstoke: Palgrave Macmillan.

Rush Wirth, S. (2017). 2017 top 500: Limited service chains. *Restaurant Business*. Available at: www.restaurantbusinessonline.com/financing/2017-top-500-limited-service-chains (accessed 10 December 2018).

Sodexo. (2017). Supplier code of conduct, 2017. Available at: www.sodexo.com/files/live/sites/sdxcom-global/files/PDF/Corporate-responsibility/Sodexo-Supplier-Code-En.pdf (accessed 10 December 2018).

Statista. (2018). Leading casual dining restaurant chains on the United States in 2017, ranked by index ranking. Available at: www.statista.com/statistics/469273/leading-casual-restaurants-by-buzz-score-us/ (accessed 10 December 2018).

Stockholm Resilience Centre. (2018). Eat-Lancet Commission on food, planet, health, 2018. Available at: https://foodplanethealth.org/ (accessed 10 December 2018).

Strom, S. (2017). Packaging food with food to reduce waste. *The New York Times*. May 30, 2017. Available at: www.nytimes.com/2017/05/30/dining/packaging-materials-food-waste.html (accessed 10 December 2018).

The Sustainable Restaurant Association. (2015). Our Sustainability Framework. Available at: https://thesra.org/framework/ (accessed 10 December 2018).

Union of Concerned Scientists. (2015). Fries, face wash, forests. scoring America's top brands on their palm oil commitments. Available at: www.ucsusa.org/global-warming/stop-deforestation/palm-oil-scorecard-2015#.WqalMegbObg (accessed 10 December 2018).

UNSCN (United Nations Standing Committee on Nutrition). (2017). Sustainable diets for healthy people and a healthy planet: nutrition. Rome: UN Standing Committee on Nutrition. Available at: www.unscn.org/uploads/web/news/document/Climate-Nutrition-Paper-Nov2017-EN-WEB.pdf (accessed 10 December 2018).

Wan, L. (2017). Investor interest in UN sustainability goals on the rise. 29 November. Available at: www.nutraingredients-asia.com/Article/2017/11/29/Investor-interest-in-UN-sustainability-goals-on-the-rise-Chr.-Hansen (accessed 10 December 2018).

Wang, Y., Chen, S., Lee, Y., & Tsai, C. (2013). Developing green management standards for restaurants: An application of green supply chain management. *International Journal of Hospitality Management*, 34, 263–273.

World Obesity Federation. (2015). Healthy venues, 2015. Available at: www.worldobesity.org/what-we-do/healthy-venues/ (accessed 10 December 2018).

9

FOOD CONSUMPTION

Food, people, and contexts

Annet Hoek, Gabrielle O'Kane and Tony Worsley

Introduction

Consumers in free market economies are compelled to make choices regarding which foods to buy: they need to decide between different types of foods and even where to buy their foods. Although action is required across the entire system of food supply and demand to make healthy and sustainable food options an easy choice, consumers' own food choices ultimately have consequences for food producers and retailers (Nestle, 2000). Accordingly, collective changes in consumers' behaviours can change demand and open pathways to healthier and sustainable food systems (Fresco, 2009).

Consumers are vital partners in achieving the goal of a healthier and more sustainable food system and therefore cannot be ignored. Whether we consider them to be engaged food citizens or less-involved consumers who make pragmatic food decisions (O'Kane, 2016a), we should consider different types of consumers in context, and use the appropriate approaches to enable behaviour change (De Bakker & Dagevos, 2012). The key question is: how?

Changing consumers' food behaviours is not an easy undertaking, and communication and awareness-raising campaigns are essential, but unlikely to be effective on their own (Garnett Mathewson, Angelides, & Borthwick, 2015; Hawkes et al., 2015). This chapter provides an overview of what can influence consumers when it comes to making healthy and sustainable food choices and will conclude with an outline of opportunities for behaviour change.

Health, sustainability and food: understanding consumer choices

It is easy to simply join the words together: a "healthy *and* sustainable diet" or "healthy *and* sustainable food choices". Although these concepts have traditionally been studied in the separate domains of health and environmental sustainability (Bailey & Harper, 2015; Van Loo, Hoefkens, & Verbeke, 2017; James, Friel, Lawrence, Hoek, & Pearson, 2018), at present, there is general consensus about their core principles: avoiding excessive food consumption beyond nutritional needs; reducing the consumption of ultra-processed foods that are energy-dense and nutrient-poor; promoting a diet comprising less animal- and more plant-derived foods; and reducing food waste (Friel, Barosh, & Lawrence, 2014; Willett et al., 2019). However, do consumers think the same way about combining health with sustainability? To understand consumers' choices and identify opportunities for change towards healthier and more sustainable food behaviours, it is important to consider the values and motives underlying health and sustainability, and how these vary between different consumers.

Health and sustainability from a consumer perspective

When consumers buy and eat foods, they know directly what price they have paid and what the foods taste like. This is notably different for the health and sustainability attributes of foods: consumers can read a label or claim, but it is not possible to directly experience the effects on their health or the environment (Aschemann-Witzel, 2015; Van Loo et al., 2017). Notwithstanding, it is important to realise they are quite different concepts to consumers. Healthy food choices give consumers private benefits, also referred to as long-term personal benefits. In contrast, sustainability is a much more abstract concept for consumers, with socially and temporally distant outcomes that do not directly benefit the individual (Van Dam & Van Trijp, 2011), which explains an attitude-behaviour gap (see Box 9.1). Health and sustainability offer consumers different benefits and are related to different motives.

BOX 9.1 MIND THE GAP

There is often a gap between what people say, or think, and their actual behaviour when it comes to sustainable food activities (e.g. Vermeir & Verbeke, 2006; McEachern, Warnaby, Carrigan, & Szmigin, 2010; Griffin & Sobal, 2013; Van Dam & Van Trijp, 2013; Garnett et al., 2015). McEachern et al. (2010), for example, interviewed self-identified "conscious consumers", who were concerned about the industrial food system, but were not as strident in their expression of these attitudes in actions compared to "ethical" consumers. These "conscious consumers" recognised inconsistencies in their own behaviour and even felt guilty about it, as they did not always make ethical choices.

This disparity, also referred to as the attitude-behaviour gap, intention-behaviour gap or the value-action behaviour gap, has been described in several studies, particularly in relation to organic foods (Aertsens, Verbeke, Mondelaers, & Van Huylenbroeck, 2009). Essentially this gap exists because other factors are prioritised at purchase, such as price, availability, taste, convenience, and habit (McEachern et al., 2010; Griffin & Sobal, 2013; Garnett et al., 2015).

In light of this effect, there is increased attention to include research approaches that are better predictors of actual behaviour, which will enable better interventions for behaviour change towards healthy and sustainable diets (Van Dam & Van Trijp, 2011; Hoek, Pearson, James, Lawrence, & Friel, 2017b).

A food choice motive such as health is generally regarded as self-centred (referring to utilitarian values and self-enhancement) while sustainable food choice motives are regarded as altruistic (referring to the value of universalism and caring for the welfare of people, animals and nature) (Aschemann-Witzel, 2015). Different consumer segments are driven by distinctive values and motives, and even at an individual level, health and sustainability motives may both be relevant but have different levels of importance.

Regardless, purely altruistic food choices are not common: consumers who make sustainable food choices often consider the food's sustainability attributes in conjunction with its health and other quality attributes, such as sensory quality (Aschemann-Witzel, 2015; O'Kane, 2016b; Van Loo et al., 2017; Sarti, Darnall, & Testa, 2018). Other research has shown that healthy and sustainable food behaviours (excluding food waste reduction behaviours) are motivated more by health than sustainability (e.g. Hoek, Pearson, James, Lawrence, & Friel, 2017a). This has led to recommendations that the health aspects of a healthy and sustainable diet should be the overarching message in communication to consumers since this could have a greater potential to support behavioural change.

Consumer segments with respect to healthy and sustainable food behaviours

Recognising individual and group differences when it comes to food, health and sustainability is also important from a behavioural change perspective. For interventions and policies to be effective, they need to be tailored towards identified target groups or consumer segments (Michie, Van Stralen, & West, 2011). While segmentation studies on both healthy *and* sustainable behaviours are still scarce, we can still draw useful insights from related studies, such as those described by Verain et al. (2012) and Sarti et al. (2018).

Verain et al. (2012) reviewed 16 segmentation studies on sustainable food behaviours and reported a pattern comprising three key consumer segments: "greens", "potential greens" and "non-greens". The smallest segment, "greens", have more favourable attitudes towards the environment and hold both individual and collective values. "Potential greens" also deem price, health and naturalness to be important. "Non-greens" have negative attitudes towards the environment and are driven by values such as security and self-enhancement. Sarti et al. (2018) examined consumer segments based on actual purchase data, which addressed the attitude-behaviour gap. The "involved" segment, which was only 7 per cent of the sample, purchased foods with both health and sustainable labels. However, the latter labels were primarily related to "organic" rather than ecological aspects.

The above examples, in line with other work (Schösler, De Boer, & Boersema, 2012; Hoek et al. 2017b) indicate that consumer segments that are primarily driven by environmental reasons are relatively small, therefore, we need to approach other consumer segments differently.

Drivers of and barriers to healthy and sustainable food choices

Healthy and sustainable food choices are related to a cluster of different behaviours, which can be associated with different foods and different consumer segments. Obviously, consumer drivers and barriers will be different depending on the area of focus. We therefore give a general overview of key drivers and barriers related to the food, the person and the physical and psycho-social context.

Food and individual-related factors

1. *Perceptions and associations* – Despite the differences between underlying motives for health or sustainable food choices, understanding which product features consumers consider as both healthy and sustainable is important. Consumer studies suggest that attributes such as "organic" and "natural" are strongly associated with both health and environmental friendliness (Tobler, Visschers, & Siegrist, 2011; Hoek et al., 2017a; Van Loo et al., 2017). Foods with these attributes are perceived to be free from pesticides and chemicals, and are believed to have positive effects on both people and the planet. Attributes that are perceived as both healthy and sustainable could be leveraged more in consumer communications (Aschemann-Witzel, 2015; Hoek et al., 2017a; Van Loo et al., 2017).

2. *Knowledge, awareness and skills* – In general, consumers seem to be less aware and have less knowledge about the environmentally sustainable aspects of foods, compared to health aspects (Lea & Worsley, 2008; Tobler et al., 2011; Hoek et al., 2017a). Consumers overestimate the environmental impact of product packaging and transport distance, while they underestimate the impact of animal-derived foods, transport mode and organic products (Lea & Worsley, 2008; Shi, Visschers, Bumann, & Siegrist, 2018). At the same time, consumers have little knowledge and awareness of the differences in environmental impact between different products and behaviours (e.g. reducing meat versus wasting less food), which indicates there is still a role for more education (Hoek et al., 2017a; Shi et al., 2018). To put healthy and sustainable behaviours into practice, consumers also need the skills and confidence to do so (i.e., self-efficacy). This is particularly relevant to encourage eating fewer animal-derived products and highly processed and packaged foods (Hoek et al,. 2017a). In contrast, highly involved consumers, such as community gardeners, have the knowledge and skills to grow their own food and to act as role models in their social spheres (O'Kane, 2016a).

3. *Attitudes and attributes* – The importance of particular product attributes is influenced by a person's attitudes and motivations, which are in turn affected by underlying values. At a general population level, numerous surveys indicate that price, convenience, taste and health, are more important factors in food choice than environmental sustainability (e.g. Lea & Worsley, 2008; Tobler et al., 2011; Van Dam & Van Trijp, 2013; Hoek et al., 2017b). Choice experiments and actual purchase data that address the attitude-behaviour gap (see Box 9.1) show that overall health and/ or sustainability food labels have relatively small effects on actual choices and behaviour (e.g. Hoek et al., 2017b; Sarti, Darnall, & Testa, 2018).

4. *The halo effect* – It is important to note that one food attribute (e.g. environmentally sustainable) might affect consumer perception of another (e.g. price). This so-called halo effect might work in a positive direction (e.g. "organic" is perceived to be healthier than conventionally grown products). However, some food attributes can also create a negative perception of another: "sustainable" products may be assumed to be more expensive by consumers (Aschemann-Witzel, 2015). These perceptions indicate that behavioural change initiatives should consider the complex interactions between different attributes.

5. *Emotions and habits* – Food choices and behaviours are also greatly influenced by feelings and emotions (affective elements of attitudes) (e.g. Desmet & Schifferstein, 2008). For example, the emotion "fear" has impacted meat purchases following various health

scares in the meat industry (Aertsens et al., 2009). Conversely, negative feelings around omitting meat from the menu act as a strong barrier to plant-based diets. Food experiences and the emotional attachment to food often stem from past experiences (O'Kane, 2016a). Some local food procurers have reported holding nostalgic memories about the way food used to be grown, which is re-created for them in local food networks, such as community gardens or farmers markets (O'Kane, 2016b). Habit is another unconscious factor, and one of the most powerful predictors of eating behaviour. This influences all healthy and sustainable food behaviours, but is particularly relevant to persistent meat consumption habits (Saba Vassallo & Turrini, 2000).

6. *Biological and demographics* – Socio-demographics are not regarded as key determinants in the choice of healthy and sustainable foods, but it appears that influencing factors are a higher income and education, and being female (e.g. Griffin & Sobal, 2013; Garnett et al., 2015).

BOX 9.2 FOOD CITIZENS AND LOCAL FOOD NETWORKS

Food citizenship is defined as: "the practice of engaging in food-related behaviours (defined narrowly and broadly) that support, rather than threaten, the development of democratic, socially and economically just, and environmentally sustainable food systems" (Wilkins 2005).

De Bakker and Dagevos (2012) argue that it is time to acknowledge the interconnection between citizens and consumers, and to develop a broader perspective on consumer alliances for change. For example, local food networks are a way for consumers to engage with healthier and more sustainable food systems and practise food citizenship.

The main local food networks used by some consumers are community gardens, community-supported agricultural enterprises (CSAs), and farmers markets (Feenstra, 1997; O'Kane, 2016a). The early discourse on the role of local food networks was that: they addressed social inequities by providing access to nutritious foods; developed bonds between farmers and their customers; allowed community members to actively participate in the food system, contributed to social cohesion; and enhanced a community's economic vitality (Feenstra, 1997).

Local food networks have been criticised as being elitist and they may not adequately address all relevant aspects to move towards a more healthful and sustainable food system. However, it is important to note that local food procurers are actively involved in trying to address the inadequacies of the dominant food system, and thereby can be considered agents of change.

Context-related factors

We describe the contextual factors along the different environmental layers of a socio-ecological model relevant to food choices (Story, Kaphingst, Robinson-O'Brien, & Glanz, 2008; O'Kane, 2016a). Overall, it is clear that most studies of healthy *and* sustainable behaviours have focused on individual-level consumer factors, such as information and labelling, but less so on the environmental context.

1. *The social environment* – Social norms are known to influence general environmental behaviours and similarly have an impact on sustainable food choices (Vermeir & Verbeke, 2006; Aertsens et al., 2009). In a study on the core healthy and sustainable food behavioural principles (Hoek et al., 2017a), the influence of others and perceived social pressure was generally relevant, but most pronounced for barriers to reduce meat consumption. Similarly, community gardeners report on the importance of drawing on others' knowledge and experience of growing their own food, while also encouraging involvement by their children and grandchildren (O'Kane, 2016a). Future behaviour change efforts should therefore take family preferences into account, and leverage role modelling by family, friends and peers.

2. *Physical environments* – Most consumers in high-income countries do their grocery shopping in supermarkets, which makes them a key factor in daily food choices. Healthy and environmentally friendly food alternatives are typically considered from what is available in their supermarket and directly visible (e.g. claims or packaging). Accordingly, consumers may feel that affordable and attractive ethical products are scarce and that there are no other options than highly processed and packaged foods (Vermeir & Verbeke, 2006; Hoek et al., 2017a). There is also a group of people who consciously avoid supermarkets and source their foods from local food markets and community gardens in a desire to reconnect with food in new ways (O'Kane, 2016a; 2016b). However, less-involved consumers experience barriers related to the pricing and scarcity of local food shops or farmers markets, which often lack the regularity and convenience demanded by consumers (Vermeir & Verbeke, 2006).

3. *Macro-level environments* – Macro-level environmental factors appear to be more distant, but have a powerful effect on people's food choices (Story et al., 2008). Where you are born and live has a major impact, as there are clear cross-cultural differences between food practices. Besides food culture, which is embedded in cultural/societal norms and values, other upstream factors determine the accessibility, affordability and acceptability of healthy and sustainable foods, e.g. food production and distribution systems, agriculture policies, and economic price structures (Bailey & Harper, 2015; Garnett et al., 2015).

Conclusion

This chapter has sought to provide an overview of the influences on consumers' food choices in relation to health *and* sustainability. Many factors play a role through interactions between the person, the food and the wider social, physical and political context. At the individual consumer level, we conclude that motives and values related to health are generally different from those underlying sustainability, with health being a stronger food choice driver. There is still a relatively low level of knowledge and awareness of the environmental impact of foods, with only a small group of consumers who are actively involved in making conscious decisions to reduce the impact of their choices. Overall, it is evident that the choice for healthy and sustainable foods should not compromise important food qualities: price, taste and convenience, which are important barriers for some consumers.

One way to approach behaviour change is to match each of the above-mentioned barriers (lower knowledge and awareness, higher price for healthy and sustainable foods) with specific behavioural change actions for each behaviour and different target groups. For example, the

Behaviour Change Wheel, a framework for designing behavioural interventions, identifies seven policy categories that are similarly relevant for healthy and sustainable food choices: Communication/Marketing, Legislation, Service provision, Regulation, Fiscal measures, Guidelines, and Environmental/Social Planning (Michie et al., 2011). This is in line with other food intervention categorizations (Garnett, 2014; Bailey & Harper, 2015). Despite this wide range of potential policy actions and interventions, it is clear that until now consumer information and various types of labelling have received more attention in research and practice, even though we know that such initiatives generally have less impact on consumer choices, compared to other measures such as taxes or subsidies (Hoek et al., 2017b).

The key to healthy and sustainable food behavioural principles (less overconsumption, less ultra-processed and packaged foods, less animal-based and more plant-based foods, less food wastage) is actually a cluster of different practices around different types of foods and behaviours. Intermediate steps and different routes to advance each of these behaviours should be defined, fitting current consumption patterns and consumer motives. For example, Schösler et al. (2012) stipulate four policy-relevant pathways for a transition towards a more plant-based diet. They include incremental changes towards more health-conscious vegetarian meals, a pathway that uses the convenience trend, smaller meat portion sizes, and a shift towards plant-based meals.

The consumer behaviour change challenge brings us back to the question: *What is the role of consumers in changing not only their own behaviours, but also changing food systems?* While some portray consumers as passive victims in a food corporate-led system, De Bakker and Dagevos (2012) point out that the potential of consumers as change agents should not be underestimated. Building on the premise that consumer demand has (partly) created the problem, it makes sense to suggest that consumers can also be part of the solution. For example, increased consumer concerns about food production, such as animal welfare, can evoke public debate and drive actual change in the industry. Although food citizens and local food networks (see Box 9.2) currently represent a minority of consumers, they have been shown to spark a wider social movement with high public presence and power to influence the development of a healthier and more ecologically sustainable food system (Levkoe, 2015).

The potential of consumers as change agents does not imply that other policy interventions can be omitted. On the contrary, what we eat and where we buy are largely influenced by the wider context, which is not under direct control by consumers. Both upstream and downstream actions are essential to create an enabling environment for healthy and sustainable food choices, on the one hand, and structural changes to the food system, on the other. This includes the involvement of government, consumers and the food industry in other policy domains, including environmental policy, urban planning, and social policy (Bailey & Harper, 2015; Garnett et al., 2015; James et al., 2018). Bailey and Harper (2015) summarised a wide range of possible interventions according to increasing "intervention" from "inform and empower" (e.g. product labelling), to "guide and influence" (e.g. healthy and sustainable food procurement in public institutions) to "incentivise, discourage or restrict" (e.g. food subsidies). While these interventions may all be useful, there is a risk of a reductionist approach leading to the selection and implementation of only those interventions that fit well with a certain ideology (Garnett, 2014). Instead, there should be focus on bringing about a longer-term cultural change, which takes into account the social and cultural influences in daily food decisions (Knott, Muers, & Aldridge, 2008). This approach supports a process in which new behaviours are normalised and are fed back into creating cultural capital. This requires measures that strengthen consumer motivations and self-efficacy, on the one hand, and incentives, regulation and legislation measures, on the other.

Overall, a holistic long-term vision, research and policy agenda is needed to drive change towards healthier and more sustainable food behaviours. This will acknowledge and leverage the fact that food choices are made at the individual level, and influenced by the social, physical and macro-level contexts of people's lives.

References

Aertsens, J., Verbeke, W., Mondelaers, K., & Van Huylenbroeck, G. (2009). Personal determinants of organic food consumption: A review. *British Food Journal*, 111(10), 1140–1167.

Aschemann-Witzel, J. (2015). Consumer perception and trends about health and sustainability: Trade-offs and synergies of two pivotal issues. *Current Opinion in Food Science*, 3, 6–10.

Bailey, R., & Harper, D. R. (2015). Reviewing interventions for healthy and sustainable diets. Research paper. London: Chatham House, The Royal Institute of International Affairs.

De Bakker, E., & Dagevos, H. (2012). Reducing meat consumption in today's consumer society: Questioning the citizen-consumer gap. *Journal of Agricultural and Environmental Ethics*, 25(6), 877–894.

Desmet, P. M., & Schifferstein, H. N. (2008). Sources of positive and negative emotions in food experience. *Appetite*, 50(2–3), 290–301.

Feenstra, G. W. (1997). Local food systems and sustainable communities. *American Journal of Alternative Agriculture*, 12(1), 28–36.

Fresco, L. O. (2009). Challenges for food system adaptation today and tomorrow. *Environmental Science & Policy*, 12(4), 378–385.

Friel, S., Barosh, L. J., & Lawrence, M. (2014). Towards healthy and sustainable food consumption: An Australian case study. *Public Health Nutrition*, 17(5), 1156–1166.

Garnett, T. (2014). Changing consumption: How can we change the way we eat? A discussion paper. Oxford: Food Climate Research Network, University of Oxford.

Garnett, T., Mathewson, S., Angelides, P., & Borthwick, F. (2015). Policies and actions to shift eating patterns: What works? A review of the evidence of the effectiveness of interventions aimed at shifting diets in more sustainable and healthy directions. London: Chatham House, Food Climate Research Network.

Griffin, M. K., & Sobal, J. (2013). Sustainable food activities among consumers: A community study. *Journal of Hunger & Environmental Nutrition*, 8(4), 379–396.

Hawkes, C., Smith, T. G., Jewell, J., Wardle, J., Hammond, R. A., Friel, S. … Kain, J. (2015). Smart food policies for obesity prevention. *The Lancet*, 385(9985), 2410–2421.

Hoek, A. C., Pearson, D., James, S. W., Lawrence, M. A., & Friel, S. (2017a). Shrinking the foodprint: A qualitative study into consumer perceptions, experiences and attitudes towards healthy and environmentally friendly food behaviours. *Appetite*, 1 08, 117–131.

Hoek, A. C., Pearson, D., James, S. W., Lawrence, M. A., & Friel, S. (2017b). Healthy and environmentally sustainable food choices: Consumer responses to point-of-purchase actions. *Food Quality and Preference*, 58, 94–106.

James, S. W., Friel, S., Lawrence, M. A., Hoek, A. C., & Pearson, D. (2018). Inter-sectoral action to support healthy and environmentally sustainable food behaviours: A study of sectoral knowledge, governance and implementation opportunities. *Sustainability Science*, 13(2), 465–477.

Knott, D., Muers, S., & Aldridge, S. (2008). Achieving culture change: A policy framework. Discussion paper. London: Cabinet Office, Strategy Unit.

Lea, E., & Worsley, A. (2008). Australian consumers' food-related environmental beliefs and behaviours. *Appetite*, 50(2–3), 207–214.

Levkoe, C. Z. (2015). Strategies for forging and sustaining social movement networks: A case study of provincial food networking organizations in Canada. *Geoforum*, 58, 174–183.

McEachern, M. G., Warnaby, G., Carrigan, M., & Szmigin, I. (2010). Thinking locally, acting locally? Conscious consumers and farmers' markets. *Journal of Marketing Management*, 26(5–6), 395–412.

Michie, S., Van Stralen, M. M., & West, R. (2011). The behaviour change wheel: A new method for characterising and designing behaviour change interventions. *Implementation Science*, 6(1), 42.

Nestle, M. (2000). Ethical dilemmas in choosing a healthful diet: Vote with your fork! *Proceedings of the Nutrition Society*, 59(4), 619–629.

O'Kane, G. (2016a). A moveable feast: Exploring barriers and enablers to food citizenship. *Appetite*, 105, 674–687.

O'Kane, G. (2016b). A moveable feast: Contemporary relational food cultures emerging from local food networks. *Appetite*, 105, 218–231.

Saba, A., Vassallo, M., & Turrini, A. (2000). The role of attitudes, intentions and habit in predicting actual consumption of fat containing foods in Italy. *European Journal of Clinical Nutrition*, 54(7), 540.

Sarti, S., Darnall, N., & Testa, F. (2018). Market segmentation of consumers based on their actual sustainability and health-related purchases. *Journal of Cleaner Production*, 192, 270–280.

Schösler, H., De Boer, J., & Boersema, J. J. (2012). Can we cut out the meat of the dish? Constructing consumer-oriented pathways towards meat substitution. *Appetite*, 58(1), 39–47.

Shi, J., Visschers, V. H., Bumann, N., & Siegrist, M. (2018). Consumers' climate-impact estimations of different food products. *Journal of Cleaner Production*, 172, 1646–1653.

Story, M., Kaphingst, K. M., Robinson-O'Brien, R., & Glanz, K. (2008). Creating healthy food and eating environments: Policy and environmental approaches. *Annual Review of Public Health*, 29, 253–272.

Tobler, C., Visschers, V. H., & Siegrist, M. (2011). Eating green. Consumers' willingness to adopt ecological food consumption behaviors. *Appetite*, 57(3), 674–682.

Van Dam, Y. K., & Van Trijp, H. C. (2011). Cognitive and motivational structure of sustainability. *Journal of Economic Psychology*, 32(5), 726–741.

Van Dam, Y. K., & Van Trijp, H. C. (2013). Relevant or determinant: Importance in certified sustainable food consumption. *Food Quality and Preference*, 30(2), 93–101.

Van Loo, E. J., Hoefkens, C., & Verbeke, W. (2017). Healthy, sustainable and plant-based eating: Perceived (mis)match and involvement-based consumer segments as targets for future policy. *Food Policy*, 69, 46–57.

Verain, M. C., Bartels, J., Dagevos, H., Sijtsema, S. J., Onwezen, M. C., & Antonides, G. (2012). Segments of sustainable food consumers: A literature review. *International Journal of Consumer Studies*, 36(2), 123–132.

Vermeir, I., & Verbeke, W. (2006). Sustainable food consumption: Exploring the consumer "attitude–behavioral intention" gap. *Journal of Agricultural and Environmental Ethics*, 19(2), 169–194.

Wilkins, J. L. (2005). Eating right here: Moving from consumer to food citizen. *Agriculture and Human Values*, 22(3), 269–273.

Willett, W., Rockström, J., Loken, B., Springmann, M., et al. (2019). Food in the Anthropocene: The EAT–Lancet Commission on healthy diets from sustainable food systems. *The Lancet*, 393(10170), 447–492.

PART III
Healthy and sustainable diets

10

HEALTHY AND SUSTAINABLE DIETS

Jennie Macdiarmid

Introduction

The current food system is unsustainable, it is contributing to the increasing prevalence of diet-related diseases and damaging the planet, and thereby posing a significant risk to food and nutrition security. Creating a new food system will need to occur against the backdrop of a changing world, with population growth, increased pressure on finite natural resources, climate change and changing lifestyles. The only way to achieve food and nutrition security is for a radical transformation of the food system, which includes changing dietary habits to diets that are healthy and environmentally, economically and culturally sustainable.

The concept of healthy and sustainable diets is not new. In 1986, Gussow and Clancy proposed that nutrition education needed go beyond a medical view of nutrition to include an understanding of the negative impact that people's food choices were having on the environment (Gussow & Clancy, 1986). Despite these earlier concerns about the impact of diets on the environment, little has been done and the food system has become more unsustainable. With growing recognition of the threat of climate change to food and nutrition security, the need for a food system and dietary habits for both health and environmental benefits has gained momentum again.

Healthy and sustainable diets have many different elements and therefore by their nature they are complex, as illustrated in the Food and Agricultural Organization (FAO) definition of sustainable diets published in 2012:

> Sustainable diets are those diets with low environmental impacts which contribute to food and nutrition security and to healthy life for present and future generations. Sustainable diets are protective and respectful of biodiversity and ecosystems, culturally acceptable, accessible, economically fair and affordable; nutritionally adequate, safe and healthy; while optimizing natural and human resources.
>
> *(Burlingame & Dernini, 2012)*

Each element described in this definition is equally important and the challenge is to understand how to bring them all together and synthesise them into dietary advice, thereby avoiding any unintended consequences. In the process of optimising each element and integrating them into a diet, conflicts and synergies will emerge, for which trade-offs and solutions need to be found (Johnston, Fanzo, & Cogill, 2014). To understand the importance and relevance of each of the different elements of healthy and sustainable diets, first, each one will be described individually, then some of the conflicts and synergies that arise when trying to combine them into a diet and the challenges faced in changing dietary habits will be discussed. Following the release of the EAT-Lancet Commission report entitled, "Food in the Anthropocene: the EAT-Lancet Commission on healthy diets from sustainable food systems", this chapter will focus on reducing meat consumption as a core consideration in achieving healthy and sustainable diets (Willett et al., 2019). However, this is not the only important component of a healthy and sustainable diet and therefore meat consumption should not be studied in isolation, rather meat consumption must be considered in the context of the whole diet. It is possible to have an unhealthy diet without eating meat. Other aspects of the diet are important in a healthy and sustainable diet, such as overconsumption of food, which is not sustainable for health or the planet. Reducing consumption of ultra-processed foods needs to be a particular focus when avoiding overconsumption of food. Producing food that is either thrown away or eaten in quantities that are greater than energy needs is wasting the finite natural resources used to produce food and generating more greenhouse gas (GHG) emissions. Reducing food waste is critically important for future food security. Diets also need to be culturally appropriate, acceptable and affordable if people are going to change their current diets.

Elements of healthy and sustainable diets

Nutritionally adequate, healthy and safe

Globally, the prevalence of diet-related disease, such as type 2 diabetes, cardiovascular disease and cancer is increasing, particularly in countries with emerging economies. Many developing countries are also starting to see the triple burden of disease (i.e. the consequences of hunger, micronutrient deficiency and obesity) co-existing within the population, households and at an individual level. It is estimated that 815 million people in the world are undernourished (e.g. have insufficient daily calories), 2 billion suffer from micronutrient deficiencies and 600 million adults are obese (FAO, 2017). The increase in obesity in developing countries is occurring faster in urban areas than in rural areas because of changing lifestyles and dietary intake. In Malawi, for example, the prevalence of obesity among woman in urban areas is estimated to be 18 per cent compared to 8 per cent in rural areas (men 4 per cent vs. 1 per cent, respectively) (Price et al., 2018).

A healthy diet is one that meets energy and nutrient requirements for human health and this varies for different subgroups of the population, according to age, sex and level of activity. They comprise achieving minimum requirements for protein, fibre and micronutrients and upper limits for nutrients, such as fat and sugar. For the intake of many micronutrients, there is not only a minimum requirement but also a safe upper limit to prevent intakes reaching a toxic level and having adverse health effects. This has implications for regulating the fortification of food or micronutrient supplements, so not to exceed the safe upper limit as part of a normal diet.

In addition to energy and nutrient requirements, there are recommended intakes of certain food groups. The World Health Organization (WHO, 2003) recommends a minimum intake of 400g per day of fruit and vegetables to reduce the risk of chronic disease (e.g. cardiovascular disease, type 2 diabetes, cancer) and micronutrient deficiency. The World Cancer Research Fund (WCRF & American Institute for Cancer Research, 2018) recommends eating no more than 500g a week of cooked red meat (e.g. beef, pork, lamb) and to eat little, if any, processed meat (e.g. ham, bacon) because of the increased risk of certain cancers (e.g. bowel, stomach cancer) from eating these foods in higher quantities. Eating oily fish is included in some national dietary guidelines because it is a good source of omega 3 fatty acids.

While these food-based recommendations are set to reduce the risk of chronic non-communicable diseases and promote good health, some can have unintended consequences for the environment. For example, in water-scarce regions of the world, irrigation of fields to grow fruit and vegetables is causing significant water stress and depleting the water available for the local population. Intensifying the production of these foods is typically sought to supply growing international markets. On one hand, while this may have a negative effect on the local water supply, on the other, it can make a huge contribution to the livelihood of the grower. With reducing fish stocks and the dietary recommendation to eat fish, an increase in aquaculture has emerged, which has its own environmental issues. These dilemmas illustrate some of the complexity of developing dietary recommendations for diets that are both healthy and sustainable, trying to avoid unintended consequences.

Food safety is an important element for healthy and sustainable diets, and that is not always given as much consideration as it needs. In 2010, the WHO estimated there were approximately 600 million cases of foodborne illnesses and 420,000 deaths globally (WHO, 2015). A disproportionate number of these is found among children under the age of 5 years and people living in developing countries (WHO, 2015). One result of foodborne diseases can be a reduction in nutrient absorption. If the illness is chronic, then in the longer term it will affect nutritional status and potentially exacerbate nutrient deficiencies.

Low environmental impact and protective of natural resources and biodiversity

There are many ways the current food system is damaging the environment, including climate change, biodiversity loss, land use change, reducing availability of freshwater, increasing pollution and soil degradation. This in turn is threatening the sustainability of food production and therefore food and nutrition security. Unlike nutrition that affects individual health, the environmental consequences of dietary habits have a global impact, and this tends to have a greater negative impact on the lives of people in low-income countries, but it is the diets eaten in developed countries that are causing most of the damage to the environment and, therefore, they need to change.

Climate change is one of the greatest threats facing the world. The food system accounts for 20–30 per cent of global GHG emissions (Vermeulen, Campbell, & Ingram, 2012). Technological advances to improve agricultural and production practices are essential but alone they are insufficient to meet the GHG reduction targets that have been set, especially within the timeframe needed to limit global warming (Bajzelj et al., 2014). Significant changes to dietary habits are needed to reduce GHG emissions to keep the "global temperature rise this century well below 2 degrees Celsius above pre-industrial levels and to pursue efforts to limit the temperature increase even further to 1.5 degrees Celsius" (UN Framework Convention on Climate Change, 2015). Climate change is not the only environmental issue associated with the food system, equally important is the impact of land use change (e.g. deforestation), the depletion of freshwater resources and degradation of soils. Land, freshwater and soil quality are all finite resources and how they are used and preserved is critical for future food and nutrition security.

Within the food system, livestock production has the greatest environmental impact and therefore consumption of animal products, particularly meat, dominates the debate around sustainable diets. Production of livestock is associated with high GHG emissions, especially ruminants, since they produce methane, which is a gas that over a 100-year time horizon has a global warming potential about 25 times greater than carbon dioxide. It is estimated that the livestock supply chain contributes about 14.5 per cent of all global anthropogenic GHG emissions and uses about 70 per cent of global agricultural land (Gerber et al., 2013). The contribution to GHG emissions is growing because of the increasing demand for animal products associated with increasing affluence in developing countries (UNFCC, 2004). Land is also needed to produce livestock feed and it is often argued that to feed the population, this land could be used more efficiently to produce food directly for human consumption. This would require a reduction in meat consumption, which in many countries is being met with some resistance.

Water is also a finite resource, but the available supply of water varies in different regions of the world. Water-intense foods, such as fruit and vegetables, often use irrigation systems for their production and if this takes place in water-scarce regions, it reduces the available water supplies for local people. Furthermore, since many of these products are exported, the impact on the local communities of water depletion is often not seen by consumers in other countries. The amount of water required to produce a food is often referred to as the water footprint. For example, it could take 15,500 litres of water to produce a kilogram of beef or 900 litres for a kilogram of tomatoes (Hoekstra, 2008). This measure is now viewed by some as too simplistic as it does not take account of whether the food is produced in a water-stressed area or the type of water that is used (e.g. from precipitation or groundwater), but it does highlight the scale of potential water demands. Livestock production has a particularly high water footprint, especially when the production of feed is included, further supporting the need for a reduction in meat consumption among many populations. A factor that is not always considered is that livestock production makes a significant contribution to many livelihoods, so alternative sources of income would need to be found where livelihoods are disrupted.

Agriculture is the biggest cause of biodiversity loss, mainly caused by the intensification of farming systems and expansion of land used for food production (i.e. deforestation) (FAO, 2016). Mass deforestation of land for plantations of monocrops, such as palm oil and animal feed, as well as for livestock production, has had devastating impacts on biodiversity (Vijay et al., 2016). Palm oil, for example, is the most traded oil globally and since it is used in most processed foods, it is difficult to avoid, despite the negative publicity of the environmental damage of deforestation. The global shift towards the production of monocrops has reduced the diversity of plants eaten, which is reducing the nutritional diversity of the diet (Ickowitz, Powell Rowland, Jones, & Sunderland, 2019). The development of agricultural production practices, such as the Green Revolution, encouraged a system that increased productivity to address hunger, but led to a shift away from traditional crops to more monocrops. The cultivars selected to grow were typically based on maximising yields for food security, but this was sometimes at the expense of the nutrient quality of traditional varieties, which increased the threat of nutrition security and health.

The focus of attention for healthy and sustainable diets has usually been on the impact of dietary choices on climate change but changing climate conditions, in turn, have the potential to reduce the nutrient density of some food commodities. Myers et al. (2014) found that increased levels of carbon dioxide in the atmosphere reduced the yield of some crops (e.g. wheat, rice, soya beans, field peas) and decreased the concentration of protein, iron and zinc. This could present a threat to nutrition security, especially in countries where these are staple crops eaten in the diet.

Cultural acceptability

The importance of food cultures and the social aspects of eating should not be underestimated or overlooked by focusing only on the health consequences of the diet. Crotty (1993) describes nutrition as a discipline divided into two domains; *pre-swallowing* nutrition (behavioural, social and cultural influences on food choices) and *post-swallowing* nutrition (biological, physiological and health consequences of the diet). The pre-swallowing nutrition is critical for understanding how to change dietary habits. Knowing what constitutes healthy and sustainable diets and developing guidelines provide the foundations for diets against which targets can be set, but the more difficult part is changing dietary habits, which are typically deeply engrained. Having a "culturally acceptable" element in the definition of a healthy and sustainable diet is important because food culture, traditions and norms vary widely and therefore recommendations need to be appropriate to the target population.

Alternative foods are being explored to replace meat in the diet. The need to eat less meat has driven a movement to find alternative sources of protein within both research communities and the food industry. There is, however, a misconception about the amount of protein people require and the amount that is eaten. For instance, in high-income countries, most people eat significantly more protein than required and even if all meat was removed from the diet, people are highly unlikely to have insufficient protein. Despite this, there is still a concern that by reducing meat consumption, you run the risk of protein deficiency and in part this is creating a market for alternative protein sources. Two alternatives that have been proposed include eating insects and manufactured meat (i.e. lab meat), since they will potentially have a lower environmental impact than livestock. Insects can also provide some essential nutrients such as zinc as well as protein but there are other aspects of eating them that need to be considered before they can be a viable option. Farming insects and feeding them on food waste could be beneficial in terms of reducing GHG emissions from decaying food, but one would need to be assured that the waste did not contain any contaminants. Insects are bio-accumulators and, depending on what they eat, they can accumulate high levels of contaminants, such as cadmium, lead and arsenic. This may be of concern for human health since large quantities of insects would be needed to make food products to be sufficient for human consumption. Another dimension is the cultural acceptability; it is common to eat insects in some populations but not in many societies that have high intakes of meat. Social and cultural norms around food, however, can change and, therefore, it is not inconceivable that insects could become a more widely acceptable food.

Food should not be seen simply as a source of fuel for the body because what someone chooses to eat can be based on pleasure, not health, or it can be used to portray an image or identity, which can vary depending on the influence of peers and social settings. In a study by Stead et al. (2011), young people said that healthy eating conflicted with being accepted by their peers and the image they associated with healthy eating was not the image that they wanted to portray. Some of the participants described feeling socially excluded by not complying with the norm of eating unhealthy food and the authors of the study concluded that "healthy eating was bad for young people's health", referring to social and mental well-being.

Accessible, economically fair and affordable

Healthy and sustainable diets not only have to be socially and culturally acceptable but also affordable and what is deemed affordable will vary widely in different populations. A US consumer spends on average $2,392 per year on food, which is 6.4 per cent of their income, by comparison, a Kenyan consumer spends on average $543 per year on food which is 46.7 per cent of their income (World Economic Forum, 2018). Healthy and sustainable diets, however, can comprise many different types of foods so, in theory, some of the different incomes could be accommodated. In high-income countries, wealthier people tend to eat more fruit and vegetables, lean meat, wholegrain and fish than people in lower-income groups. Drewnowski observed that people on lower incomes could achieve food security, that meets energy requirements, for less money by eating energy-dense foods (e.g. high fat and high sugar foods) rather than lower-density food (e.g. fruits and vegetables) (Drewnowski & Eichelsdoerfer, 2010). Pulses, potatoes and root vegetables tend to be cheaper than most meat, fish and fruits and have the added benefit that they have a lower environmental impact. However, for many people, high fat and high sugar foods are very palatable and pleasurable to eat, as well as being cheap, which makes them more attractive than many more nutritious foods. Foods high in sugar and vegetable fats can also have a lower environmental impact than food derived from animal products.

The problem of meat consumption

Meat is a good example of the complexity of trying to satisfy all the different elements of a healthy and sustainable diet, particularly in terms of how to provide consistent dietary advice. It has dominated discussions about environmentally sustainable diets, since the evidence shows that diets need to have less meat and more plant-based foods (Willett et al., 2019). As described in the previous sections, livestock production has a high environmental impact, regardless of whether it is produced using an extensive (e.g. grazing) or intensive production system. From a nutrition perspective, eating meat can have positive and negative health consequences. While eating large amounts of red and processed meat can increase the risk of diet-related chronic diseases, when it is eaten in appropriate quantities, it is a good source of bioavailable micronutrients (e.g. iron, zinc) (Hurrell & Egli, 2010). Most of the research in this area has focused on high-income countries, where meat consumption is high and on average could be reduced with few negative health consequences. However, diets in many low- and middle-income countries tend to be nutritionally inadequate and micronutrient deficiencies are common, so eating a small amount of animal products would improve the nutrient density of the diet. To achieve a slight increase in animal products in the diet would require mechanisms to be put in place to make the food accessible and affordable to people, especially those with the lowest income.

Furthermore, from an environmental perspective, if meat is to continue to be part of the diet, then the whole animal should be eaten, not just selected cuts of meat. This would mean eating more fatty meats, which would be unhealthy and eating parts of the animal that many people view as undesirable, such as offal, despite being nutrient-dense.

The most challenging consideration here is how to persuade people to eat less meat especially when in many cultures it has a high status and traditionally is a central part of the diet. People typically enjoy eating meat and studies have shown a high level of reluctance to eat less meat (Graça, Calheiros, & Oliveira, 2015; Macdiarmid, Douglas, & Campbell, 2016). Reasons given include enjoying the taste of meat, not knowing what to eat in place of meat, concern about protein deficiency or not wanting to be different to their peers and going against the social norm to eat meat. Food also gives people an identity and is intertwined with social behaviour, which is very much the case in terms of eating meat. Eating patterns that deviate from the norm can be associated with other non-food-related characteristics, which can create negative perception of that person by others and create a fear of stigmatisation if someone chooses to change their diet. The label of being vegetarian or vegan can stop some people from changing their diets (Markowski & Roxburgh, 2019).

Reducing meat will not guarantee an improvement in the diet or a lower environmental damage because it depends on which food replaces the meat. Vieux et al. (2012) modelled the effect of reducing the amount of meat to less than 50g/day in the average French diet. Replacing the calories with dairy products reduced GHG emissions by about 7 per cent compared with a reduction of 12 per cent when no foods were substituted. Replacing the calories with selected fruit and vegetables (e.g. those produced in heated greenhouses, air-freighted) increased emissions by 2.7 per cent. This was due to the large amount of fruit and vegetables that was needed to replace the calories since they have a low energy density. This demonstrates that the whole diet is important, not just meat, and replacement foods must be considered carefully to avoid a rebound effect. This study, however, only included GHG emissions and if water stress had been incorporated, the results would change.

Most studies have used hypothetical substitutions for meat but currently very little is known about what people would choose to eat in place of meat. Whatever the food, it must be considered in the context of the whole diet. It is unlikely that meat would be the only food to change in the diet and the composition of a meal could be altered. In the case of a meal comprising meat, potatoes and vegetables, it is unlikely that the meat would simply be swapped with pulses or other vegetables, rather the whole composition of the meal would change and may not include any vegetables (e.g. pasta and cheese). The type of substitutions and alternative meals eaten will determine the magnitude of the change, which may be smaller than anticipated.

Healthy and sustainable diets in practice

After establishing a framework linking the different elements of healthy and sustainable diets, the next step is to translate this into dietary guidelines with key principles that can be applied in practice. There are several considerations, first, to realise that no single exemplar diet exists, as there are multiple combinations of foods that will meet the criteria of a healthy and sustainable diet. Second, it cannot be assumed that healthy diets will necessarily be more sustainable and for this reason dietary guidelines do need to be revised to include environmental sustainability. It is possible for a healthy diet to have a high environmental impact or an unhealthy diet to be more environmentally sustainable than a healthy diet. For example, the GHG emissions associated with sugar production are relatively low compared to livestock production, therefore, if the sole aim is to have a diet with lower GHG emissions, this could comprise a lot of sugar, but this would not be recommended for health.

Researchers have used mathematical models to create diets that combine the different elements of healthy and sustainable diets. One of the early studies illustrated the consequence of just using mathematical modelling and not including all the different elements of the diet, for example, cultural acceptability (Macdiarmid et al., 2012). Using computer modelling, it was possible to create a diet that achieved energy and nutrient requirements for a healthy diet and a reduction in GHG emissions of 90 per cent. This model only had to achieve nutrient and energy requirements and a reduction in GHG emissions, which resulted in an optimised diet that comprised only seven food items (i.e. wholegrain breakfast cereal, pasta, peas, fried onions, brassicas, sesame seeds and confectionery). Clearly it is unrealistic to think people would eat this diet. Social and economic elements were then incorporated into the modelling to make the diet more realistic and culturally acceptable, and so foods commonly eaten by the population, realistic quantities and combining foods that were typically eaten together (e.g. breakfast cereal and milk) as well as affordable to the target population were added. The diet still had to meet energy and nutrient requirements and with these added constraints the new diet had a greater number of foods but the reduction in GHG emissions was only 36 per cent lower than currents diets. This demonstrated the types of compromise and trade-offs in practice that are needed when trying to bring together the different elements of what comprises healthy and sustainable diets.

Conclusion

It is commonly agreed that the current food system is unsustainable, it is causing poor health and environmental damage and therefore dietary habits need to change. The definition of healthy and sustainable diets is complex but ignoring it is not an option, and will need nutritional, environmental, economic and social scientists to work together to find viable answers. Work has progressed in the last few years with dietary guidelines in Sweden, The Netherlands, Germany, Qatar, China and Brazil revised to incorporate elements of environmental sustainability (Fischer & Garnett, 2016). These revisions are typically to reduce consumption of animal products, to consume more plant-based foods, intakes not to exceed energy requirements and to reduce consumption of energy-dense, nutrient-poor, ultra-processed food products. With dietary guidelines gradually being revised and a greater recognition of the problem of climate change as well as other environmental issues associated with the food system, realistic pathways must be found to help change dietary habits to achieve healthy and sustainable diets. Key will be to consider social and economic factors that drive food choice. The complexity and challenge to create a healthy and sustainable food system that can deliver food and nutrition security are immense. However, diets need to be radically changed and the pace of change needs to be picked up if the pending irreversible environmental damage is to be slowed down and further public health problems are not to be minimised.

The chapters that follow in Part III will elaborate on the healthy and sustainable diet characteristics described in this chapter. In particular, each of the chapters will focus on one of the following prominent challenges for achieving healthy and sustainable diets to improve both human and planetary health: animal-based versus plant-based diets; overconsumption; consumption of junk food; as well as the issue of food waste, which is a major threat to food security.

References

Bajzelj, B., Richards, K. S., Allwood, J. M., et al. (2014). Importance of food-demand management for climate mitigation. *Nature Climate Change*, 4(10), 924–929.

Burlingame, B., & Dernini, S. (2012). *Sustainable diets and biodiversity: Directions and solutions for policy, research and action.* Rome: FAO.

Crotty, P. (1993). The value of qualitative research in nutrition. *Annual Review of Health Social Science*, 3(1), 109–118.

Drewnowski, A., & Eichelsdoerfer, P. (2010). Can low-income Americans afford a healthy diet? *Nutrition Today*, 44(6), 246–249.

FAO (Food and Agriculture Organization). (2016). The state of the world's forests 2016. Forests and agriculture: land-use challenges and opportunities. Rome: FAO. www.fao.org/3/a-i5588e.pdf

FAO. (2017). The state of food security and nutrition in the world 2017: Building resilience for peace and food security. Rome: FAO.

Fischer, C. F., & Garnett, T. (2016). Plates, pyramids, planet. Developments in national healthy and sustainable dietary guidelines: A state of play assessment. Rome: FAO. Available at: www.fao.org/3/a-i5640e pdf

Gerber, P. J., Steinfeld, H., Henderson, B., et al. (2013). *Tackling climate change through livestock: A global assessment of emissions and mitigation.* Rome: FAO.

Graça, J., Calheiros, M. M., & Oliveira, A. (2015). Attached to meat? (Un)willingness and intentions to adopt a more plant-based diet. *Appetite*, 95, 113–125.

Gussow, J. D., & Clancy, K. L. (1986). Dietary guidelines for sustainability. *Journal of Nutrition Education*, 18(1), 1–5.

Hoekstra, A. Y. (2008). The water footprint of food. Available at: http://waterfootprint.org/media/downloads/Hoekstra-2008-WaterfootprintFood pdf. 2008

Hurrell, R., & Egli, I. (2010). Iron bioavailability and dietary reference values. *The American Journal of Clinical Nutrition*, 91(5), 1461S–1467S.

Ickowitz, A., Powell, B., Rowland, D., Jones, A., & Sunderland, T. (2019). Agricultural intensification, dietary diversity, and markets in the global food security narrative. *Global Food Security*, 20, 9–16.

Johnston, J.L., Fanzo, J. C., & Cogill, B. (2014). Understanding sustainable diets: A descriptive analysis of the determinants and processes that influence diets and their impact on health, food security, and environmental sustainability. *Advances in Nutrition*, 5(4), 418–429.

Macdiarmid, J. I., Douglas, F., & Campbell, J. (2016). Eating like there's no tomorrow: Public awareness of the environmental impact of food and reluctance to eat less meat as part of a sustainable diet. *Appetite*, 96, 487–493.

Macdiarmid, J. I., Kyle, J., Horgan, G. W., et al. (2012). Sustainable diets for the future: Can we contribute to reducing greenhouse gas emissions by eating a healthy diet? *American Journal of Clinical Nutrition*, 96, 632–639.

Markowski, K. L., & Roxburgh, S. (2019) "If I became a vegan, my family and friends would hate me:" Anticipating vegan stigma as a barrier to plant-based diets. *Appetite*, 135, 1–9.

Myers, S. S., Zanobetti, A., Kloog, I., *et al.* (2014). Increasing CO2 threatens human nutrition. *Nature*, 510(7503), 139–142.

Price, A. J., Crampin, A. C., Amberbir, A., *et al.* (2018). Prevalence of obesity, hypertension, and diabetes, and cascade of care in Sub-Saharan Africa: A cross-sectional, population-based study in rural and urban Malawi. *The Lancet Diabetes & Endocrinology*, 6(3), 208–222.

Stead, M., McDermott, L., MacKintosh, A. M., & Adamson, A. (2011). Why healthy eating is bad for young people's health: Identity, belonging and food. *Social Science & Medicine*, 72, 1131–1139.

UNFCC. (2004). Information on global warming potentials. FCCC/TP/2004/3. Available at: https://unfccc.int/resource/docs/tp/tp0403.pdf

United Nations Framework Convention on Climate Change. (2015). The Paris agreement. Available at: https://unfccc.int/files/meetings/paris_nov_2015/application/pdf/paris_agreement_english_.pdf (accessed 11 May 2018).

Vermeulen, S., Campbell, B., & Ingram, J. (2012). Climate change and food systems. *Annual Review of Environment and Resources*, 37, 195–222.

Vieux, F., Darmon, N., Touazi, D., & Soler, L. (2012). Greenhouse gas emissions of self-selected individual diets in France: Changing the diet structure or consuming less? *Ecological Economics*, 75, 91–101.

Vijay, V., Pimm, S. L., Jenkins, C. N., & Smith, S.J. (2016). The impacts of oil palm on recent deforestation and biodiversity loss. *PLOS One*, 11(7), e0159668.

WHO (World Health Organization). (2015). *Estimates of the global burden of foodborne diseases*. Geneva: WHO Foodborne Disease Burden Epidemiology Reference Group, 2007–2015.

WHO/FAO. (2003). Diet, nutrition and the prevention of chronic diseases. WHO Technical Report Series 916. Geneva: WHO.

Willett, W., Rockström, J., Loken, B., Springmann, M., et al. (2019). Food in the Anthropocene: The EAT-Lancet Commission on healthy diets from sustainable food systems. *The Lancet*, 393(10170), 447–492.

World Cancer Research Fund/American Institute for Cancer Research. (2018). Diet, nutrition, physical activity, and cancer: A global perspective. continuous update project expert report 2018. Available at: www.dietandcancerreport.org

World Economic Forum. (2018). Which countries spend the most on food? Available at: www.weforum.org/agenda/2016/12/this-map-shows-how-much-each-country-spends-on-food/ Updated 2018. (accessed 11 May 2018).

11

OVERCONSUMPTION AND THE GLOBAL SYNDEMIC

Boyd Swinburn and Sarah Gerritsen

Introduction

At one level, overconsumption is an easy concept to grasp because it implies that people or populations consume more energy than they expend and therefore they gain weight. However, there are complex societal, environmental, psychological and biological interactions that underpin the energy balance, and these need to be reconciled with broader nutrition issues, such as under-nutrition. Since all population nutrition problems are created and sustained by the current food systems and the political economies within which they operate, we need to take a wider view of overconsumption. In this chapter, we will first deal with the concept of energy overconsumption itself and then broaden the discussion to consider the current construct of malnutrition in all its forms and then draw on the work of the Lancet Commission on Obesity (Swinburn et al., 2019).

The flipping point into overconsumption

The concept of the flipping point (Swinburn et al., 2011) serves to illustrate the inter-relationship between the changing societal drivers of energy consumption and biological responses (Figure 11.1). A century ago, high levels of physical activity were needed just for daily living, for example, through transportation, food preparation and household chores. Since then, labour-saving mechanisation, computerisation and motorisation have progressively decreased the need for that level of exercise. Yet it is only in the last 40 years that the obesity epidemic has exploded across the world. Why did obesity prevalence not rise substantially until the 1970s and 1980s, when the energy demands of daily living have been dropping for at least a century?

From 1910 to the 1970s, total per-person energy available in the US food supply (food production plus imports minus exports and non-human use) (Gerrior et al., 2004) fell, pre-sumably through reducing food energy intake to match the decreasing demand of physical activity energy expenditure. This is energy balance mechanisms working as expected through appetite systems – less need for energy expenditure, less appetite activation, less energy intake. This "pull" process allows changes in energy expenditure demands to be met without major changes in body energy stores.

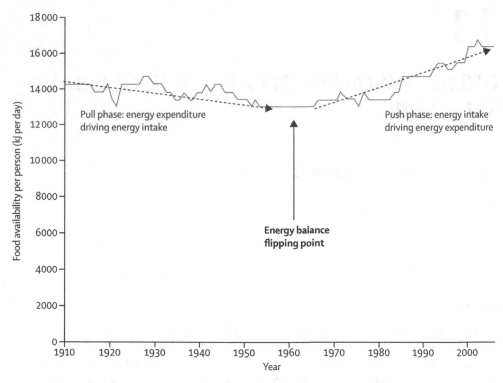

FIGURE 11.1 The flipping point into overconsumption
Source: Swinburn et al. (2011).

The period since the 1970s has been characterised as a "push" phase with a striking rise in the quantity of refined carbohydrates and fats in the US food supply (Putnam, 2000), a rise in the available calories per capita, and consequent rises in obesity prevalence. This push phase from a greater food supply drove up energy intakes and also created a 50 per cent increase in food waste since the 1970s (Hall, Guo, Dore, & Chow, 2009). So what was the flipping point in energy balance that occurred? Increasing energy intake leads to increasing body weight and total energy expenditure due to the increases in lean mass (as well as fat mass) during weight gain. It is not widely appreciated that the state of obesity is a state of relatively higher energy expenditure. So the energy balance mechanisms have now flipped from balancing energy intake to match energy expenditure through appetite mechanisms, to balancing energy expenditure to match energy intake through the mechanism of weight gain.

Obesogenic food environments and passive overconsumption

Since people and populations do not purposefully set out to become obese, Blundell and Macdiarmid (1997) coined the term "passive overconsumption" to acknowledge the fact that when people live in an obesogenic food environment (Egger & Swinburn, 1997) – surrounded by highly palatable, convenient, heavily marketed, affordable and ultra-processed foods – they naturally tend to overconsume total energy beyond requirements and gain weight.

Modern food systems have become more industrialised and globalised. They are dominated by large, often transnational, actors, capable of economies of scale and of maintaining long supply chains. The driving force for the move to this type of food system is the added-profit value of ultra-processed foods compared to unprocessed foods. In addition, transnational food companies have gained such concentrated power that they can manipulate political processes to create the regulatory and economic conditions most favourable to their profitability. These modern food systems are not only present in wealthy countries but also dominate in most middle-income countries and, increasingly, in low-income countries. In low- and middle-income countries, the mix of traditional and modern food systems, and the regulatory and economic conditions they operate within, are not only sustaining an unacceptably high level of undernutrition but also a rapidly rising burden of obesity and non-communicable diseases (NCDs), such as cardiovascular disease, diabetes and cancer.

From calorie-centrism to more unifying concepts

To address the underlying causes of malnutrition in all its forms, new paradigms and concepts are needed. In particular, the 'calorie-centric' paradigm needs to change from not enough or too many calories, to food quality, variety and sustainability. This chapter will take this broader approach to overconsumption and consider it in the context of malnutrition in all its forms and the Global Syndemic.

Malnutrition in all its forms: the result of failing food systems

In 2015, the United Nations Sustainable Development Goals (SDGs) enshrined the objective of "ending all forms of malnutrition" by 2030, urging a common definition of malnutrition which included undernutrition, micronutrient deficiencies and obesity. This definition recognises that undernutrition and obesity are both due to poor diet quality and a low variety of healthy foods. Other connections between undernutrition and obesity are the effects of undernutrition in utero and infancy on increasing the risks of subsequent obesity and NCDs in adulthood, and that both are related to poverty and food environments where access to healthy foods is low and/or access to unhealthy foods is high. Both undernutrition (including stunting and micronutrient deficiencies) and obesity often coexist within populations, households and individuals and across the life course. The convergence of distinct nutritional policy areas in one policy construct has been helpful to coordinate action, reframing these issues as systemic level failings requiring systemic solutions, as opposed to individual failings.

The highest global burden of disease is from malnutrition

Malnutrition in all its forms is compiled as a single risk factor from three nutrition sub-risks and is by far the biggest cause of ill health and premature death in every country in the world by a substantial margin (Figure 11.2) (Afshin et al., 2017). The contribution from undernutrition reduces proportionally and the proportion from high body-mass index (BMI) and dietary risks for NCDs increases proportionally from low-income countries to high-income countries.

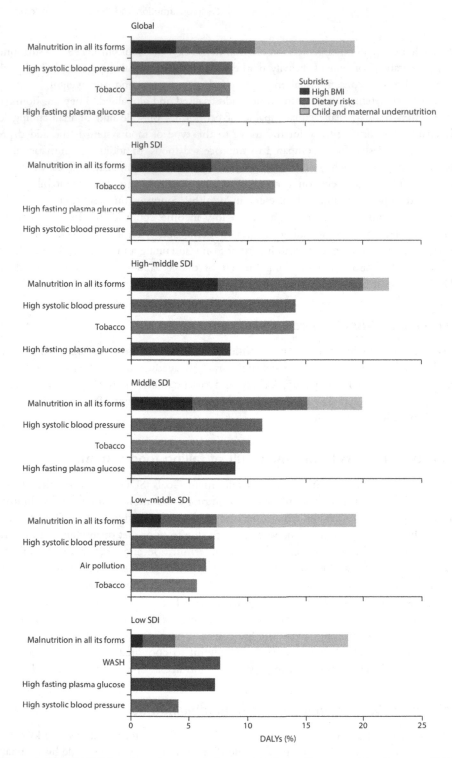

FIGURE 11.2 The DALYs lost from the top risk factors globally and by stage of development (SDI).
Note: DALY Disability-Adjusted Life Years; SDI Sustainable Development Indicator.
Source: Afshin et al. (2017).

Globally, undernutrition has been gradually decreasing in a linear fashion but is still highly prevalent in many African and Asian countries and progress has recently stalled (Von Grebmer et al., 2017). Obesity is increasing almost linearly in all countries but with less of an apparent relationship with a country's economic status, except that prevalence is still low in the lowest-income countries (NCD Risk Factor Collaboration, 2017). In high- and middle-income countries, obesity is more prevalent among the more disadvantaged sub-populations.

The global food system has never been more advanced, and yet its failures have never been more evident. Although sufficient food is produced to meet the dietary energy requirements of the global population, 815 million people are undernourished, lacking access to that food (FAO, 2013) and micronutrient deficiencies affect an estimated 2 billion people globally (FAO, 2013). On the other hand, energy-rich, nutrient-poor, ultra-processed foods are cheap, widely available and aggressively marketed – a key driving force in the global obesity pandemic with nearly 2 billion people with overweight or obesity. At the same time, the increasingly industrialised and globalised food system is driving unprecedented environmental damage, contributing up to 29 per cent of anthropogenic greenhouse gas (GHG) emissions, rapid deforestation and massive biodiversity loss (Jägerskog & Jønch Clausen, 2012; Vermeulen, Campbell, & Ingram, 2012).

The Global Syndemic

The 2019 report by the Lancet Commission on Obesity argued that the three global pandemics of obesity (encompassing dietary risks for NCDs), undernutrition (including micronutrient deficiencies) and the health impacts of climate change should be characterised collectively as the Global Syndemic (Swinburn et al., 2019). A syndemic is a synergy of epidemics (in this case, global epidemics or pandemics), which co-occur in time and place, negatively interact with each other and have common societal drivers. The three pandemics have shared systemic drivers and, consequently, fundamental changes within the food systems (alongside action in the other major systems of transport, urban design and land use) can serve as double-duty or triple-duty actions by improving the trajectories of two or three of the pandemics together.

The Systems Outcomes framework

The Systems Outcomes Framework is shown in Figure 11.3a–d (Swinburn et al., 2019). The sequence of figures (a–d) shows progressively zoomed-in views from the Global Outcomes view of the consequences of intersecting natural and human systems (a); to the Global Syndemic view of the interaction and common drivers of obesity, undernutrition, and climate change (b); to the five feedback loops view (c); and the individual view (d). The Global Outcomes view (Figure 11.3a) is the most zoomed-out view of the global system, showing the four major global goals of ecological health and well-being, human health and well-being, social equity, and economic prosperity emanating from the human-created systems and the natural systems that determine these outcomes. This framework is, in essence, an inside-out version of the socio-ecological model which originated from the child development theories of Bronfenbrenner in the 1970s (Bronfenbrenner, 1992) and contributed to paradigms for public health through the work of Dahlgren and Whitehead (1991). However, in the Systems Outcomes framework, the individual is no longer at the centre. Instead, the natural ecosystems are at the centre since everything on the planet is sustained by the natural world. Next is the important Governance layer, which is how humans make the decisions and set the rules for how society operates. The major levers of governance – rules and policies, economic

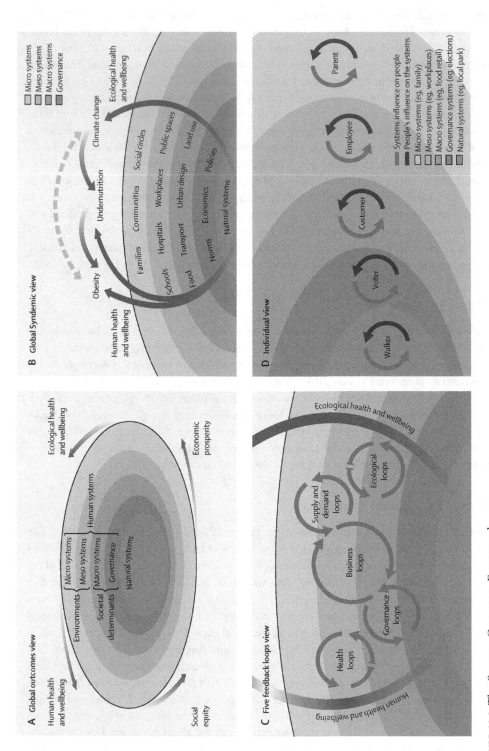

FIGURE 11.3 The Systems Outcomes Framework.
Source: Swinburn et al. (2019).

incentives and disincentives, and norms – set the conditions for the human systems that create societies, businesses and built environments. Then come the macro-systems that are the dominant sectors of society (e.g. the education system, the healthcare system, the social protection system). Mesosystems are the settings through which people interact (e.g. homes, schools, shops, workplaces) and the microsystems are social networks through which people interact with each other.

Interactions and common drivers of the Global Syndemic

Figure 11.3b zooms in to show the Global Syndemic view with the interactions between obesity, undernutrition and climate change and their common drivers from the natural systems through the layers of human systems. In terms of interactions, some are clear and some are less clear. The food systems is a major (25–30 per cent) contributor to GHGs through livestock methane emissions, food waste, deforestation, manufacturing, and transport (Vermeulen et al., 2012). Climate change will clearly exacerbate undernutrition through increased food insecurity (Haugen, Schug, Collman, & Heindel, 2015), with poorer people and poorer countries being the worst affected. Foetal and infant undernutrition is an established risk factor for obesity (Gillman et al., 2007). The impact of obesity on climate change and vice versa is uncertain at this stage.

Governance structures and the levers of power set the operating conditions for the major systems driving the Global Syndemic, which are: food and agriculture systems, transportation, urban design and land use. Since the 1980s, core policy and economic incentives have been focused on increasing GDP, company profits and shareholder wealth (Stiglitz, Sen, & Fitoussi, 2010), with little attention given to the external costs of damage to human health and the health of the planet. Consequently, some wealth goals have been achieved while health, equity and the environment have suffered.

Common driver examples

Food, transport, land use and urban design systems are emphasised as drivers in the Systems Outcomes Framework (Figure 11.3b). These drivers create the environments which to a large extent shape our behaviours, such as our car use and food choices. For example, a food supply system dominated by cheap, energy-dense, micronutrient-poor, processed foods promotes obesity and/or undernutrition depending on people's contexts (High Level Panel of Experts on Food Security and Nutrition, 2017); a car-dominated transport system promotes low physical activity (Tranter, 2010) and generates 24 per cent of global GHG emissions (International Energy Agency, 2017); and a largely animal-based food production system is a highly inefficient way to create nutritious foods to feed the world's undernourished population (Ranganathan et al., 2016), creates 9 per cent of GHG production (Ripple et al., 2013) and increases the risk of diseases like obesity and cancer (Lippi et al., 2016; You & Henneberg, 2016). Regulatory systems that allow the marketing of breastmilk substitutes contribute to low breastfeeding rates (Piwoz & Huffman, 2015), which is a risk for undernutrition (David & David, 1984) and obesity (Arenz, Ruckerl, Koletzko, & Von Kries, 2004; Arenz, Ruckerl, Koletzko, & Von Kries, 2012) and infant formula manufacturing creates considerably more GHG than breastfeeding (Linnecar, Gupta, Dadhich, & Nupur, 2014). Systems are socio-cultural in nature as well. A population's values, beliefs, attitudes, religious expectations and social practices shape the types of foods people eat, how they use food for hospitality, the status attributed to particular foods, vulnerability to commercial marketing, and are powerful determinants of a population's diet.

Five critical sets of feedback loops

Figure 11.3c zooms in further to show more explicitly the five main sets of feedback loops which define modern food systems. Why do we have the food systems we have? The central engine in all food systems is the business model, which is a series of positive feedback loops along the food value chain with foods (and related services) being exchanged at each step for money so that providers and receivers get what they want in an efficient manner. Business operates under the conditions set by the governance loops, and the supply and demand feedback loops operate along the chain to the final consumer level. This broadly explains why we have the food systems we have. For example, processing foods creates extra profit and extra shelf-life and convenience so that the products can be marketed more heavily and demand increased. Therefore, ultra-processed foods increasingly dominate the food systems because they reinforce the business feedback loops of greater profits and they reinforce the demand feedback loops for consumers through taste, value for money, and long shelf-life.

Why must food systems change? Our modern food systems have worked well to feed populations, from the centre of mega-cities to remote rural outposts, but their fundamental flaws are now driving the Global Syndemic. The reason why the food systems must change is that they are destroying the planet and creating the world's biggest health problem of malnutrition in all its forms. In Figure 11.3c, the parallel lines across the return arrows from the environment and health to the food system represent delays in feedback. A ruined local environment, an overheated planet and unhealthy populations will have negative impacts on food producers and sellers but only after considerable delay.

Why is it so hard to change food systems? If governments, guided by the science, want to change food systems for better health and environmental outcomes, why do they struggle to do so? The answer lies in the systemic responses to interventions within systems. Consider interventions, such as taxes on sugary drinks, removal of subsidies for cattle and dairy farming, the inclusion of methane production in carbon-pricing schemes, labelling foods so that consumers understand their health and environmental impacts, or regulations on marketing unhealthy foods to children. When any of these interventions are proposed, there is immediate, strong, and often successful push-back from the business and, sometimes, consumer demand feedback loops. The public will push back against rising food costs or a perceived reduction in food choice, especially if the reasons are not well explained and the poor are disproportionately affected. Businesses whose profits are threatened will react against such proposals and attack the government. Large food corporations will lobby politicians who will get cold feet and favour short-term popularity over longer-term outcomes. In the end, the power balance within the governance structures determines who will benefit and who will lose from the subsidies, taxes, regulations, information disclosures, and so on. Too often, it is large corporations and their shareholders who benefit and the consumers and the environment who suffer.

The roles for individuals

Figure 11.3d shows where individuals fit into the systems: everywhere. Individuals interact at each of the systems levels in two main ways. First, those systems influence the choice environments for individuals – what food is available, where, at what price, in what condition, with what information. Second, individuals have varying degrees of agency within each of those systems – as a parent, worker, shopper, voter, and so on. Individuals, therefore, are not merely passive victims of the systems but also agents within the systems, with the opportunity to act to bring about change.

What actions can be taken within the food system to combat the Global Syndemic?

A fundamental re-orientation of food systems is required. Superficial repairs at the edges will not deliver the global outcomes needed for the twenty-first century (High Level Panel of Experts on Food Security and Nutrition, 2017). Momentum at the global and local level is building for this fundamental change, including through conceptualising the current food systems as a major driver of the Global Syndemic.

Creating double-duty and triple-duty actions

Many of the actions needed to reduce undernutrition, obesity and climate change are already known and well documented. However, their implementation has been slow and patchy (Roberto et al., 2015). This 'policy inertia' needs to be seen as part of the problem and addressed by:

- fortifying governments to act on the evidence-based consensus recommendations in front of them;
- reducing the power of the vested-interest private food sector within the governance systems;
- increasing the demand from the public and civil society for policy action to transform food systems.

The Lancet Commission on Obesity (Swinburn et al., 2019) used the concept of double- or triple-duty actions to identify actions that address two or three aspects of the Global Syndemic. A simple example of a triple-duty action would be to have sustainable dietary guidelines as the policy document underpinning nutrition education, healthy food policies and sustainable agriculture. Only Sweden, Germany, Qatar, and Brazil have included sustainability in their national dietary guidelines. When Australia and the US governments attempted to do the same, they were defeated by pressure from the food industry. Further examples of triple-duty actions are outlined below.

The Framework Convention on Food Systems (FCFS)

A global framework convention that creates the regulatory framework for action to transform food systems towards being healthier, more sustainable and more equitable would fortify governments to implement the existing recommendations for better nutrition. The Framework Convention on Tobacco Control (FCTC) and the UN Framework Convention on Climate Change (FCCC) are the key models to draw upon. In particular, it would address conflicts of interest, as is achieved through Article 5.3 of the FCTC, by excluding vested-interest industry players from policy development participation. There is extensive backing for a FCFS among civil society organisations (Consumers International and World Obesity Federation, 2014), but not yet from national governments.

Collective civil society action to demand policy action

Civil society, non-governmental organisations, professional and community organisations, academia and the general public are rarely coordinated and united enough to exert sufficient power to create systemic change. They are also resource-poor and have multiple agendas. However, the experience of civil society pressure in Mexico to achieve food policies, such as taxes on sugary drinks and unhealthy food, is instructive. Bloomberg Philanthropies invested in Mexican civil society and research organisations over several years to raise public awareness of the need for policy actions to reduce diabetes, to work with legislators and to collect the evidence of effectiveness of the policies (Donaldson, 2017). The Lancet Commission on Obesity suggested that an investment fund of US$1 billion from philanthropic and other sources could plausibly support 100 countries to apply the "Mexican approach" for food policy action.

Business models for the twenty-first century

In economic terms, the current business models represent a clear case of commercial success (companies and shareholders making profits) but market failure (consumers and the environments suffering the negative consequences) (Moodie, Swinburn, Richardson, & Somaini, 2006). While some businesses are becoming more socially and environmentally responsible, these responsibilities need to be as embedded in the ethos and regulation of business as much as financial responsibility currently is. The negative health and environmental costs of food products and practices need to be part of the costs of doing business and not passed on to current and future taxpayers to pay for. Additionally, massive global agricultural subsidies of about half a trillion dollars a year predominantly support the production of beef and dairy and a small number of grains such as corn, wheat and rice used for animal feed or as the basis of ultra-processed foods (Dangour et al., 2013). It is clear that these incentive structures in our current food systems do not support the radical transformation that is required to achieve better social and environmental outcomes.

Conclusion

Overconsumption of energy leading to obesity is a massive global problem, but it is only one aspect of a broader group of pandemics that are the inevitable outcomes of modern food systems. Fundamental transformations are needed within global food systems, and the economic and regulatory environments they operate in, if we are to achieve food systems that promote human health, social equity, environmental sustainability and economic prosperity.

References

Afshin, A., Sur, P. J., Fay, K. A., Cornaby, L., Ferrara, G., Salama, J. S., et al. (2019) Health effects of dietary risks in 195 countries, 1990–2017: A systematic analysis for the Global Burden of Disease Study 2017. *The Lancet*, 393, 1958–1972.

Arenz, S., Ruckerl, R., Koletzko, B. & Von Kries, R. (2004). Breast-feeding and childhood obesity: A systematic review. *International Journal of Obesity and Related Metabolic Disorders*, 28, 1247–1256.

Blundell, J. E. & Macdiarmid, J. I. (1997). Passive overconsumption, fat intake and short-term energy balance. *Annals of the New York Academy of Sciences*, 827, 392–407.

Bronfenbrenner, U. (1992). Ecological systems theory. In R. Vasta (ed.), *Six theories of child development: Revised formulations and current issues*. New York: Jessica Kingsley Publishers Ltd.

Consumers International & World Obesity Federation. (2014). *Recommendations towards a global convention to protect and promote healthy diets*. London: Consumers International, World Obesity Federation.

Dahlgren, G., & Whitehead, M. (1991). *Policies and strategies to promote social equity in health*. Stockholm: Institute for Futures Studies.

Dangour, A. D., Hawkesworth, S., Shankar, B., et al. (2013). Can nutrition be promoted through agriculture-led food price policies? A systematic review. *BMJ Open*, 3.

David, C. B., & David, P.H. (1984). Bottle-feeding and malnutrition in a developing country: The 'bottle-starved' baby. *Journal of Tropical Pediatrics*, 30, 159–164.

Donaldson, E. (2017). Advocating for sugar-sweetened beverage taxation: A case study of Mexico. Baltimore, MD: Johns Hopkins Bloomberg School of Public Health.

Egger, G., & Swinburn, B. (1997). An "ecological" approach to the obesity pandemic. *BMJ*, 315, 477–480.

FAO (Food and Agriculture Organization). (2013). The state of food and agriculture 2013. Rome: FAO.

Gerrior, S., Bente, L., & Hiza, H. (2004). Nutrient content of the U.S. Food Supply. 1909–2000. Washington, DC: US Department of Agriculture, Center for Nutrition Policy and Promotion.

Gillman, M. W., Barker, D., Bier, D., et al. (2007). Meeting report on the 3rd International Congress on Developmental Origins of Health and Disease (DOHaD). *Pediatric Research*, 61, 625–629.

Hall, K. D., Guo, J., Dore, M., & Chow, C. C. (2009). The progressive increase of food waste in America and its environmental impact. *PLoS One*, 4, e7940.

Haugen, A. C., Schug, T. T., Collman, G., & Heindel, J. J. (2015). Evolution of DOHaD: the impact of environmental health sciences. *Journal of Developmental Origins of Health and Disease*, 6, 55–64.

High Level Panel of Experts on Food Security and Nutrition. (2017). Nutrition and food systems. A report by the High Level Panel of Experts on Food Security and Nutrition of the Committee on World Food Security. Rome: High Level Panel of Experts on Food Security and Nutrition.

International Energy Agency. (2017). CO_2 emissions from fuel combustion. Paris: International Energy Agency.

Jägerskog, A., & Jønch Clausen, T. (2012). Feeding a thirsty world: Challenges and opportunities for a water and food secure future. Report no. 31. Stockholm: Stockholm International Water Institute.

Linnecar, A., Gupta, A., Dadhich, J. P., & Nupur, B. (2014). Formula for disaster: Weighing the impact of formula feeding vs breastfeeding on environment. Asia: Breastfeeding Promotion Network of India/Stockholm: International Baby Food Action Network.

Lippi, G., Mattiuzzi, C., & Cervellin, G. (2016). Meat consumption and cancer risk: A critical review of published meta-analyses. *Critical Reviews in Oncology/Hematology*, 97, 1–14.

Moodie, R., Swinburn, B., Richardson, J., & Somaini, B. (2006). Childhood obesity: A sign of commercial success, but a market failure. *International Journal of Pediatric Obesity*, 1, 133–138.

NCD Risk Factor Collaboration. (2017). Worldwide trends in body-mass index, underweight, overweight, and obesity from 1975 to 2016: A pooled analysis of 2416 population-based measurement studies in 128.9 million children, adolescents, and adults. *The Lancet*, 390, 2627–2642.

Oddy, W. H. (2012). Infant feeding and obesity risk in the child. *Breastfeed Review*, 20, 7–12.

Piwoz, E. G. , & Huffman, S. L. (2015). The impact of marketing of breast-milk substitutes on WHO-recommended breastfeeding practices. *Food Nutrition Bulletin*, 36, 373–386.

Putnam, J. (2000). Major trends in the U.S. food supply, 1909–1999. *Food Reviews*, 23, 8–15.

Ranganathan, J., Vennard, D., Waite, R., *et al.* (2016). Shifting diets for a sustainable food future. Working Paper, Instalment 11 of Creating a Sustainable Food Future. Washington, DC:World Resource Institute.

Ripple, W. J., Smith, P., Haberl, H., Montzka, S. A., Mcalpine, C., & Boucher, D. H. (2013). Ruminants, climate change and climate policy. *Nature Climate Change*, 4, 2.

Roberto, C. A., Swinburn, B., Hawkes, C., *et al.* (2015). Patchy progress on obesity prevention: Emerging examples, entrenched barriers, and new thinking. *The Lancet*, 385, 2400–2409.

Stiglitz, J. E., Sen, A. , & Fitoussi, J. (2010). *Mismeasuring our lives: Why GDP doesn't add up. The report by the Commission on the Measurement of Economic Performance and Social Progress*. New York: The New Press.

Swinburn, B. A., Kraak, V. I., Allender, S., Atkins, V. J., Baker, P. I., Bogard, J. R., ... Devarajan, R. (2019). The global syndemic of obesity, undernutrition, and climate change: The Lancet Commission report. *The Lancet*, doi:10.1016/S0140–6736(18)32822–32828.

Swinburn, B. A., Sacks, G., Hall, K. D., McPherson, K., Finegood, D. T., ... Gortmaker, S. L. (2011). The global obesity pandemic: Shaped by global drivers and local environments. *The Lancet*, 378, 804–814.

Tranter, P. J. (2010). Speed kills: The complex links between transport, lack of time and urban health. *Journal of Urban Health*, 87, 155–166.

Vermeulen, S. J., Campbell, B. M., & Ingram, J. S. I. (2012). Climate change and food systems. *Annual Review of Environment and Resources*, 37, 195–222.

Von Grebmer, K., Bernstein, J., Hossain, N., *et al.* (2017). *2017 Global Hunger Index: The inequalities of hunger*. Washington, DC/Bonn/Dublin: International Food Policy Research Institute, Welthungerhilfe, and Concern Worldwide.

You, W., & Henneberg, M. (2016). Meat consumption providing a surplus energy in modern diet contributes to obesity prevalence: An ecological analysis. *BMC Nutrition*, 2(30).

12

CO-BENEFITS FOR CLIMATE AND HEALTH OF SHIFTING TOWARDS PLANT-BASED DIETS

Cristina Tirado-von der Pahlen

Introduction

Globally, dietary patterns are changing towards the consumption of more animal foods and this is a key determinant of health that plays a significant role in environmental degradation and climate change. Diets high in meat and low in vegetables and fruits are associated with adverse health outcomes, such as cancer, heart disease, obesity and type 2 diabetes. Current dietary patterns in most high-income countries are not sustainable and the extent of their adverse environmental impact will only worsen as they expand into low- and middle-income countries (Nelson, Hamm, Hu, Abrams, & Griffin, 2016; Springmann, Clark, & Mason-D'Croz, 2018a).

The food system is responsible for up to 30 per cent of human-induced greenhouse gas (GHG) emissions. Animal-based foods are the main contributor (Vermeulen, Campbell, & Ingram, 2012; Tubiello et al., 2015; Niles et al., 2018), with livestock production accounting for approximately 14.5 per cent of GHG emissions (FAO, 2013a). Emissions from agriculture could rise by as much as 80 per cent in 2050 due to the increased demand for animal products (Popp, Lotze-Campen, & Bodirsky, 2010; Hedenus, Wirsenius, & Johansson, 2014; Tilman & Clark 2014; Springmann, Godfray, Rayner, & Scarborough, 2016b).

The Paris Climate Change Agreement aims to keep the global temperature rise this century well to below 2 degrees Celsius above pre-industrial levels and to pursue efforts to limit the temperature increase even further to 1.5 degrees Celsius. The Intergovernmental Panel on Climate Change (IPCC) Special Report 1.5 C highlights the need for mitigation options limiting the demand for land, including dietary changes away from land-intensive animal products (IPCC, 2018).

If not addressed properly, food-related GHG emissions could account for half of all emissions allowed by targets for keeping the global rise in temperature to less than 2 degrees Celsius by 2050, and could exceed total permissible levels by 2070 (Hedenus et al., 2014; Springmann et al., 2016b). Dietary shifts that include a reduction in meat and animal-based foods – particularly in groups with high per capita meat consumption in high-income countries – are necessary to reach the 2 degrees Celsius climate goal (Hedenus et al., 2014) and to avoid the irreversible impacts of climate change. However, dietary changes may not be appropriate for everyone and are dependent on nutrition status, culture, and other considerations. For example, consumption of animal foods is an important aspect of some indigenous cultures.

This chapter explores current knowledge about the co-benefits for health and sustainability of lowering the ratio of animal:plant foods in our diets, and outlines actions that can be taken to reduce animal foods consumption and increase plant food consumption to promote healthy and sustainable diets.

Current consumption patterns and future trends for animal- and plant-based diets

Current diets with high intakes of meat, fat and sugar, and inadequate intakes of fruits, vegetables and grains, represent a major risk to health, social systems and environmental life support systems (Lim et al., 2010; Aleksandrowicz et al., 2016; GLOPAN, 2016).

Socio-economic and demographic changes have a key role in the medium- to long-term evolution of food consumption and dietary patterns. Rising incomes in low- and middle-income countries and rapid urbanisation, particularly in Asia, are creating changes in food demand. Dietary patterns are changing towards the consumption of more foods of animal origin (FAO, 2013b). The IMPACT model has projected that for most regions, per capita levels of meat and milk consumption in 2030 will rise with additional per capita income, while consumption of cereals will decrease (Msangi & Rosegrant, 2011).

Figure 12.1 shows the projection of per capita meat consumption to 2030. Meat consumption in high-income countries such as the US is far beyond the world average, while the growth in dynamic economies, such as China and Brazil, accounts for much of what is observed in East Asia and the Latin American region. East Asian economies such as China show substantial growth in meat consumption over the 2000–30 period, though the projected levels of per capita consumption remain below Latin America's 2030 levels. The total per capita consumption levels and growth in Sub-Saharan Africa and the South Asian regions are relatively small (Msangi & Rosegrant, 2011).

Red meat consumption has declined everywhere in recent years, except East Asia, where it has risen by nearly 40 per cent, suggesting that it is possible to reduce meat consumption if the appropriate drivers are in place (GLOPAN, 2016). This may reflect a shift in dietary pattern as countries become wealthier and prefer healthier components found in higher-quality diets.

Figure 12.2 shows the change of per capita consumption of fruits and vegetables to 2030. A projection of how fruit and vegetable consumption changes over time shows that within this commodity group, East Asia, the Middle East and the North Africa region have the strongest tendencies towards future growth in intake of the nutrient-rich foods within this category (Msangi & Rosegrant, 2011).

Environmental impacts of animal- versus plant-based foods

Global demand for beef is projected to increase by 95 per cent, and global demand for animal-based foods in general by 80 per cent, between 2006 and 2050 (WRI, 2016). This growth is expected to be concentrated in urban areas of emerging economies, particularly

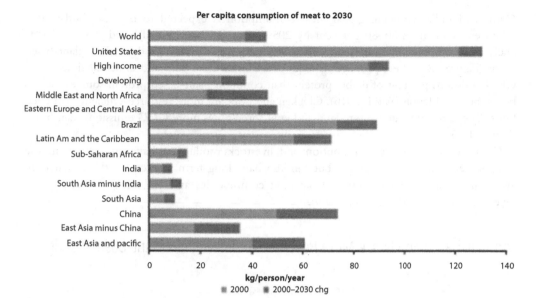

FIGURE 12.1 Projection of per capita consumption of meat to 2030
Source: Msangi & Rosegrant (2011). Reproduced with permission from the International Food Policy Research Institute www.ifpri.org. The original paper in which these figures appear is available online at http://ebrary.ifpri.org/utils/getfile/collection/p15738coll2/id/124834/filename/124835.pdf

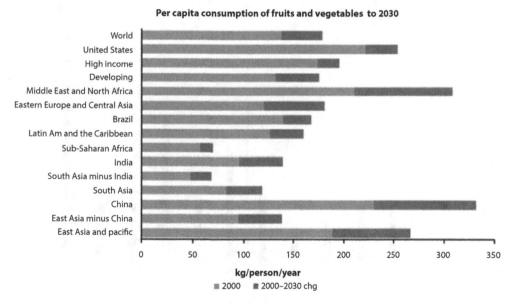

FIGURE 12.2 Change of per capita consumption of fruits and vegetables to 2030
Source: Msangi & Rosegrant (2011). Reproduced with permission from the International Food Policy Research Institute www.ifpri.org. The original paper in which these figures appear is available online at http://ebrary.ifpri.org/utils/getfile/collection/p15738coll2/id/124834/filename/124835.pdf.

China and India. Growing global meat consumption is expected to increase food-related GHG emissions from 30–80 per cent by 2050 (WRI, 2016). Animal-based foods are generally more resource-intensive and environmentally impactful to produce than plant-based foods (Figure 12.3). Beef production requires 20 times more land and emits 20 times more GHG emissions per unit of edible protein than common plant-based protein sources such as beans, peas and lentils (WRI, 2016). Chicken and pork are more resource-efficient than beef, but still require three times more land and emit three times more GHG emissions than beans (Figure 12.3).

Global trends in meat consumption and livestock production have an impact on the environment and climate change, but can also have long-term impacts on the production, availability, and pricing of certain basic food commodities and on access to nutritionally diverse food sources (Friel et al., 2009).

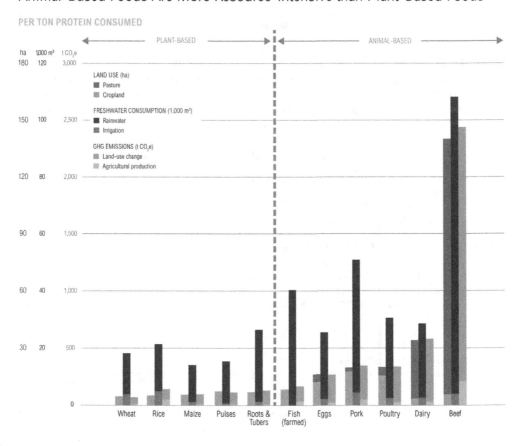

FIGURE 12.3 Food-related land and water resource use and greenhouse gas emissions (plant-based versus animal based)

Source: WRI (2016).

Opportunities for dietary shifts away from animal foods for high meat consumers

Lowering the level of animal-sourced foods in the diets of high meat-consuming countries, needs to become a key element of climate mitigation strategies (Hedenus et al., 2014; Smith et al., 2014; Tirado, 2017; IPCC, 2018). For example, the average US citizen could cut their diet-related environmental impacts by nearly one half just by eating less meat and dairy products (WRI, 2016). When applied to the average US diet in 2009, an animal protein reduction scenario (which cut people's meat/dairy/fish/egg consumption in half) can reduce per person land use and agricultural GHG emissions by nearly one-half, or almost as much as a vegetarian scenario (which eliminated meat and fish, but increased dairy consumption relative to the average American) (WRI, 2016). The beef reduction scenarios reduced per person land use and greenhouse gas emissions by 15 per cent (replacing one-third of beef consumption with other meats or legumes) to 35 per cent (reducing beef consumption by 70 per cent, down to the world average level) (WRI, 2016).

Co-benefits for health and sustainability by lowering the ratio of animal: plant foods in current diets

Diets high in vegetables, fruits, whole grains, pulses, nuts, and seeds, with modest amounts of meat and dairy, promote health and well-being. A number of studies have shown that reduction of red meat to help reduce the risk of cardiovascular disease and the risk of colorectal cancer and increased consumption of fruits and vegetables can reduce the risk of cardiovascular disease, cancer, and all causes of mortality (WHO, 2015).

The IPCC is the international body for assessing the science related to climate change. The IPCC Fifth Assessment Report (AR5) highlighted the co-benefits that can be achieved from actions that reduce emissions and also improve health in high meat-consuming countries, by shifting consumption away from animal products, especially from ruminant sources, towards less emission-intensive diets (Smith et al., 2014). In very low-income settings, however, better access to animal protein can be essential to improve nutrition for groups lacking diverse food sources.

Many studies have examined how shifting current animal-based dietary patterns towards plant-based patterns as recommended in the EAT-Lancet Commission report (Willett et al., 2019) may result in reduced GHG emissions and other environmental benefits. These diets can improve public health and nutritional outcomes, while also helping to reduce GHG emissions (Friel et al., 2009; Tilman & Clark, 2014; Green et al., 2015; Springmann et al., 2016b; Milner et al., 2017; IPCC, 2018, Willet et al., 2019).

Comparisons of omnivorous diets to more sustainable alternatives, such as Mediterranean, pescetarian and vegetarian diets, have shown the latter to reduce emissions from food production (Tilman & Clark, 2014) (Figure 12.4a). Similar comparisons have shown a decrease in disease risk globally. For instance, incidence rates of type 2 diabetes were reduced by 16–41 per cent and of cancer by 7–13 per cent, while relative mortality rates from coronary heart disease were 20–26 per cent lower and overall mortality rates for all causes combined were cut by 0–18 per cent (Tilman & Clark, 2014) (Figure 12.4b).

A transition to more nutritious and diverse diets (with fewer processed foods and more fruit and vegetables) is frequently projected to result in reduced GHG emissions, as well as likely reductions in NCDs (Green et al., 2015; Milner, Green, & Dangour, 2015). For example, if the average adult

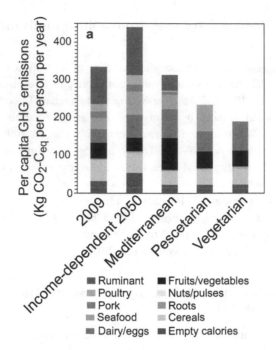

FIGURE 12.4a Per capita food production GHG emissions for five diets (2009 global-average, 2050 global income-dependent, Mediterranean, pescetarian and vegetarian)

Source: Tilman & Clark (2014).

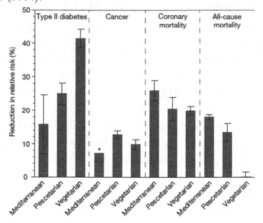

FIGURE 12.4b Diet-dependent percentage reductions in relative risk of type 2 diabetes, cancer, coronary heart disease mortality and of all-cause mortality when comparing each alternative diet (Mediterranean, pescetarian and vegetarian) to its region's conventional omnivorous diet

diet in the UK conformed to WHO recommendations, its associated GHG emissions would be reduced by 17 per cent (Green et al., 2015). Further emission cuts of around 40 per cent could be achieved by making realistic modifications to diets so that they contained fewer animal products and processed snacks, and more fruit, vegetables and cereals (Green et al., 2015). In India, dietary changes in line with nutritional guidelines (lower amounts of wheat, dairy, and poultry, and increased amounts of legumes) could help to address projected reductions in the availability of freshwater for irrigation in 2050 and, simultaneously reduce diet-related GHG emissions and improve diet-related health outcomes (Milner et al., 2017).

Globally, it is estimated that transitioning to more plant-based diets, in line with WHO recommendations on healthy eating (WHO, 2015) and the guidelines on human energy requirements and recommendations by the World Cancer Research Fund, could reduce global mortality by 6-10 per cent and food-related GHG emissions by 29-70 per cent compared with a reference scenario for 2050 (Springmann et al., 2016b). Yet, less than half of all regions meet, or are projected to meet, dietary recommendations for the consumption of fruit, vegetables and red meat, while also exceeding the optimal total energy intake. Therefore, significant changes in the global food system would be necessary for regional diets to match these global healthy dietary patterns (Springmann et al., 2016b).

Following public health objectives by adopting energy-balanced, low-meat dietary patterns that are in line with available evidence on healthy eating has been shown to lead to an adequate nutrient supply for most nutrients, and large reductions in premature mortality (Springmann et al., 2018b). This approach has led to a substantial reduction of environmental impacts globally (reducing GHG emissions by 54–87 per cent) in most regions, except for some environmental domains (cropland use, freshwater use, and phosphorus application) in low-income countries (Springmann et al., 2018b).

The EAT-Lancet Commission Report concluded that a transformation to healthy diets by 2050 will require substantial dietary shifts (which differ regionally) including a greater than 50 per cent reduction in global consumption of unhealthy foods, such as red meat and sugar, and a 100 per cent increase in consumption of healthy foods, such as nuts, fruits, vegetables, and legumes (Willett et al., 2019). This could prevent up to 11.1 million deaths per year in 2030, a 19.9 per cent reduction of all premature mortality due to prevention of CVD, diabetes and cancer, among other diseases (Willett et al., 2019).

Shifting current dietary patterns to more plant-based alternatives

Strategies, policies and measures to promote healthier, more plant-based, and sustainable diets, include economic interventions, changes to the production and consumption, education and other transformative approaches.

Economic incentives

Positive shifts in dietary patterns towards more plant-based diets can be brought about by economic incentives that align the marketing practices of retailers and processors with public health and climate goals. Public-sector incentives for food service companies, retailers and distributors are another potential way of promoting sustainable and healthy dietary patterns with higher plant-based diets. Food procurement is also a key area to promote dietary shifts to plant protein. Governments are often the largest buyers of food products, for example, for schools, state institutions such as universities, hospitals, government, and the military, etc. Such incentives can encourage food labelling (for nutritional content, carbon and water footprints) in a way that helps consumers achieve nutritional requirements while meeting environmental goals (Tirado, 2017).

Production: supporting production of fruits, vegetables and pulses

On the production side, eliminating agricultural subsidies for foods that adversely affect human health and supporting the local production of fruits, vegetables and pulses have the potential to make these healthy foods more accessible to lower-income communities, as well as support environmental goals (Jacoby et al., 2014). The promotion of healthy diets based on the local, seasonal production of agro-ecological foods, along with the promotion of short marketing circuits, have been proposed as opportunities to increase produce added value and forge closer ties between farmers, consumers and the land (Jacoby et al., 2014).

Consumption: taxation

On the consumption side, taxing food-related emissions and creating economic incentives could make diets more sustainable and healthier (Springmann, Mason-D'Croz, & Robinson, 2017). Modelling studies show that the climate change mitigation potential of pricing emissions that result from food commodities could be substantial. A GHG emissions tax on foods (corresponding to their emissions intensities), if properly designed, could be a powerful health-promoting climate policy affecting health improvements worldwide. Sparing food groups known to be beneficial for health – such as fruits and vegetables – from taxation, selectively compensating for income losses associated with tax-related price increases, and using a portion of tax revenues for health promotion are potential policy options that could help avert most of the negative health impacts experienced by vulnerable groups, while still promoting changes towards diets which are more environmentally sustainable (Springmann et al., 2017).

Food-based dietary guidelines

The inclusion of sustainability criteria in food-based dietary guidelines is a key means of encouraging healthy, sustainable diets with a higher content of plant protein foods. To date, only a few countries (notably Brazil, Germany, Qatar and Sweden) have included sustainability criteria in their national dietary guidelines (FAO/FCRN, 2016). Broadly speaking, the advice issued by these countries focuses on reducing meat consumption, choosing seafood from non-threatened stocks, eating more plants and plant-based products, reducing energy intake and reducing food waste. Sweden and its Nordic neighbours have emphasised the environmental impact of diet in their sustainability criteria. Brazil's guidelines also address the social and economic aspects of sustainability and urge people to avoid ultra-processed foods that damage traditional food cultures and health. Investment in interdisciplinary research and action to address the broader social and economic dimensions of sustainable diets is needed, especially in developing countries (FAO/FCRN, 2016). Updating food-based national dietary guidelines to reflect the latest evidence on healthy eating can by itself be critical to improve health and reduce climate and environmental impacts while complementing the broader criteria of sustainability (Springmann et al., 2018b).

Transformative approaches to dietary shifts

Effective transformative approaches for shifting towards healthy and sustainable diets are those that are evidence-based, socio-culturally and geographically appropriate, sustainable, integrated, equitable, ethical, and embraced by the communities and the institutions that have shaped them (Nordic Food Policy Lab, 2018). These approaches may include, for example, establishing healthy and sustainable institutional food procurement and urban food services, promoting traditional and local food cultural heritage, biodiversity, gastronomy, local and regional identity, rural development and eco-tourism, innovative cooperatives of producers and consumers, urban, community and school gardens and public meals, among others (Nordic Food Policy Lab, 2018).

Policies, including food, agriculture, health, and nutrition, dietary guidance, environment, water, trade, transportation and economics, need to be integrated via a multi-stakeholder process to promote dietary shifts to plant-based diets. Governments should work with industry to encourage investment in the research and development of alternatives to animal-based protein, including plant-based proteins, and develop a regulatory environment to support such innovation. This may bring numerous challenges and need for behavioural change. Educational initiatives to increase consumer knowledge and informed decision-making, as well as incentives to make healthier foods such as fruits and vegetables more affordable and accessible are critical.

Conclusion

Globally, dietary patterns are changing towards the consumption of more animal foods and this has a significant role in environmental degradation and climate change. At the same time, diets that are high in meat and low in vegetables and fruits, are associated with adverse health outcomes.

There are opportunities to achieve co-benefits from actions that reduce climate-altering emissions and also improve health in high meat-consuming countries, by shifting consumption away from animal products towards less emission-intensive diets, rich in fruits, vegetables, pulses and cereals. A general transition to more plant-based diets could lead to lower GHG emissions and likely reductions in diet-related non-communicable diseases. It is important to highlight, however, that in regions affected by undernutrition, where people often rely on few staple crops and poor-quality diets, higher meat intake could be nutritionally beneficial. Approaches to sustainable diets are context-specific and can result in reductions in environmental and health impacts globally and in most regions, particularly in high-income and middle-income countries, but they can also increase resource use in low-income countries when diets diversify.

Transformative approaches to more plant-based diets may involve subsidising or providing economic incentives for the production and consumption of more fruits, vegetables and pulses, the inclusion of sustainability criteria in dietary guidelines, taxing excessive meat consumption, conducting public education campaigns and educational programmes in schools, labelling, promoting collaboration and shared agreements among others.

Positive shifts towards more plant-based diets can be brought about by economic incentives that align the marketing practices of retailers and distributors with public health and climate goals. Public-sector incentives for food service and food procurement companies are a potential way of promoting dietary shifts to plant protein.

Food-based dietary guidelines that include sustainability criteria are key to changing dietary patterns to more sustainable, healthier diets. Transitioning to more plant-based diets in line with WHO and other international dietary guidelines could decrease global mortality, shrink the global food gap and substantially reduce diet-related GHG emissions. Updating national dietary guidelines to reflect the latest evidence on healthy eating can by itself be critical for improving health and reducing environmental impacts and contributing to sustainability.

Investment in multidisciplinary research is needed to collect the evidence necessary to promote a shift to sustainable and healthy diets in different socio-economic and cultural environments, particularly in low-income countries.

Dietary and nutritional considerations should be integrated into climate-change mitigation and adaptation. In this context, it is critical to promote demand-side climate mitigation options for the agriculture and food sector, such as changes in dietary patterns and food procurement towards less GHG-intensive, healthier, more plant-based alternatives.

References

Aleksandrowicz, L., Green, R., Joy, E. J. M., Smith, P., & Haines, A. (2016). The impacts of dietary change on greenhouse gas emissions, land use, water use, and health: A systematic review. *PLoS ONE*, 11(11), e0165797.

FAO (Food and Agriculture Organization). (2013a). Tackling climate change through livestock: A global assessment of emissions and mitigation opportunities. Rome: FAO.

FAO. (2013b). The state of food and agriculture, 2013. Rome: FAO.

FAO/FCRN. (2016). Plates, pyramids and planets. Available at: www.fao.org/3/a-i5640e.pdf

Friel, S., Dangour, A. D., Garnett, T., Lock, K., Chalabi, Z., & Roberts, I.et al. (2009). Public health benefits of strategies to reduce greenhouse-gas emissions: Food and agriculture. *The Lancet*, 374, 2016–2025.

GLOPAN. (2016). Food systems and diets: Facing the challenges of the 21st century. London: GLOPAN.

Green, R., Milner, J., Dangour, A. D., Haines, A., Chalabi, Z., Markandya, A., ... Wilkinson, P. (2015). The potential to reduce greenhouse gas emissions in the UK through healthy and realistic dietary change. *Climate Change*, 129, 253–265. doi:10.1007/s10584–10015–1329-y.

Hedenus, F., Wirsenius, S., & Johansson, D. J. A. (2014). The importance of reduced meat and dairy consumption for meeting stringent climate change targets. *Climate Change*, 124, 79–91.

IPCC. (2018). Global warming of 1.5 °C. IPCC special report on the impacts of global warming of 1.5 °C above pre-industrial levels and related global greenhouse gas emission pathways, in the context of strengthening the global response to the threat of climate change, sustainable development, and efforts to eradicate poverty. Available at: www.report.ipcc.ch/sr15/pdf/sr15_spm_final.pdf

Jacoby, E., Tirado, C., Diaz, A., Pena, M., Sanches, A., & Coloma, M. (2014). Family farming, food security and public health in the Americas. *World Nutrition*, 5(6), 537–551.

Lim, S. S., Vos, T., Flaxman, A. D., Danaei, G., Shibuya, K., & Adair-Rohani, H. (2010). A comparative risk assessment of burden of disease and injury attributable to 67 risk factors and risk factor clusters in 21 regions, 1990–2010:A systematic analysis for the Global Burden of Disease Study. *The Lancet*, 380(9859), 2224–2260.

Milner, J., Green, R., & Dangour, A. D. (2015). Health effects of adopting low greenhouse gas emission diets in the UK. *BMJ Open*, 5, e007364. doi:10.1136/bmjopen-2014-007364.

Milner, J., Joy, E. J., Green, R., Harris, F., Aleksandrowicz, L., Agrawal, S., ... Dangour, A.D., (2017). Projected health effects of realistic dietary changes to address freshwater constraints in India: A modelling study. *The Lancet Planetary Health*, 1(1), e26–e32.

Msangi, S., & Rosegrant, M. W. (2011). Feeding the future's changing diets: implications for agriculture. markets, nutrition, and policy. Available at: www.foresightfordevelopment.org

Nelson, M. E., Hamm, M. W., Hu, F. B., Abrams, S. A., & Griffin, T. S. (2016). Alignment of healthy dietary patterns and environmental sustainability: A systematic review. *Advances in Nutrition*, 7(6), 1005–1025.

Niles, M., Ahuja, R., Barker, T., Esquivel, J., Gutterman, S., Heller, M. ... Vermeulen, S. (2018). Climate change mitigation beyond agriculture: A review of food system opportunities and implications. *Renewable Agriculture and Food Systems*, 33(3), 297–308.

Nordic Food Policy Lab. (2018). Available at: www.norden.org/en/nordic-food-policy-lab

Popp, A., Lotze-Campen, H., & Bodirsky, B. (2010). Food consumption, diet shifts and associated non-CO_2 greenhouse gases from agricultural production. *Global Environmental Change*, 20, 451–462.

Smith, K. R., Woodward, A., Campbell-Lendrum, D., et al. (2014). Human health: impacts, adaptation, and co-benefits. In: C. B. Field, et al. (eds), *Climate change 2014: Impacts, adaptation, and vulnerability. Part A: global and sectoral aspects. Contribution of Working Group II to the Fifth Assessment Report of the Intergovernmental Panel on Climate Change.* Cambridge: Cambridge University Press, pp. 709–754.

Springmann, M., Clark, M. D., Mason-D'Croz, M., *et al.* (2018a). Options for keeping the food system within environmental limits. *Nature*, 562, 519–525.

Springmann, M., Godfray, H. C. J., Rayner, M., & Scarborough, P. (2016b). Analysis and valuation of the health and climate change co-benefits of dietary change, *Proceedings of the National Academy of Sciences of the United States (PNAS)*, 113(15), 4146–4151.

Springmann, M., Mason-D'Croz, D., & Robinson, S. (2017). Mitigation potential and global health impacts from emissions pricing of food commodities. *Nature Climate Change*, 7, 69–74.

Springmann, M., Mason-D'Croz, D., Robinson, S., Garnett, T., Godfray, H. C. J., Gollin, D., ... Scarborough, P. (2016a). Global and regional health effects of future food production under climate change: A modelling study. *The Lancet*, 387, 1937–1946.

Springmann, M., Wiebe, K., Mason-D'Croz, D., Sulser, T. B., Rayner, M., & Scarborough, P.(2018b). Health and nutritional aspects of sustainable diet strategies and their association with environmental impacts: A global modelling analysis with country-level detail. *The Lancet Planetary Health*, 2(10), e451–e461.

Tilman, D., & Clark, M. (2014). Global diets link environmental sustainability and human health. *Nature*, 515(7528), 518–522. doi:10.1038/nature13959.

Tirado, M. C. (2017). *Sustainable diets for healthy people and a healthy planet.* Rome: United Nations Standing Committee on Nutrition.

Tubiello, F. N., Salvatore, M., Ferrara, A. F., House, J., Federici, S., ... Smith, P. (2015). The contribution of agriculture, forestry and other land use activities to global warming, 1990–2012. *Global Change Biology*, 21(7), 2655–2660.

Vermeulen, S. J., Campbell, B. M., & Ingram, J. S. I. (2012). Climate change and food systems. *Annual Review of Environment and Resources*, 37, 195–222. Available at: www.annualreviews.org/doi/abs/10.1146/annurev-environ-020411-130608

WHO (World Health Organization). (2015). Healthy diet fact sheet, no.°394. Geneva: WHO. Available at: www.who.int/mediacentre/factsheets/fs394/en/

Willett, W., Rockström, J., Loken, B., Springmann, M., Lang, T., Vermeulen, S., ... Murray, C. J. L. (2019). Food in the Anthropocene: The EAT-Lancet Commission on healthy diets from sustainable food systems. *The Lancet*, 393(10170), 447–492

World Cancer Research Fund/American Institute for Cancer Research. (2007). Food, nutrition, physical activity, and the prevention of cancer: A global perspective. Washington, DC: AICR. Available at: www.aicr.org/assets/docs/pdf/reports/Second_Expert_Report.pdf

WRI. (2016). Shifting diets for a sustainable food future: Creating a sustainable food future. Available at: www.wri.org/sites/default/files/Shifting_Diets_for_a_Sustainable_Food_Future_0.pdf

13

THE UNTENABLE ROLE OF "JUNK FOOD" IN A HEALTHY AND SUSTAINABLE FOOD SYSTEM

Michalis Hadjikakou and Phillip Baker

Introduction

Achieving a healthy and sustainable food system necessitates interventions throughout the food supply chain. This entails concurrent change in production practices and consumption patterns, the combination of which can accelerate positive transformation. There has been growing awareness over recent years of the importance of promoting diets that are both healthy and sustainable as one of the key strategies to safeguard human and environmental health (Tilman & Clark, 2014; Development Initiatives, 2017). National dietary guidelines, traditionally focused solely on health outcomes, are now being revised in several countries to explicitly include environmental sustainability recommendations (Ritchie, Reay, & Higgins, 2018).

While there remain data gaps and uncertainty with respect to the environmental implications of diverse food products in different geographic locations, studies highlight the significant co-benefits of curbing excess caloric intakes and reducing the intake of animal products (Tilman & Clark, 2014; Poore & Nemecek, 2018). However, serious consideration must be given to other ways of reducing diet-related environmental impacts. Reducing the consumption of junk foods, which are both detrimental to health and use scarce planetary resources, must also be seen as a key component of maximising health and sustainability outcomes (Friel, Barosh, & Lawrence, 2014; van Dooren, Marinussen, Blonk, Aiking, & Vellinga, 2014; Hadjikakou, 2017).

The aim of this chapter is to explore the importance of limiting the amount of junk food produced and consumed as a key premise towards a truly healthy and sustainable global food system. In developing this argument, alternative nomenclatures for junk food products are considered in relation to their sustainability implications. Consumption trends are then illustrated with a brief review of the evidence base for the health and sustainability implications of these foods, including current data gaps and related uncertainty. This chapter closes by discussing potential policy responses to reduce the production and consumption of these foods.

What are junk foods? Alternative definitions

Junk food is "a colloquial term for palatable but unwholesome food that is high in fat, salt, or sugar but deficient in protein, fiber, and vitamins" (Stedman, 2012). This definition emphasises that these food products are highly unhealthy but attract consumers because of their "hyper-palatable" nature. Segen (2012) offers specific examples: "Junk foods are often highly salted—e.g., potato chips/crisps, pretzels—high in refined carbohydrates (empty calories)—e.g., candy, soft drinks—and high in saturated fats—e.g., cake, chocolates." This demonstrates that junk foods are a heterogeneous group of food products and beverages characterised by a high degree of processing, palatability, ease and convenience of access, and the potentially adverse consequences to health associated with their frequent consumption (Bell, Kremer, Magarey, & Swinburn, 2005; Monteiro et al., 2013).

The term "junk food" is inherently colloquial. The metaphor "junk" traditionally only refers to the problematic health implications of these foods. However, as is argued throughout this chapter, the production and consumption of junk food also have significant environmental impacts.

In thinking about junk foods from both a health and sustainability perspective, it is necessary to consider the scientific nomenclature used in the medical and public health literature to describe food products of a similar nature. Table 13.1 offers a more nuanced perspective of how the term chosen to describe this class of products can have implications with respect to the actual products being considered, the way they relate to notions of health and sustainability, and the burden of responsibility placed on producers or consumers. Table 13.1 is also intended to serve as a reference to readers of this chapter, as junk food is interpreted in

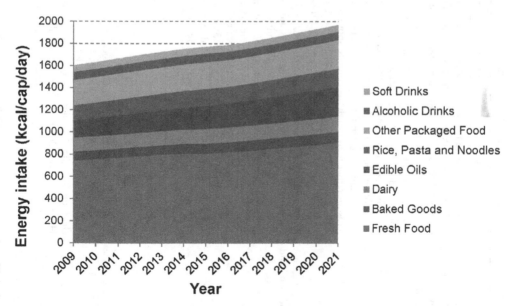

FIGURE 13.1 Average global caloric intake from processed and fresh foods
Note: The 2009–2016 period is based on actual data while 2017–2021 is based on a Euromonitor trend forecast. "Other Packaged Food" includes the following: breakfast cereals, confectionery, ice cream and frozen desserts, processed fruit and vegetables, processed meat and seafood, ready meals, sauces, dressings and condiments, soup, spreads, sweet biscuits, snack bars and fruit snacks.
Source: Based on data from Euromonitor (2018).

TABLE 13.1 Alternative overlapping definitions for junk food products

Term group	Definition and usage	Examples of food products	Sustainability relevance	Policy implications
Nutrition-related terms such as: "non-core" or "discretionary", or "energy-dense, nutrient poor" (EDNP)	Foods or beverages that do not belong to the core (nutritious) food groups and should only be consumed sometimes or in small amounts (Bell et al., 2005); these foods are also referred to as "other foods" or "extras", and are eaten for pleasure rather than health	Cakes and biscuits; confectionery and chocolate; pastries and pies; ice confections, butter, cream, and spreads high in saturated fats; processed meats and fattier/salty sausages; potato chips, crisps and other fatty or salty snack foods; sugar-sweetened soft drinks and cordials, sports and energy drinks and alcoholic drinks (Friel et al., 2014)	Non-core and discretionary are compatible with the notion of discretionary consumption used in economics in reference to purchased goods and services that are considered non-essential; EDNP foods are associated with poor sustainability performance in relation to their nutrient density (Drewnowski et al., 2015)	Terms such as "non-core" and "discretionary" imply consumer-oriented responsibility because they emphasise the notion of necessity and choice; EDNP is a more neutral term in this sense
Terms relating to the degree of processing: "processed" and "ultra-processed"	Processed foods are derived from unprocessed or minimally processed foods and industrially produced ready-to-eat or ready-to-heat food products resulting from the processing of several food substances; ultra-processed foods are a subgroup of processed foods that are ready-to-consume, mostly made from industrial ingredients and additives (Monteiro et al., 2019)	Burgers, frozen pasta, pizza and pasta dishes, nuggets and sticks, crisps, biscuits, confectionery, cereal bars, carbonated and other sugared drinks, and various snack products (Monteiro et al., 2013); these terms are often used interchangeably with "junk food"	The degree of processing implies additional environmental impacts (e.g. energy, packaging and transport) compared to fresh food choices (Friel et al., 2014; Friel et al., 2017); unlike the category above, more of these products can be meal replacements hence their consumption is not strictly discretionary	These terms are associated with producer-oriented responsibility; the high degree of processing and packaging puts emphasis on the production stage of the supply chain, where profitability incentives dominate
Terms relating to convenience aspect: "Convenience" or "ready-to-eat"	Food products that can save time and effort in preparation, consumption, or clean-up (Brunner, van der Horst, & Siegrist, 2010)	Packaged chips, canned vegetables, bread, commercialised fruit juices. salt, sugar, flour. Frozen meals/pre-packaged foods; not all products in this category are junk foods	Overlaps with the above as these foods are mostly processed and packaged and can often replace meals; their long shelf-life and large-scale production can create some environmental efficiencies	Imply more consumer-oriented responsibility as it emphasises the notion of ease and potential for time saving; associated with household production and convenience orientation framing (Schubert, Jennaway, & Johnson, 2010)

this chapter as encompassing dimensions from all three categories shown and the terms are used interchangeably depending on their incidence in the literature.

Global consumption trends of junk food: a cause for concern

Trends in junk food consumption are intrinsically linked to profound changes in global diets, characterised by both an increase in total caloric energy (the "expansion effect") and a shift in the composition of food consumed (the "substitution effect"); these two effects are illustrated in Figure 13.1. These changes are best described as a "nutrition transition" – a shift in dietary patterns and nutrient intakes as populations move from traditional diets to those associated with more modern and more "westernised" lifestyles (Kearney, 2010). This generally entails a shift away from traditional diets featuring predominantly staple cereals and starchy vegetables, towards those higher in animal products, caloric sweeteners and fat (especially from vegetable oils), with an increased share of ultra-processed food identified as a central feature of the transition (Monteiro et al., 2013; Baker & Friel, 2014; Tilman & Clark, 2014). A combination of drivers has been linked to these changes, including rising incomes, urbanisation, technological and labour market changes – all giving rise to changing tastes and attitudes with respect to food (Kearney, 2010).

Figure 13.1 depicts recent and near future trends in average global energy intakes from fresh and processed foods, highlighting a concurrent increase in fresh and processed foods, with processed foods already accounting for more than 1000 kcal/cap/day (equivalent to more than 50 per cent of total caloric intake). The energy share from edible oils, mostly comprised of vegetable oils, such as soybean and palm oil commonly found in junk foods (Lee, Koh, & Wilcove, 2016), appears to be growing at the highest rate over this period. These globally averaged trends show how calorie intake from different processed foods is increasing steadily alongside fresh foods. However, in reality, increases in unhealthy dietary patterns are outpacing increases in healthy patterns in most world regions (Imamura et al., 2015).

In recent years, the nutrition transition appears to be occurring at a faster rate, as evidenced in rapidly transitioning countries, such as China, Mexico, South Africa and Brazil (Kearney, 2010; Monteiro et al., 2013; Popkin, 2017). This is highlighted in Figure 13.2, especially in the case of lower middle-income countries (LMICs) where energy intake from processed foods (see Box 13.1) is forecast to reach 750 kcal/cap/day by 2021, compared to just over 500 kcal/cap/day in 2009. Stuckler et al. (2012) found that the growth in consumption of snacks and soft drinks accounts for a large part of the increase in LMICs. Upper middle-income countries (UMICs) are also experiencing a slower yet sustained energy increase from processed foods, forecast to reach around 1,150 kcal/cap/day by 2021, up from around 1,000 kcal/cap/day in 2009. This is in contrast to high-income countries where the already high energy intake from processed foods appears to be remaining constant at around 1,600–2,000 kcal/cap/day, depending on the region.

BOX 13.1 EUROMONITOR DATASET DETAILS

Processed food categories: alcoholic drinks; *baked goods; breakfast cereals; confectionery; dairy; edible oils; ice cream and frozen desserts; processed fruit and vegetables; processed meat and seafood; ready meals; rice, pasta and noodles; sauces, dressings and condiments; soup; spreads, sweet biscuits, snack bars and fruit snacks;* soft drinks

Categories in italic are foods classified as "packaged food" in Euromonitor (2018). Euromonitor countries are categorised as follows on the basis of World Bank country income classifications.

- *High-income countries*: Australia, Austria, Belgium, Canada, Chile, Czech Republic, Denmark, Finland, France, Germany, Greece, Hong Kong, Hungary, Ireland, Israel, Italy, Japan, Netherlands, New Zealand, Norway, Poland, Portugal, Saudi Arabia, Singapore, Slovakia, South Korea, Spain, Sweden, Switzerland, Taiwan, United Arab Emirates, the United Kingdom, the United States
- *Upper middle-income countries*: Argentina, Brazil, Bulgaria, China, Colombia, Malaysia, Mexico, Peru, Romania, Russia, South Africa, Thailand, Turkey, Venezuela
- *Lower middle-income countries*: Egypt, India, Indonesia, Morocco, the Philippines, Ukraine, Vietnam

Since most LMICs and UMICs are located in the Middle East, Africa and the Asia Pacific, home to the majority of the world's population, the trends shown in Figure 13.2 and also documented elsewhere (Baker & Friel, 2014; Popkin, 2017,) are concerning. While different regions have experienced the effects of the nutrition transition in different ways and at different rates, food cultures and associated consumption patterns have been permanently altered across the world (Kearney, 2010; Monteiro et al., 2013). As a result of these changes, and in combination with the attractive pricing of junk food products, lower socio-economic groups are increasingly acquiring much of their dietary energy from these foods (Hadjikakou, 2017; Popkin, 2017). This latter point is critical when considering equitable ways to reduce the production and consumption of these products in exchange for healthier alternatives.

How do junk foods relate to healthy and sustainable diets?

Health implications

Junk food consumption is an established risk factor for overweight/obesity and several diet-related non-communicable diseases (NCDs) (Basu, McKee, Galea, & Stuckler, 2013; Imamura et al., 2015). These adverse health impacts are a direct result of excessive consumption of sugar, fats, and salt, all of which are found in abundance in junk foods. High levels of processed food consumption correlates with obesity prevalence across countries of different income levels (Stuckler et al., 2012). Excess sugar consumption, particularly when a significant portion comes from sugar-sweetened beverages (SSBs), is linked to diabetes mellitus, even after controlling for body mass index (Basu et al., 2012). Increased consumption of saturated and trans-fatty acids, from animal fats and vegetable oils, and high levels of dietary sodium, much of it due to the high salt content of most processed foods, is associated with cardiovascular disease (Mozaffarian, Katan, Ascherio, Stampfer, & Willett, 2006). The consumption of processed meats, prevalent in junk food meals, is also associated with increased risk of colorectal cancer (Bouvard et al., 2015).

The long-term public health impacts arising from high levels of overweight/obesity are far-reaching and diverse: premature mortality, increased morbidity from NCDs, reduced

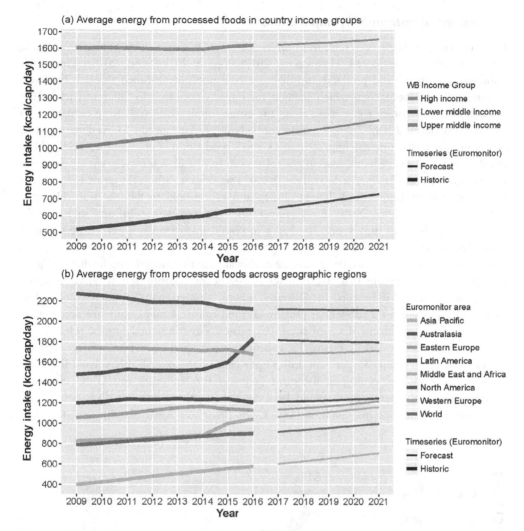

FIGURE 13.2 Trends in caloric energy from processed food consumption for (a) different World Bank country income groups, and (b) Euromonitor geographic areas.

Note: The 2009–2016 period is based on historical data while 2017–2021 is based on a Euromonitor trend forecast.

Source: Based on data from Euromonitor (2018) and World Bank (2018).

productivity at school and work and, ultimately, a reduced quality of life. By 2030, the combined medical costs resulting from the treatment of diet-related NCDs are projected to add to annual public healthcare costs by US$48–66 billion in the USA and £1.9–2 billion in the UK (Wang, McPherson, Marsh, Gortmaker, & Brown, 2011). Current trends in junk food consumption in many low- and middle-income countries are expected to contribute to similar public health impacts and associated costs, even as the incidence of obesity increases alongside persistent levels of undernutrition (Stuckler et al., 2012; Monteiro et al., 2013; Baker & Friel, 2014).

Environmental sustainability implications

While the negative impacts of junk food on health are well documented, the environmental impacts remain underexplored (Hadjikakou, 2017; Popkin, 2017; Scott, 2018). The environmental impacts of food products and diets are commonly determined through life cycle assessment (LCA) approaches, which account for impacts occurring in different parts of the production process, or, in some cases, along the entire supply chain (i.e., from farm-to-fork) (Poore & Nemecek, 2018). There is a growing body of product-specific LCAs demonstrating the significant environmental impact of junk food production. For example, studies have found that confectionery items, such as chocolate, can have a high life cycle energy footprint (Carlsson-Kanyama, Ekström, & Shanahan, 2003), a significant carbon footprint as a result of their milk content (Jungbluth & König, 2014), and strong links to deforestation (Higonet, Bellantonio, & Hurowitz, 2018). Land conversion associated with palm and soybean oils, both key ingredients of junk foods, has had a profound impact on tropical deforestation in recent decades (Lee et al., 2016).

Studies have recently considered the national-scale environmental implications of junk food production, showing that it can make a significant contribution to environmental impacts across several indicators. In Australia, where "discretionary" foods (as defined in Table 13.1) account for a substantial portion of total caloric intakes, they are accordingly responsible for a significant share of total diet-related environmental impact (Hendrie et al., 2016; Hadjikakou, 2017). Figure 13.3 shows how discretionary products account for 35 per cent, 39 per cent, 35 per cent and 33 per cent of the overall diet-related life cycle water use, energy use, ecological footprint (a proxy for land use) and GHG emissions respectively. Similar percentages would be expected in other countries with comparable food consumption patterns, such as the USA (Blair & Sobal, 2006) and the UK

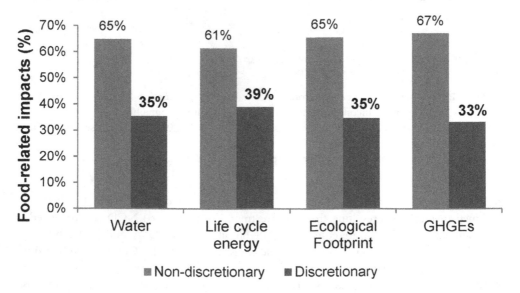

FIGURE 13.3 Contribution of discretionary products to total food-related environmental impact across four indicators for an average household in Australia

Source: Based on data from Hadjikakou (2017).

(Monteiro et al., 2018), although quantitative estimates of overall environmental impacts are lacking. Further research is needed on the environmental impacts associated with the significant degree of processing, refining, packaging, transportation, and refrigeration of junk foods, which can be expected to be high for many products.

While it is clear that junk food production may have significant environmental implications, we should consider this impact relative to that of healthier, less processed foods. Current imitations of LCAs (see Box 13.2) make such comparisons challenging; caution is therefore warranted when interpreting such results. To illustrate, while Carlsson-Kanyama et al. (2003) find significantly larger life cycle energy inputs for chocolate on a per portion basis compared to the majority of fruits, vegetables and grains, Hadjikakou (2017) finds that, when spending is shifted away from baked goods and confectionery towards fruit and/or vegetables, the environmental impacts could actually increase across indicators other than energy. This is true only if considering environmental intensity per dollar of food product, rather than per 100g. However, it has been strongly argued that food LCAs must also consider environmental intensity in relation to nutrient density (Drewnowski et al., 2015). It could be argued that junk foods, thanks to certain attributes such as large economies of scale, lower perishability and reduced time-cost of sourcing, preparing and consuming food, can deliver energy and certain macronutrients "efficiently" in a pure environmental sense. Nonetheless, their questionable contribution to nutrient adequacy must be factored into any meaningful sustainability assessment against fresh nutritious foods.

BOX 13.2 FOOD LCA CAVEATS

A detailed discussion of the methodological aspects of LCA is outside the scope of this chapter. However, two important shortcomings are worthy of note in the context of modelling shifts to healthier diets with less junk food. First, there is an enormous diversity in agricultural and industrial production systems and local environmental settings (Poore & Nemecek, 2018). The environmental implications of very similar food products can therefore differ widely, depending on the context and definition of environmental impact. Second, modelling the environmental impacts of hypothetical dietary changes, such as a shift towards diets lower in junk food, is highly complex because of the assumptions entailed in different units of comparison, inevitable product category-level aggregation, and the considerable uncertainty ranges in environmental intensities of individual products (Ridoutt, Hendrie, & Noakes, 2017).

More LCA studies to improve the evidence base on environmental impacts of diverse processed foods are certainly required. Nonetheless, focusing solely on quantifying and reducing the environmental impacts of mostly unhealthy products through increased efficiency and more sustainable sourcing strategies is problematic for a number of reasons. First, in a world where achieving food and nutrition security is an utmost priority, any food consumption beyond metabolic needs constitutes an unnecessary and potentially avoidable environmental burden – it is essentially a form of waste (Blair & Sobal, 2006). Second, the use of otherwise nutritious raw ingredients, such as potable water, meat, dairy, eggs and cereals to produce highly processed foods high in sugar, salt and fat, using processes that often entail considerable additional energy and packaging, should also be considered a suboptimal use of planetary resources. Less junk food would mean that, either more of these ingredients would be directly available for consumption in an unprocessed form, or that, alternatively, their production could be reduced in the absence of discretionary food demand, thus benefiting society and the environment (Hadjikakou, 2017). Third, over-emphasis on LCAs and incremental reductions in the environmental impacts of junk food risk further legitimising the emphasis placed by food corporations on sustainable sourcing as the main approach to framing food system sustainability (Scott, 2018). This could potentially detract from more fundamental questioning of the existence of such foods in the first place, leading to the maintenance of a status quo that emphasises profit maximisation over health and long-term food system sustainability (Hadjikakou & Wiedmann, 2017, Mason & Lang, 2017).

Measures to reduce the production and consumption of junk food

Junk food in the context of a healthy and sustainable food system

Despite the need for further research on the environmental intensities of different types of junk foods, it is clear that the production of these foods uses increasingly scarce planetary resources to produce unnecessary calories. When coupled with the overwhelming evidence of junk food's impact on an increased incidence of NCDs, and their strong association with corporate power (see Chapter 15), the expanding global production and consumption of junk food are antithetical to a healthy and sustainable food system. It follows that policy measures to curtail the consumption of junk food must therefore target the root causes of this consumption in the current food system model, namely, the dominance of a small number of large food corporations, the erosion of traditional food cultures and food environments, and the prioritisation of profit, convenience and artificial palatability over nutrition (IPES-Food, 2017). Previous attempts to tackle this issue have highlighted the systemic nature of the challenge and the need for a package of holistic interventions in combination with specific interventions that target different parts of the system, from production to consumption (Kearney, 2010; Poore & Nemecek, 2018).

The NOURISHING framework (Hawkes, Jewell, & Allen, 2013), aimed primarily at reducing overweight and obesity, emphasises the importance of combining policies to create lasting behavioural change, build a healthier food environment, and improve food supply chains. Terms such as "discretionary" and "non-core" highlight the importance of empowering consumers (see Table 13.1). National dietary guidelines have an important role to play, offering an appropriate medium to align health and sustainability objectives (Mason & Lang, 2017; Ritchie, Reay, & Higgins, 2018). However, any attempts to promote healthy and sustainable diets must not detract from the need to fundamentally transform food environments and food supply chains, as this could de-emphasise the responsibility of food businesses in policy responses.

Long-term shifts in consumer behaviour can only be sustained when complemented by positive changes in the food environment to ensure that healthy food options remain accessible and affordable relative to junk foods. This can be achieved through implementing a synergistic package of interventions including, for example, marketing restrictions on unhealthy foods and beverages, pricing interventions (as seen in the taxation of SSBs), nutrition labels and food composition requirements. Such measures are likely to be most effective when designed to shift behaviours across the population, as well as interventions to protect vulnerable groups (e.g. lower socio-economic segments and children) (Bell et al., 2005). Terms such as "processed" and "ultra-processed" (see Table 13.1) rightly place an important share of the responsibility on the food industry. More LCAs of products with a view to maximising supply chain efficiency may result in marginal environmental intensity improvements for individual food products but changes in industry practices must extend well beyond this (Scott, 2018). Actively engaging with the food industry and major investors in agri-food sectors not only to reformulate junk foods but also to ultimately "divest" away from them must be promoted as the more sustainable long-term business model (Hadjikakou, 2017).

Conclusion

This chapter has reviewed alternative definitions of junk food, explored current consumption trends and briefly considered evidence of its health and environmental impacts. It has argued strongly that the use of scarce environmental resources to create profitable but highly discretionary or ultra-processed products can no longer be justified in a world faced with the formidable challenge of ensuring sustainable food and nutrition security for growing populations. Junk food is therefore incompatible with the notion of a sustainable food system that does not prioritise short-term gains over long-term losses (Mason & Lang, 2017). For this reason, significant reductions in the production and consumption of junk food should be seen as highly complementary to mainstream food system health and sustainability agendas of tackling the overconsumption of meat and reducing food waste. To paraphrase Lee et al. (2016), it makes absolutely no sense to junk the planet for junk food.

References

Baker, P., & Friel, S. (2014). Processed foods and the nutrition transition: Evidence from Asia. *Obesity Reviews*, 15(7), 564–577.

Basu, S., McKee, M., Galea, G., & Stuckler, D. (2013). Relationship of soft drink consumption to global overweight, obesity, and diabetes: A cross-national analysis of 75 countries. *American Journal of Public Health*, March, e1–e7.

Basu, S., Stuckler, D., McKee, M., & Galea, G. (2012). Nutritional determinants of worldwide diabetes: An econometric study of food markets and diabetes prevalence in 173 countries. *Public Health Nutrition*, 13, 1–8.

Bell, A. C., Kremer, P. J., Magarey, A. M., & Swinburn, B. A. (2005). Contribution of 'noncore' foods and beverages to the energy intake and weight status of Australian children. *European Journal of Clinical Nutrition*, 59(5), 639–645.

Blair, D., & Sobal, J. (2006). Luxus consumption: Wasting food resources through overeating. *Agriculture and Human Values*, 23(1), 63–74.

Bouvard, V., Loomis, D., Guyton, K. Z., Grosse, Y., Ghissassi, F. E., Benbrahim-Tallaa, L., … Straif, K. (2015). Carcinogenicity of consumption of red and processed meat. *The Lancet Oncology*, 16(16), 1599–1600. doi:10.1016/S1470–2045(15)00444–00441.

Brunner, T. A., van der Horst, K., & Siegrist, M. (2010). Convenience food products: Drivers for consumption. *Appetite*, 55(3), 498–506.

Carlsson-Kanyama, A., Ekström, M. P., & Shanahan, H. (2003). Food and life cycle energy inputs: Consequences of diet and ways to increase efficiency. *Ecological Economics*, 44(2–3), 293–307.

Development Initiatives. (2017). Global nutrition report 2017: Nourishing the SDGs. Bristol: Development Initiatives.

Drewnowski, A., Rehm, C. D., Martin, A., Verger, E. O., Voinnesson, M., & Imbert, P. (2015). Energy and nutrient density of foods in relation to their carbon footprint. *The American Journal of Clinical Nutrition*, 101(1), 184–191. doi:10.3945/ajcn.114.092486.

Euromonitor. (2018). Nutrition: Energy from fresh and packaged food. Available at: www.portal.eurom onitor.com (accessed 30 May 2018).

Friel, S., Barosh, L. J., & Lawrence, M. (2014).Towards healthy and sustainable food consumption: An Australian case study. *Public Health Nutrition*, 17(5), 1156–1166.

Hadjikakou, M. (2017). Trimming the excess: Environmental impacts of discretionary food consumption in Australia. *Ecological Economics*, 131, 119–128.

Hadjikakou, M., & Wiedmann, T. (2017). Shortcomings of a growth-driven food system. In P. A. Victor, & B. Dolter (eds), *Handbook on growth and sustainability*. Cheltenham: Edward Elgar Publishing, pp. 256–276.

Hawkes, C., Jewell, J., & Allen, K. (2013). A food policy package for healthy diets and the prevention of obesity and diet-related non-communicable diseases: The NOURISHING framework. *Obesity Reviews*, 14(S2), 159 168.

Hendrie, G., Baird, D., Ridoutt, B., Hadjikakou, M., & Noakes, M. (2016). Overconsumption of energy and excessive discretionary food intake inflates dietary greenhouse gas emissions in Australia. *Nutrients*, 8(11), 690.

Higonet, E., Bellantonio, M., & Hurowitz, G. (2018). *Chocolate's dark secret: How the cocoa industry destroys national parks*. Washington, DC: Mighty Earth.

Imamura, F., Micha, R., Khatibzadeh, S., Fahimi, S., Shi, P., Powles, J., & Mozaffarian, D. (2015). Dietary quality among men and women in 187 countries in 1990 and 2010: A systematic assessment. *The Lancet Global Health*, 3(3), e132–e142.

IPES-Food. (2017). *Too big to feed: Exploring the impacts of mega-mergers, consolidation, concentration of power in the agri-food sector*. London: International Panel of Experts on Sustainable Food Systems.

Jungbluth, N., & König, A. (2014). Life cycle assessment of Swiss chocolate. Paper presented at SETAC Europe 24th Annual Meeting, 11–15 May 2014, Basel.

Kearney, J. (2010). Food consumption trends and drivers. *Philosophical Transactions of the Royal Society of London B: Biological Sciences*, 365(1554), 2793–2807.

Lee, J. S. H., Koh, L. P., & Wilcove, D. S. (2016). Junking tropical forests for junk food? *Frontiers in Ecology and the Environment*, 14(7), 355–356.

Mason, P., & Lang, T. (2017). *Sustainable diets: How ecological nutrition can transform consumption and the food system*. Abingdon: Routledge.

Monteiro, C. A., Cannon, G., Lawrence, M., Costa Louzada, M. L., & Pereira Machado, P. (2019). Ultra-processed foods, diet quality, and health using the NOVA classification system. Rome: FAO. Available at: www.fao.org/3/ca5644en/ca5644en.pdf

Monteiro, C. A., Moubarac, J. C., Cannon, G., Ng, S. W., & Popkin, B. (2013). Ultra-processed products are becoming dominant in the global food system. *Obesity Reviews*, 14, 21–28.

Monteiro, C. A., Moubarac, J.-C., Levy, R. B., Canella, D. S., Louzada, M. L. D. C., & Cannon, G. (2018). Household availability of ultra-processed foods and obesity in nineteen European countries. *Public Health Nutrition*, 21(1), 18–26.

Mozaffarian, D., Katan, M. B., Ascherio, A., Stampfer, M. J., & Willett, W. C. (2006). Trans fatty acids and cardiovascular disease. *New England Journal of Medicine*, 354(15), 1601–1613.

Poore, J., & Nemecek, T. (2018). Reducing food's environmental impacts through producers and consumers. *Science*, 360(6392), 987–992.

Popkin, B. M. (2017). Relationship between shifts in food system dynamics and acceleration of the global nutrition transition. *Nutrition Reviews*, 75(2), 73–82.

Ridoutt, B. G., Hendrie, G. A., & Noakes, M. (2017). Dietary strategies to reduce environmental impact: A critical review of the evidence base. *Advances in Nutrition: An International Review Journal*, 8(6), 933–946.

Ritchie, H., Reay, D. S., & Higgins, P. (2018). The impact of global dietary guidelines on climate change. *Global Environmental Change*, 49, 46–55.

Schubert, L., Jennaway, M., & Johnson, H. (2010). Explaining patterns of convenience food consumption. In G. Lawrence, K. Lyons, & T. Wallington (eds), *Food security, nutrition and sustainability*. London: Earthscan, pp. 130–144.

Scott, C. (2018). Sustainably sourced junk food? Big food and the challenge of sustainable diets. *Global Environmental Politics*, 18(2), 93–113.

Segen, J. (2012). *Segen's medical dictionary*. Huntingdon Valley: Farlex.

Stedman, T. L. (2012). *Stedman's medical dictionary for the health professions and nursing*. Philadelphia, PA: Wolters Kluwer Health/Lippincott Williams & Wilkins.

Stuckler, D., McKee, M., Ebrahim, S., & Basu, S. (2012). Manufacturing epidemics: The role of global producers in increased consumption of unhealthy commodities including processed foods, alcohol, and tobacco *PLOS Medicine*, 9(6), e1001235.

Tilman, D., & Clark, M. (2014). Global diets link environmental sustainability and human health *Nature*, 515(7528), 518–522.

van Dooren, C., Marinussen, M., Blonk, H., Aiking, H., & Vellinga, P. (2014). Exploring dietary guidelines based on ecological and nutritional values: A comparison of six dietary patterns *Food Policy*, 44, 36–46.

Wang, Y. C., McPherson, K., Marsh, T., Gortmaker, S. L., & Brown, M. (2011). Health and economic burden of the projected obesity trends in the USA and the UK. *The Lancet*, 378(9793), 815–825.

World Bank. (2018). *World development indicators: Data*. Washington, DC: World Bank. Available at: http://data.worldbank.org/indicator (accessed 30 May 2018).

14

FOOD WASTE

Liza Barbour and Julia McCartan

Introduction

The food system produces food for consumption, together with a number of outputs that are returned to the natural environment, including: greenhouse gas (GHG) emissions; packaging; and food waste, each of which contributes to environmental degradation (Friel, Barosh, & Lawrence, 2014). The United Nation's Sustainable Development Goals (SDGs) Target 12.3 calls to halve per capita global *food waste* at the retail and consumer levels and reduce *food losses* along production and supply chains by 2030 (UN, 2015). Food loss and food waste are defined by the Food and Agriculture Organization (FAO) as two distinct concepts. "Food loss" arises predominantly in the production and distribution stages of the food supply chain and is caused mainly by the functioning of the food production and supply system or its institutional and legal framework. Conversely, "food waste" refers to the removal from the food supply chain of food which is otherwise fit for consumption, by choice, or which has spoiled or expired, and is mainly a consequence of economic or social behaviour, poor stock management, or neglect (FAO, 2014). The key drivers of food waste and loss vary among low-, middle- and high-income countries (Papargyropoulou, Lozano, Steinberger, Wright, & Ujang, 2014). This chapter will focus on food wasted in high-income countries at the retail and consumption stages.

The extent of food waste globally

The world is currently experiencing unprecedented levels of food waste. The FAO estimates that, globally, 1.3 billion tonnes of food are wasted or lost every year, which is one-third of food produced for human consumption (Gustavsson, Cederberg, Sonesson, van Otterdijk, & Meybeck, 2011). This has consequences for global food security. There are 795 million people who are undernourished globally yet approximately one in every four food calories is wasted and is not consumed by humans (Searchinger, Hanson, Ranganathan, & Lipinski, 2014). It is estimated that 88 million tonnes of food waste are generated in the 28 European Union member states annually, equating to approximately 173 kilograms of food waste per person (Stenmarck, Jensen, Quested, & Moates, 2016).

Agricultural production, post-harvest handling and storage are responsible for 54 per cent of global food wastage while processing, distribution, retail and consumption contribute approximately 46 per cent to global wastage volumes (FAO, 2013). Figure 14.1 demonstrates the distribution of food waste at each stage of the food supply chain across the globe. The difference is most apparent at the consumption stage; with 31–39 per cent of food wastage occurring at this stage in high-income regions, compared with just 4–16 per cent in low-income regions (FAO, 2013). In Europe and North America, per capita food wasted at the consumer level is approximately 95–115 kilograms per year, while in South and Southeast Asia and Sub-Saharan Africa, this figure is much less, approximately 6–11 kilograms per year (Gustavsson et al., 2011). This suggests that in higher-income countries, households are responsible for the majority of food waste.

There are marked variations among food groups in their proportional contribution to food waste. Figure 14.2 illustrates the weight of avoidable, possibly avoidable and unavoidable household food and drink waste by food group generated in the UK each year. *Avoidable food waste* is food that could have been eaten at some point prior to being thrown away, *possibly avoidable food waste* is food that is eaten in some situations but not others (e.g. potato skins) and *unavoidable food waste* is food that is not, and has not been, edible under normal circumstances (e.g. eggshells or chicken bones) (Quested et al., 2011). Fresh vegetables and salads are responsible for the highest proportion of food waste (by weight) of all food groups (Quested et al., 2011).

Food waste and healthy and sustainable diets

There are four key associations between food waste and healthy and sustainable diets:

1. *Essential nutrients are lost as food waste* – Spiker, Hiza, Siddiqi and Neff (2017) demonstrate that nutritional deficits in the typical American diet correlate with nutrients lost when food goes to waste, in particular, fibre, calcium, magnesium, potassium and

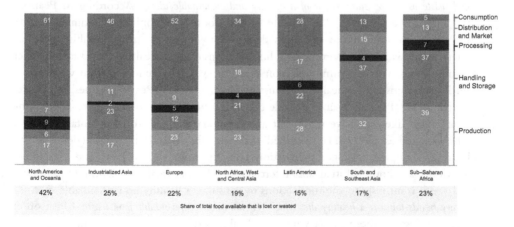

FIGURE 14.1 Food loss and waste across the food supply chain by region
Source: Lipinski, Clowes, Goodwin, & Hanson (2017), World Resources Institute analysis based on (Gustavsson et al., 2011).

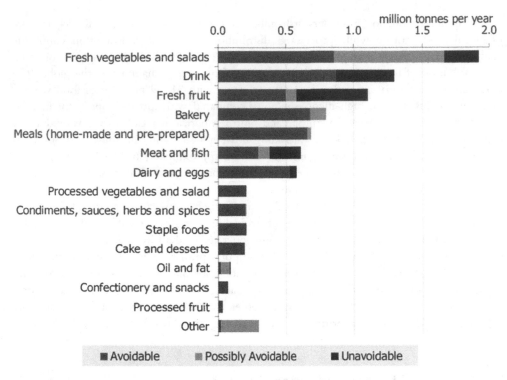

FIGURE 14.2 Weight of food and drink waste by food group in the UK
Source: Quested et al. (2011) and Quested and Johnson (2009).

vitamins A, C, D and E. In 2012, American women under-consumed dietary fibre by 8.9g per day and the daily amount of fibre lost via food waste is enough to fill this nutrition gap for as many as 1.3 million adult women. Other nutrients lost include calories (1,217kcal per capita per day) and protein (33g per capita per day).

2. *Food waste as a core characteristic of a healthy and sustainable diet* – According to Pearson, Friel and Lawrence (2014) "Behaviours around food provisioning, including reducing food waste are one of the principles described to ensure a strong, healthy and just society living within its environmental limits." Consuming a healthy and sustainable diet is synonymous with waste minimisation strategies, whereby reducing food waste is the fourth characteristic of a healthy and sustainable diet (Hoek, Pearson, James, Lawrence, & Friel, 2017). Pearson et al. (2014) describe how waste minimisation behaviour changes are most likely to have significant and immediate impacts on the sustainability of diets. Quested et al. (2011) identified that wasteful behaviour is embedded in the planning, shopping, storage, preparation and consumption of food and that these behaviours are both habitual and intertwined. The personal conviction to minimise food waste is intrinsic to the motivations to consume a healthy and sustainable diet.

3. *Dietary trends towards a healthy diet which generates more unavoidable food waste* – Pearson et al. (2014) describe the paradox whereby a healthy diet reliant on fresh fruit, vegetables, dairy and meat is contributing greater to food waste due to: (a) the generation of organic household waste; and (b) the fact that these food items are the most susceptible

to spoilage. See also Figure 14.2 which illustrates fresh vegetables and salads as generating the highest food waste by weight of all the food groups (Quested et al., 2011).

4. *Metabolic food waste through overconsumption* – Burlingame has referred to "metabolic food waste", a concept of food waste which she describes as the consumption of food in excess of nutritional requirements and which manifests as overweight and obesity (Institute of Medicine, 2014). This concept aligns with the first characteristic of a healthy and sustainable diet, as articulated by Friel et al. (2014) which recognises that excess food consumed above a person's nutritional requirements represents an avoidable environmental burden.

The economic costs of food waste

Food that is produced but then not consumed represents a wasted investment in agricultural production and consumer expenses. The economic cost of global food waste is estimated to be approximately US$936 billion per year (FAO, 2013). The annual cost of food waste has been estimated to be US$166–218 billion in the United States (Benson, Daniell, & Otten, 2017), 143 billion Euros in the EU 28 states (Stenmarck et al., 2016) and AU$30 billion in Australia (Australian Government, 2017). These figures do not account for the environmental impacts and wider social costs that influence health and livelihoods. The FAO full cost accounting framework predicts that global food waste costs US$2.6 trillion annually (US$1 trillion in economic costs, US$700 billion in environmental costs and US$900 billion in social costs) – roughly proportional to the gross domestic product of France (FAO, 2014).

The environmental consequences of food waste

Food loss and waste are responsible for approximately 8 per cent of global GHG emissions annually (FAO, 2015). With an annual global carbon footprint at 3.3 Gtonnes of CO_2 equivalent, if food waste were a country, it would rank third for GHG emissions, after China and the United States (FAO, 2013). Almost 28 per cent of the world's agricultural land area is used to produce food that is never eaten (FAO, 2013). The production of lost and wasted food accounts for approximately one-quarter of total freshwater use (Hall, Guo, Dore, & Chow, 2009). Wasted food is a major component of municipal landfills in high-income countries. In the United States, food waste decomposing in landfills accounts for 16 per cent of US methane emissions; a GHG with 25-fold global warming potential compared to carbon dioxide (Benson et al., 2017).

The drivers behind food waste

In low-income countries, upstream factors in the food supply chain are responsible for the majority of food loss and waste (FAO, 2013). Most food lost at the post-harvest and processing levels can be attributed to poor infrastructure for storage, processing and transport which leads to food spoilage (Chalak, Abou-Daher, Chaaban, & Abiad, 2016). In contrast, the drivers behind food waste in high-income countries tend to lie downstream, and largely relate to the retail and consumption stages. These are shaped by a series of political, economic, behavioural and sociocultural drivers.

Political and economic drivers

In an industrialised system, food is recognised as a commodity. The liberalisation of international trade has shaped the global food environment by increasing the total volume of food available for consumption (Friel et al., 2013). Evidence suggests that exposure to large food and drink portion sizes has become routine and is a key driver of excess energy intake (Livingstone & Pourshahidi, 2014). Additionally, advertising and price discounts have a major influence on food purchasing habits (Chandon & Wansink, 2012) and foods sold in smaller quantities are often higher in price per kilogram (Roodhuyzen, Luning, Fogliano, & Steenbekkers, 2017). These factors encourage consumers to purchase more food than originally intended or needed. This "push effect" is a contributor towards food waste, as consumers find it difficult at times to control their food intake due to the oversupply of readily available, relatively inexpensive and often aggressively marketed food (Hall et al., 2009).

In terms of food loss, the retail sector sets rigorous quality standards regarding the shape, size, weight and aesthetics of crops (Gustavsson et al., 2011). Retailers use these arbitrary standards to reject produce from the farm gate, meaning that some crops never reach the marketplace. An Australian study found that between 10–30 per cent of the north Queensland banana crop is discarded on-farm, equating to 37,000 tonnes per annum (White, Gallegos, & Hundloe, 2011). A waste audit revealed that 78 per cent of the discarded bananas were considered to be edible and were instead rejected for minor blemishes and other characteristics such as size and shape (White et al., 2011).

Behavioural and sociocultural drivers

Roodhuyzen et al. (2017) have categorised several behavioural factors which contribute to the generation of household food waste. These include practices relating to meal planning (e.g. not checking existing stock in the household), shopping practices (e.g. impulse buying and not sticking to a shopping list), storing practices (e.g. storing food for too long or in inappropriate packaging or under suboptimal temperatures), preparation and serving practices (e.g. preparing and serving large portions) and consumption practices (e.g. failure to consume leftovers). Personal factors, such as having the knowledge and skills to manage food appropriately, can also influence food waste behaviours and motivation to minimise food waste.

Sociocultural factors can also shape individual attitudes towards food waste. Reduced social and emotional linkages to food can reduce the perceived "value" of food and normalise food waste behaviours (Roodhuyzen et al., 2017). Other sociocultural factors include unpredictable lifestyles and limited time availability which can compromise one's ability to manage food. Consumers with busy schedules may opt to purchase takeaway meals instead of preparing meals from already bought ingredients. Such competing demands can lead to a series of trade-offs which influence an individual's motivation to prevent or minimise food waste (Van Geffen, van Herpen, & van Trijp, 2016).

Actions to reduce food waste

Papargyropoulou et al. (2014) have proposed *the food waste hierarchy* (Figure 14.3) to identify and prioritise the most appropriate options for the prevention and management of food waste.

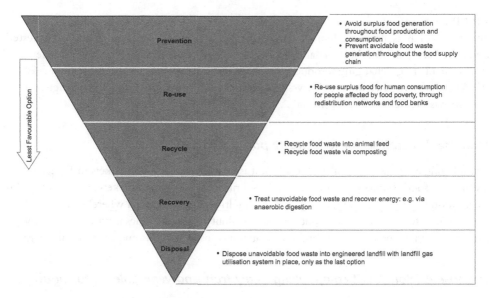

FIGURE 14.3 The food waste hierarchy
Source: Papargyropoulou et al. (2014).

As illustrated in Figure 14.3, the prevention of food waste (i.e. avoiding the production of surplus food and preventing avoidable food waste), is the most advantageous option within this food waste hierarchy. Despite this, an Australian investigation revealed that most food waste assessments relate to waste by consumers, with very little data on pre-farm gate or post-harvest losses (Mason, Boyle, Fyfe, Smith, & Cordell, 2011). Resources currently focus on the diversion of wasted food, rather than prevention, as demonstrated by these examples of responses from across the globe.

Response 1: Development of a National Food Waste Strategy (Australia and Canada)

There is an economic imperative for governments to address food waste. Mason and Lang (2017) suggest that reducing consumer food waste globally could save $300 billion annually, thereby supporting political interest in addressing the issue. Canada and Australia have invested in dedicated national food waste strategies that have the potential to prevent food waste. Canada's strategy is built on three pillars: policy change, innovation and behaviour change (National Zero Waste Council, 2017), which encourage donations to food charities through a tax incentive, improving "best before" and food expiry regulations and banning organic materials from entering landfills. Australia's strategy has four key areas: policy support, business improvements, market development and behaviour change (Australian Government, 2017).

Response 2: Waste and Resources Action Programme (United Kingdom)

WRAP (the Waste and Resources Action Programme) was established in 2000 to promote sustainable waste management and has evidentially reduced household food waste in the UK.

WRAP raises consumer awareness and modifies behaviours via the Love Food Hate Waste initiative which is now implemented in Australia, New Zealand and Canada (Quested, Ingle, & Parry, 2013). WRAP also works with the food industry to change the retail environment (e.g. changing products, packaging and labelling) (Quested et al., 2013). WRAP largely focuses on the "recycle" option in the food waste hierarchy (Figure 14.3) but also has elements of "prevention".

Response 3: Retail sector food waste policy (France)

Exemplifying a "re-use" action (Figure 14.3), it is now illegal for supermarkets in France to discard unused food (Barilla Center for Food & Nutrition, 2017). Supermarkets are encouraged to donate food to rescue organisations, as part of a multi-strategy approach whereby (1) schools are now required to teach students about food sustainability; (2) companies must report food waste statistics in environmental reports; and (3) restaurants must offer consumers take-home bags.

Response 4: Non-profit co-op selling "ugly fruit and vegetables" (Portugal)

A novel "preventative" approach (Figure 14.3) is Fruta Feia (ugly fruit), a non-profit co-op in Portugal which facilitates the purchase and sale of fruit and vegetables excluded from conventional food supply chains due to aesthetic standards. Ribeiro, Sobral, Peças, and Henriques (2017) analysed the economic, environmental and social impacts of this project and demonstrated the success and sustainability of this business model. Despite these benefits, this response has been criticised on the grounds that lower prices for "ugly" produce neglect the labour required to produce and harvest crops, and perpetuate a food system where food is undervalued (Turner, 2014).

Response 5: Food rescue and redistribution

Food rescue operations remain the predominant response to food waste where food destined to landfill is diverted to emergency food relief agencies who feed people experiencing hardship. This "re-use" approach (Figure 14.3) has also been widely criticised (McIntyre, Tougas, Rondeau, & Mah, 2016) as compromising moral and (in many countries) legal obligations to fulfil the Human Right to Adequate Food, it provides governments with a "band-aid" solution to the issue of food waste. On a positive note, food rescue agencies are more commonly adopting policies which encourage healthier food redistribution and the delivery of emergency food relief via more dignified, socially inclusive strategies (Ford, 2004; Campbell, Ross, & Webb, 2013).

In addition to the responses presented here, technological advances continue to stimulate innovative responses. For example, novel food packaging can lengthen shelf-life and minimise food spoilage when food is distributed and stored (Verghese, Lewis, Lockrey, & Williams, 2013), streamlined hospital-setting food service can minimise plate waste (e.g. hotel room-service-style menu selection) and web-based technology programs such as Yume can link food producers with wholesale redistribution channels.

Conclusion

Food waste significantly impacts the environment, and the ability of our growing population to consume a healthy and sustainable diet. Globally, 1.3 billion tonnes of food are wasted or lost every year, which equates to one-third of food produced for human consumption. Increasingly, governments and non-governmental organisations are investing in concerted and collaborative efforts to halve food waste by 2030, in line with the UN SDG's Target 12.3. The definition of food waste remains problematic in relation to quantifying and monitoring progress to reduce waste. At a household level, the adoption of waste minimisation strategies is intrinsic to the consumption of a healthy and sustainable diet. At a systems level, the prevention rather than diversion of food waste remains most advantageous.

References

Australian Government. (2017). National Food Waste Strategy: Halving Australia's food waste by 2030. Available at: www.environment.gov.au/system/files/resources/4683826b-5d9f-4e65-9344-a9000609 15b1/files/national-food-waste-strategy.pdf (accessed 14 September 2019).

Barilla Center for Food & Nutrition. (2017). Food Sustainability Index 2017. Available at: http://food sustainability.eiu.com/wp-content/uploads/sites/34/2016/09/FoodSustainabilityIndex2017GlobalEx ecutiveSummary.pdf (accessed 14 September 2019).

Benson, C., Daniell, W., & Otten, J. (2017). A qualitative study of United States food waste programs and activities at the state and local level. *Journal of Hunger & Environmental Nutrition*, 13(4),553–572. doi:10.1080/19320248.2017.1403408.

Campbell, E. C., Ross, M., & Webb, K. L. (2013). Improving the nutritional quality of emergency food: A study of food bank organizational culture, capacity, and practices. *Journal of Hunger & Environmental Nutrition*, 8(3), 261–280.

Chalak, A., Abou-Daher, C., Chaaban, J., & Abiad, M. G. (2016). The global economic and regulatory determinants of household food waste generation: A cross-country analysis. *Waste Management*, 48, 418–422.

Chandon, P., & Wansink, B. (2012). Does food marketing need to make us fat? A review and solutions. *Nutrition Reviews*, 70(10), 571–593.

FAO (Food and Agriculture Organization). (2013). Food wastage footprint impact on natural resources: Summary report. Available at: www.fao.org/docrep/018/i3347e/i3347e.pdf (accessed 20 May 2018).

FAO. (2014). Food wastage footprint full cost accounting: final report. Available at: www.fao.org/3/a -i3991e.pdf (accessed 14 September 2019).

FAO. (2015). Food wastage footprint and climate change. Available at: www.fao.org/3/a-bb144e.pdf (accessed 14 September 2019).

Ford, D. (2004). The Greater Boston Food Bank spotlights nutritious food distribution to the hungry as part of the U.S. fight against obesity.

Friel, S., Barosh, L. J., & Lawrence, M. (2014). Towards healthy and sustainable food consumption: An Australian case study. *Public Health Nutrition*, 17(5), 1156–1166.

Friel, S., Hattersley, L., Snowdon, W., Thow, A. M., Lobstein, T., Sanders, D., … Kelly, B. (2013). Monitoring the impacts of trade agreements on food environments. *Obesity Reviews*, 14, 120–134.

Gustavsson, J., Cederberg, C., Sonesson, U., van Otterdijk, R., & Meybeck, A. (2011). Global food losses and food waste: Extent, causes and prevention. Available at: www.fao.org/docrep/014/m b060e/mb060e00.pdf (accessed 14 September 2019).

Hall, K. D., Guo, J., Dore, M., & Chow, C. C. (2009). The progressive increase of food waste in America and its environmental impact. *PloS One*, 4(11), e7940.

Hoek, A., Pearson, D., James, S., Lawrence, M., & Friel, S. (2017). Shrinking the food-print: A qualitative study into consumer perceptions, experiences and attitudes towards healthy and environmentally friendly food behaviours. *Appetite*, 108, 117–131.

Institute of Medicine. (2014). *Sustainable diets: Food for healthy people and a healthy planet: Workshop summary*. Washington DC: The National Academies Press.

Lipinski, B., Clowes, A., Goodwin, L., & Hanson, C. (2017). SDG Target 12.3 on Food Loss and Waste: 2017 PROGRESS REPORT.

Livingstone, M. B. E., & Pourshahidi, L. K. (2014). Portion size and obesity. *Advances in Nutrition*, 5(6), 829–834.

Mason, L., Boyle, T., Fyfe, J., Smith, T., & Cordell, D. (2011). National food waste data assessment: Final report. Available at: www.environment.gov.au/system/files/resources/128a21f0-5f82-4a7d-b49c-ed0d2f6630c7/files/food-waste.pdf (accessed 14 September 2019).

Mason, P., & Lang, T. (2017). *Sustainable diets: How ecological nutrition can transform consumption and the food system*. New York: Routledge.

McIntyre, L., Tougas, D., Rondeau, K., & Mah, C. L. (2016). "In"-sights about food banks from a critical interpretive synthesis of the academic literature. *Agriculture and Human Values*, 33(4), 843–859.

National Zero Waste Council. (2017). National Food Waste Reduction Strategy. Available at: www.nzwc.ca/focus/food/national-food-waste-strategy/Documents/NFWRS-Strategy.pdf (accessed 14 September 2019).

Papargyropoulou, E., Lozano, R., Steinberger, J., Wright, N., & Ujang, Z. (2014). The food waste hierarchy as a framework for the management of food surplus and food waste. *Journal of Cleaner Production*, 76, 106–115. doi:10.1016/j.jclepro.2014.04.020.

Pearson, D., Friel, S., & Lawrence, M. (2014). Building environmentally sustainable food systems on informed citizen choices: Evidence from Australia. *Biological Agriculture & Horticulture*, 30(3), 183–197. doi:10.1080/01448765.2014.890542.

Quested, T., Ingle, R., & Parry, A. (2013). Household food and drink waste in the United Kingdom 2012. Available at: www.wrap.org.uk/sites/files/wrap/hhfdw-2012-main.pdf.pdf (accessed 14 September 2019).

Quested, T., & Johnson, H. (2009). Household food and drink waste in the UK. Available at: www.wrap.org.uk/sites/files/wrap/Household_food_and_drink_waste_in_the_UK_-_report.pdf (accessed 14 September 2019).

Quested, T., Parry, A., Easteal, S., & Swannell, R. (2011). Food and drink waste from households in the UK. *Nutrition Bulletin*, 36(4), 460–467. doi:10.1111/j.1467–3010.2011.01924.x.

Ribeiro, I., Sobral, P., Peças, P., & Henriques, E. (2017). A sustainable business model to fight food waste. *Journal of Cleaner Production*, 177, 262–275.

Roodhuyzen, D., Luning, P. A., Fogliano, V., & Steenbekkers, L. (2017). Putting together the puzzle of consumer food waste: Towards an integral perspective. *Trends in Food Science & Technology*, 68, 37–50.

Searchinger, T., Hanson, C., Ranganathan, J., & Lipinski, B. (2014). The Great Balancing Act. Working Paper, Installment 1 of Creating a Sustainable Food Future.

Spiker, M. L., Hiza, H. A. B., Siddiqi, S. M., & Neff, R. A. (2017). Wasted food, wasted nutrients: Nutrient loss from wasted food in the United States and comparison to gaps in dietary intake. *Journal of the Academy of Nutrition and Dietetics*, 117(7), 1031–1040.e1022. doi:10.1016/j.jand.2017.03.015.

Stenmarck, A., Jensen, C., Quested, T., & Moates, G. (2016). Estimates of European food waste levels. Available at: www.eu-fusions.org/phocadownload/Publications/Estimates%20of%20European%20food%20waste%20levels.pdf (accessed 14 September 2019).

Turner, B. (2014). Food waste, intimacy and compost: The stirrings of a new ecology. *Journal of Media Arts Culture*, 11(1), 1–11.

UN (United Nations). (2015). Sustainable Development Goals. Available at: https://sustainabledevelopment.un.org/sdgs

Van Geffen, L., van Herpen, E., & van Trijp, H. (2016). Causes and determinants of consumers' food waste: A theoretical framework.

Verghese, K., Lewis, H., Lockrey, S., & Williams, H. (2013). The role of packaging in minimising food waste in the supply chain of the future. Melbourne: RMIT University.

White, A., Gallegos, D., & Hundloe, T. (2011). The impact of fresh produce specifications on the Australian food and nutrition system: A case study of the north Queensland banana industry. *Public Health Nutrition*, 14(08), 1489–1495. doi:10.1017/s1368980010003046.

PART IV

Creating healthy and sustainable food systems: Politics, policy, people and practitioners

15

THE POLITICAL ECONOMY OF HEALTHY AND SUSTAINABLE FOOD SYSTEMS

Phillip Baker and Alessandro Demaio

Introduction

The food systems we inherit today are among the greatest of human achievements. Over the past century, we have witnessed massive increases in worldwide food production and steady declines in undernutrition and food insecurity. Paradoxically, we have never been more aware of the threats that unsustainable food systems pose for human and planetary health. Against a backdrop of rapid economic and social transition, many countries are now experiencing a double burden of undernutrition and overweight/obesity. Malnutrition in all its forms is today the leading contributor to the global burden of disease. At the same time, food systems are a leading driver of global environmental degradation, including deforestation and biodiversity loss, water scarcity and pollution, and climate change (Garnett, 2013: 23). As the world's population grows to 10 billion by 2050, becomes more affluent and urbanised, and increasingly consumes energy-dense and resource-intensive foods, these challenges will only become more pressing.

In recent decades, the idea of "sustainable food systems" – those that deliver "food security and nutrition for all in such a way that the economic, social and environmental bases to generate food security and nutrition for future generations are not compromised" (HLPE, 2014) – has jumped into the scientific and policy lexicon. Notably, in 2019, the EAT-Lancet Commission on Food, Planet and Health released its landmark report, "Food in the Anthropocene" (Willett et al., 2019), highlighting the threat that unsustainable food systems pose to human and planetary health. It defines safe operating boundaries for food production and consumption, sets out scientific targets to achieve healthy and sustainable food systems, and defines a universal reference diet that "meets nutritional requirements, within planetary boundaries to minimise damage to Earth's systems". It calls for a Great Food Transformation in order to sustainably nourish a projected world population of 10 billion people by 2050 (Willett et al., 2019). The message is clear: if we are committed to sustainable development, food systems cannot continue in their present form. We need transformative, even radical, change.

However, achieving food systems sustainability presents an immense political challenge of great complexity. It is a "wicked problem" involving many public and private stakeholders, often with competing interests, worldviews and beliefs. Globalisation has pushed many of the productive and regulatory activities relating to food systems outside of national jurisdictions, while the expanding scope of international trade rules has diminished the regulatory autonomy of governments to act within them. Neoliberal free market thinking has given rise to more market-orientated forms of food governance. With this has come an expansion in the size and reach of transnational food corporations, and the power they wield in relation to both state and non-state actors, globally and nationally.

In this chapter, this complexity is explored. The aim is to outline the web of political economy factors driving the unsustainable nature of today's food systems. *Political economy* in this regard means the interplay between political, economic and social forces in society, the distribution of power and resources between different individuals and groups within and surrounding food systems, and the processes that generate, sustain and transform these relationships over time (Corduneanu-Huci, Hamilton, & Ferrer, 2012). Although political economy factors do not directly cause unhealthy and unsustainable food systems, they significantly influence (i.e. drive change or retain the status quo) policy responses that can exacerbate or mitigate the problem and are therefore essential to investigate.

This chapter is divided into two sections First, food system actors are identified by considering who deploys and accrues power within food systems in relation to whom. Second, the concept of power is explored as it relates to food systems, as arguably the single most important variable to consider in political economy analysis. Understanding the complexity of sustainable food systems necessarily requires a trans-disciplinary approach (IPES-Food, 2015). Therefore, themes from the food policy and governance, public health, political science and regulatory studies literatures are engaged with. In doing so, a richer understanding is provided rather than drawing upon one disciplinary perspective alone.

Who exercises power in relation to whom within and surrounding food systems?

The starting point for understanding the political economy of food systems is to consider *who exercises power* and *in relation to whom*. Food systems typically comprise highly complex actor networks that evolve as food systems develop from traditional (more local/national and rural) to mixed and modern (i.e. more globally integrated and urban) over the course of a country's economic development. To understand who is within this scope we require a holistic conceptualisation of a food system encompassing both constitutive and political economy elements (IPES-Food, 2015). On this basis, food systems comprise a broad range of actors with the power to influence: (1) market transactions within food supply chains; (2) food environments and consumer behaviour; and (3) institutions, knowledge systems and regulatory frameworks that influence those systems (HLPE, 2017; IPES-Food, 2017). The political economy of healthy and sustainable food systems also encompasses a broad range of issues. Actors may contest or act collectively to address singular or multiple issues simultaneously including social (e.g. labour, fair trade, occupational health, nutrition, food security), environmental (e.g. biodiversity, pesticides, air pollution), consumer (e.g. information, choice, price), economic (e.g. food production, trade, marketing, subsidies, taxation) and cross-cutting (e.g. governance, integrated food policy) (IPES-Food, 2015; Mason & Lang, 2017).

Given this complexity, categorising food system actors into discrete types risks over-simplification. Others have used "actor triangle" models to categorise actors and understand relationships of policy contestation (Lang, 2006), and regulatory governance (Abbott & Snidal, 2009; Havinga, van Waarden, & Casey, 2015). The latter defines three main actor types – state, market and civil society – and four hybrid types comprising various combinations of the main types. These models adapted and have had added a multi-level conceptualisation, acknowledging that food actors may operate at or across different levels: transnational, national and sub-national. Figure 15.1 presents this as a "food actor pyramid". The term "state" refers to national and sub-national governments, and inter-governmental organisations. "Market actors" refers to private-interest for-profit organisations, including highly capitalised transnational corporations through to medium and small businesses operating at national and local levels. "Market" is used instead of "supply chain actors" to acknowledge the importance of firms operating outside of supply chains (e.g. financiers, consultancies). "Civil actors" are public interest, non-governmental organisations, social movements, research organisations and academics, communities and consumers. "Hybrid" actors are those with characteristics of more than one type, including multi-stakeholder and public private partnerships (MSPs/PPPs), and philanthropic organisations with private and public interests.

The pyramid represents the total space in which these actors contest food systems issues and/or act collectively to address them (Lang, 2006; Abbott & Snidal, 2009). It provides a framework for understanding relationships of power, i.e. state actors may exercise power in relation to state, market and civil actors; market actors in relation to market, state and civil, and so on (Table 15.1). The term "power imbalances" therefore refers to disproportionate relations of power between food actor types (e.g. government and market actors), within types (e.g. market actors at different segments in the supply chain), or between levels of actors (e.g. transnational corporations and national governments).

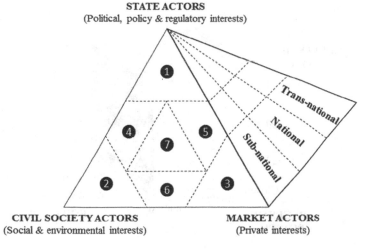

STATE ACTORS
(Political, policy & regulatory interests)

CIVIL SOCIETY ACTORS
(Social & environmental interests)

MARKET ACTORS
(Private interests)

FIGURE 15.1 Food actor pyramid model showing actor types
Source: Adapted from Abbott & Snidal (2009) and Lang (2005).

TABLE 15.1 Food actor types

Actor type	Examples
(1) State	Inter-governmental organisations, international financial and trade organisations; national and sub-national governments, including political leaders, parliamentarians, courts, government agencies and bureaucrats
(2) Market	Financiers, consultancies, standard setters, input suppliers, food producers, manufacturers, wholesalers, distributors, supermarkets, food service providers, advertisers, waste disposers
(3) Civil society	Public interest non-governmental organisations (e.g. labour, health, consumer, professional, environmental, religious), social movements (e.g. food sovereignty, farmers, local), communities, households and citizens
(4–7) Hybrid	(4) State-funded NGOs and service providers; state-funded research institutions and academics; (5) State-owned businesses; public-private partnerships involving state and market actors only; (6) Private interest non-governmental organisations (i.e. business associations and front groups), privately funded research institutions and academics, philanthropic organisations; (7) Multi-stakeholder and public-private partnerships involving all types

Where, at what levels and in what forms is power deployed and accrued within food systems?

Although useful, a broad description of food actors does not provide a complete understanding as to where and at what levels power manifests and in what forms it is deployed and accrued. Nor does it reveal how different dimensions of power have changed empirically (i.e. in terms of observable or indicative changes). This section achieves this by adapting and drawing upon Gaventa's three-dimensional Powercube model (Gaventa, 2006). This model, shown in Figure 15.2, is useful for understanding the interrelationships between different dimensions of power as it relates to complex food actor power relations. It depicts the levels (global, national, subnational), spaces (closed, invited, claimed), and forms (instrumental, structural, discursive) of

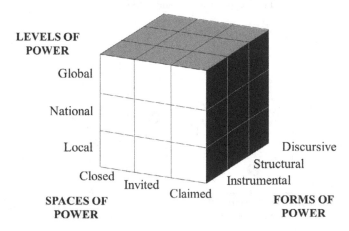

FIGURE 15.2 The Powercube model showing levels, spaces and forms of power
Source: Adapted from Gaventa (2006) .

power that food actors can deploy or draw upon. Each side of the cube represents a continuum rather than a static set of possible categories (Gaventa, 2006).

Levels of power: a shift upwards and downwards

The first dimension of the model is consistent with a 'multi-level' conceptualisation of food governance whereby power can manifest at a given level (i.e. horizontally) and/or across multiple levels (i.e. vertically) from the local to the global (Brons & Hospes, 2016). There is no doubt that in recent decades the loci of food systems power has shifted *upwards* from the national to the global level, underpinned by processes of globalisation.

Trade liberalisation has systematically reduced barriers to cross-border food trade and investment, binding governments to international trade laws and limiting the scope of regulatory options they have available to achieve domestic objectives (Baker, Kay, & Walls, 2014). The inclusion of agriculture in the General Agreement on Tariffs and Trade 1994, the establishment of the World Trade Organization (WTO) in 1995, and since then an explosion of regional and bilateral trade agreements have markedly widened the scope of global trade rules. These rules not only encompass barriers to cross-border commodity trade, but also food-related services, foreign investment, and intellectual property rights, among others (McMichael, 2009). In parallel, many countries have liberalised their economies unilaterally alongside the spread of neoliberal free-market thinking and economic policies emphasising market liberalisation, privatisation of state-owned enterprises, and market-orientated approaches to governance. At the same time, phenomenal growth in the financialisation of the global food economy has provided capital for accelerated food industry expansion (McMichael, 2009; Clapp, 2014).

These globalisation processes have helped facilitate an unprecedented increase in the number, size and reach of transnational food corporations (TFCs) and in turn the expansion of cross-border food production and supply chain networks (Clapp & Fuchs, 2009; IPES-Food, 2017). The expanded ability of TFCs to shift capital and locations of productive activities across borders has increased their power to influence government policy agendas, as states must increasingly compete to attract and retain the investments and jobs they provide. With this has come the expansion of global food marketing and advertising activities as TFCs enter new markets throughout the Global South, powerfully shaping beliefs about which foods are considered normal and socially desirable (Hawkes, 2006). Increasing distances between localities of production and consumption reduce the visibility of the social and environmental externalities of production processes and economic relationships in globalised supply chains, thereby rendering harmful production practices invisible to government regulators and consumers (Dauvergne, 2010; Clapp, 2014).

In this new context, the role of inter-governmental organisations in food governance remains prominent, if not more important than ever. This includes the policy-making and standard-setting roles of the specialised United Nations (UN) agencies, such as the Food and Agriculture Organization (FAO), the World Health Organization (WHO) and the UN Environmental Programme (UNEP). As largely normative and technical agencies, they operate from a weaker power base relative to the financial and rule-making power of the international development banks and the WTO. Nonetheless, the recent adoption of the Sustainable Development Goals (SDGs), the Paris Climate Change Accord and the Decade of Action on Nutrition present important UN-led frameworks for integrating action on sustainable food systems (IFPRI, 2017). The Codex Alimentarius Commission (Codex), the UN food-standard setting body, also plays a prominent role in standards areas, such as food labelling and food composition, as well as its risk analysis procedures and outcomes informing aspects of the arbitration of certain food trade disputes considered at the WTO. At the same time, and partly in response to weak state-led responses on sustainability, a multitude of new non-state actors have emerged (Mason & Lang, 2017). This includes new expert bodies (e.g. International Panel of Expert on Sustainable Food Systems), public-private partnerships (e.g. Scaling Up Nutrition), multi-stakeholder forums (e.g. EAT), and philanthropic foundations (e.g. Bill and Melinda Gates Foundation).

As power has shifted upwards away from national governments it has also shifted *downwards* to the sub-national level. In response to rapid urbanisation and decentralisation of authority underway in many countries, sub-national actors (especially municipal governments) are taking on more prominent roles in food governance. Increasing recognition of the important role of cities has led to the establishment of international (e.g. the Milan Food Policy Pact involving ~140 signatory cities) and national (e.g. the UK's Sustainable Food Cities) city networks to foster commitment, cooperation and learning. Many sub-national governments have established food policy councils as structures for multi-stakeholder engagement and have developed urban food policies targeting single or multiple sustainability issues (Hawkes & Halliday, 2017). As the world becomes more urbanised, and as mega-cities become new centres of economic and political power, this shift downwards will likely become increasingly important.

Spaces of power: closed, invited and claimed

As power has shifted upwards and downwards, it has also shifted *outwards* as non-state actors have come to play increasingly important roles in food governance. Here the Powercube concept of spaces can be engaged, the institutional channels and arenas in which food system actors interact, make decisions and take action. Power determines who participates and who does not in decision-making and sets boundaries for potential action (Gaventa, 2006). Invited spaces are inclusive, where actors can participate to inform decision-making, although the powerful may pre-determine agendas. Closed spaces are exclusionary, where the powerful make decisions behind closed doors. Spaces are claimed when actors capture existing or create newly autonomous arenas for engagement and action. Spaces can vary in issue focus, rules governing conduct (i.e. from informal norms to formalised laws), and so on. They may be institutionalised and ongoing (e.g. government bodies) or more transient and temporary (e.g. consultations, conferences), or represent spaces of material exchange in food supply chains. They can be interconnected and change dynamically, e.g. at any given stage of a policy process, spaces may be invited for some but closed to others.

The concept of invited spaces aligns closely with "participatory" and "reflexive" forms of governance viewed by many as crucial to fostering dialogue, learning and accountability among food actors, and to formulating integrated and adaptable policies that address the dynamic complexity of food systems challenges (Marsden, 2013; IPES-Food, 2015). Given this complexity and the breadth of issues relevant to healthy and sustainable food systems, there are many spaces of governance spanning many policy sectors, both public and private, from local to global levels. The institutional complexity and breadth of issues involved raise the challenge of "institutional ownership" of sustainable food systems, whereby it can become the "responsibility of all but the mandate of none". In this regard, strengthening capacities and creating institutional spaces for cross-sectoral coordination and dialogue underpin *policy coherence* – achieving food systems' sustainability's objectives through synergistic actions across sectors (horizontal coherence) and levels (vertical coherence) of governance, while ensuring actions in one sector do not undermine those in others (Hawkes, 2015).

A diversity of state-anchored institutional designs have emerged at global, national and sub-national levels as invited spaces for sustainable food governance. For example, the Committee on World Food Security is the world's foremost inclusive intergovernmental and multi-stakeholder platform for coordinating food security and nutrition actions. At national and (mostly) sub-national levels, food policy councils have emerged since the early 1980s to convene actors and coordinate action. These range from addressing singular (e.g. food security, nutrition) to more integrated and multi-issue approaches (Hawkes & Halliday, 2017). At the national level, some countries have developed inclusive state-anchored governance models. Brazil's National System of Food Security and Nutrition is an example of a multi-sectoral/multi-level institutional framework of this nature. In this system, the National Council on Food and Nutrition Security (CONSEA), and similar councils established sub-nationally, convene stakeholders and formulate/monitor policy. Civil society provides direct input through a range of legal, institutional and informal mechanisms, thereby improving accountability and responsiveness. Enabling legislation mandates national whole-of-government cooperation. This has underpinned Brazil's success in driving down malnutrition rates in the context of strong social policy reform and economic growth (Meija-Costa & Fanzo, 2012).

In many (mostly high-income) countries, and globally, public-private and multi-stakeholder partnerships (MSP) have emerged as new spaces since the early 2000s, as governments have adopted preferences for more market-orientated approaches to governance (Clapp & Scrinis, 2017). For example, Scaling Up Nutrition is an MSP involving the UN, donor, civil society and business networks operating across 60 countries. Another is the UN Global Compact as the world's largest corporate social responsibility (CSR) initiative involving more than 8,000 corporate entities across 170 countries, including many of the world's largest food companies. At the national level, Australia's Healthy Food Partnership and the UK's Public Health Responsibility Deal are examples of PPPs to address unhealthy diets. As governance models, some of these have given rise to concerns, including conflicts between private and public interests, lack of transparency and public accountability, power asymmetries between corporate and civil actors in decision-making and their focus on 'nutrient-centric' approaches to nutrition (see Chapter 6 by Scrinis in this volume). The participation of corporate actors in policy decision-making may at the same time "depoliticise" food problems by enrolling others in negotiations, resulting in compromise and weaker outcomes (e.g. voluntary rather than mandatory regulation) (Clapp & Scrinis, 2017).

Businesses have also increasingly claimed new spaces by establishing private consortia and multi-stakeholder alliances to set private sustainability standards, often in unison with civil society groups and completely outside of government involvement, e.g. the Roundtable on Sustainable Palm Oil. The entry of food industry groups into global food and nutrition policy fora and regulatory bodies is another example of claiming (or attempts at claiming) invited spaces. For example, the Second International Conference on Nutrition was attended by over 90 private sector representatives who participated in industry-sponsored side-events and provided input into the final outcome documents (Clapp & Scrinis, 2017). Codex is another space where food industry representatives have comprised large proportions of member country delegations. As governments have reduced social safety nets, and in many cases failed to address sustainability challenges, civil society organisations have also claimed new spaces by taking on regulatory and service-delivery functions usually performed by governments. These include, for example, initiatives on sustainable fisheries (e.g. the Marine Stewardship Council), trade (e.g. Fair Trade), and food banks as a response to food insecurity in urban localities (Clapp & Fuchs, 2009; Mason & Lang, 2017). Strongly grounded in the principles of food sovereignty and democracy, food movements in many countries have also developed "alternative" institutional spaces and policies for governing healthy and sustainable food systems, e.g. establishing "people's" food policies in the UK and Australia.

Forms of power

The third dimension of the Powercube refers to the forms of power that actors exercise within and across levels and spaces. Here, instrumental, structural and discursive concepts of power are adopted, given their comprehensive theoretical development and application in the food and political science literatures. Drawing on political science theories on power, Doris Fuchs and Jennifer Clapp have developed and applied a framework that extensively conceptualises these three interacting forms of power. Although they apply this framework to the study of the growing power of agri-food businesses in food governance worldwide, it provides a useful lens through which to understand the power of other actor types and power relations between actors across levels and spaces. This is a different conceptualisation to the visible, hidden and invisible forms of power in Gaventa's original Powercube model.

Instrumental power refers to the direct influence of one actor over another to affect decision-making and outcomes (Clapp & Fuchs, 2009). This includes, for example, having access to decision-makers (e.g. through lobbying, or shared social networks), and possessing material resources (e.g. financial, organisational, human) and intrinsic capacities (e.g. leadership, strategic skills) to influence others. Much of the food politics literature refers to the instrumental power of 'Big Food' in undermining political commitment for action and shaping food and nutrition policies through corporate lobbying activities. This includes forming cohesive international lobby groups, directly engaging with political decision-makers, making political donations, financing large-scale media campaigns to influence public opinion, and financing research to skew scientific evidence in favour of corporate interests (IPES-Food, 2015; Clapp & Scrinis, 2017). Participation in MSPs further expands the instrumental power of industry by facilitating direct input into the policy processes (Clapp & Scrinis, 2017).

Structural power is a more diffuse form that manifests through the imposition of limits on the range of choices available to others (Clapp & Fuchs, 2009). It manifests through, for example, the establishment of formal processes and institutional structures (e.g. laws, regulations), the shaping of informal norms and decision-making biases within policy-making institutions (i.e. which beliefs and practices are considered (un)acceptable), and through commanding a structurally important position within a given organisational process or economic arrangement. This form of power shapes both the decisions of actors but also their "non-decisions" by implicitly selecting alternative courses of action and pre-defining preferences before any actual or visible decision-making process begins.

An obvious example of structural power is the growth in the number and diversity of private standards and self-regulatory schemes initiated by corporate actors in recent decades.

These have overlain and, in many instances, supplanted government regulation across a diversity of sustainability issues (e.g. sustainable sourcing, human rights, nutrition). Private standards have emerged for several reasons. This includes the need for TFCs to coordinate more complex and globally integrated supply chains (e.g. through imposing supplier standards), to respond to increasing pressure from civil society and regulators, to delay the adoption of state regulation, and to achieve competitive advantages (e.g. as forms of product differentiation) (Henson & Reardon, 2005; Challies, 2013). At the same time, many governments have, as a reflection of neoliberal free-market thinking, adopted "cutting red-tape" agendas that act as an institutionalised deterrent to new state regulation.

Another example of structural power is the increasing size and economic importance of food corporations in global and national economies (IPES-Food, 2017). 'Big Food', as providers of jobs, investments and tax revenues, can command substantial bargaining power with governments. This can result in policy concessions that serve corporate interests while enabling and reinforcing an industrial food systems paradigm (IPES-Food, 2017). Economic globalisation expands this power by making it easier to shift investments and productive activities across borders, meaning governments must compete to attract and retain TFC investments. Governments may even make policy concessions voluntarily without corporations expressing their preferences in the first place. Market concentration, which has increased markedly at the global and national levels since the 1980s, further expands this form of power. This is when market share increasingly consolidates in the hands of a declining number of firms operating within and across segments of the food supply chain, largely through company mergers and acquisitions. Market power readily converts into political power as firms leverage their expanding structural importance to influence policy decision-making, which in turn creates a favourable environment for ongoing consolidation (IPES-Food, 2017).

The third form, *discursive power*, is the power to shape underlying values, belief-systems (i.e. ideologies) and social norms, and the surface-level "frames" through which food problems are interpreted and communicated (Clapp & Fuchs, 2009). This more hidden form of power precedes and surrounds decision-making and non-decision-making processes. It is the power to socialise others into accepting "truths" about a given problem and what problem interpretations and solutions are considered normal, acceptable and desirable. For example, the terms "discretionary" and "ultra-processed" as descriptors imply different forms of responsibility for making "junk food" choices – the former emphasises consumer responsibility, the latter industry culpability (see Chapter 13). Actors can exercise discursive power through, for example, media engagement, public relations efforts and advertising. It can manifest further through shaping deeper values, beliefs and norms within political systems, policy-making institutions and in society-at-large, e.g. the neoliberal belief in an expanded role for markets in governance, and the view that government should have no or a minimal role in regulating free enterprise. Discursive power also underpins collective action – those who can agree on a common interpretation of a given problem (i.e. internal frame coherence) are more likely to mobilise supporters, counter opposition and influence decision-makers (Baker et al., 2018).

Achieving frame coherence is not easy, given the complexity of sustainable food systems, and the many ways in which different actors can frame, contest or act collectively to address a broad range of singular or integrated issues. Defining sustainability, which issues should be prioritised (or ignored), and what trade-offs between issues are (un)desirable is, in this way, deeply political. Some view sustainability as a "non-problem", as overly complex or too costly to deal with; as the responsibility of individuals alone, or as a lesser priority relative to other objectives (e.g. hunger reduction) (Mason & Lang, 2017). A prominent "productivist" view is that producing more food more efficiently to feed a rapidly growing population should be the primary (and potentially only) objective. Some focus on shaping consumer demand through information provision (e.g. labelling) or by using below-the-radar approaches focused on choice-editing or nudging. Others advocate for multi-issue and integrated approaches that mainstream sustainability into multiple policy areas, including dietary guidelines (Garnett, 2013; Mason & Lang, 2017). A final view is that sustainability problems arise because of the unequal balance of power between different food system actors, requiring stronger state-anchored and participatory models of governance (Garnett, 2013).

Whose interpretations predominate and whose do not, within and across difference levels and spaces, is ultimately a reflection of power, including the capacity to couple discursive with instrumental and structural forms (Clapp & Fuchs, 2009). For example, corporate actors can draw upon their monetary resources and public relations networks (i.e. instrumental power) to exercise discursive power within and across numerous spaces at global and national levels, influencing the interpretation and framing of issues within and across several policy discourses simultaneously. Private standards and self-regulatory schemes (i.e. structural power) within broader CSR programmes can portray corporations as "good corporate citizens", legitimising their role in food governance and the belief that self-regulation is more efficient and effective than state intervention (Challies, 2013). Discursive power also manifests in the productive and marketing activities of the food companies themselves. The development and extensive advertising of "fortified, functionalised and reformulated" foods is a direct response to rising concerns regarding the health impacts of industrial food. The appropriation of alternative food movement discourses through, for example, organic, Fair Trade or animal welfare-compliant product offerings, is another example of the adaptive capacity of TFCs to exercise discursive power (Clapp & Scrinis, 2017).

Moving forward

The EAT-Lancet Commission has established scientific targets for healthy and sustainable food systems, and sets out a cogent set of policy actions for achieving the ambition of a Great Food Transformation in the twenty-first century (Willett et al., 2019). This chapter has taken the position that this will require the active pursuit of new food systems' political economies, in short, the reconfiguration of food systems power relations. On this point, the Lancet Obesity Commission report, released almost in parallel to the EAT-Lancet report, brings *the* central political economy challenge into focus – the need to redefine the fundamental goals of the system (Swinburn et al., 2019). The practices, structures and ideological frameworks that underpin capitalism in its present form (i.e. neoliberal, extractive, materialist) entrench a set of political economy drivers that prioritises never-ending growth – and hence consumption – as the primary objective. Environmental, social and economic harms are considered problems to be managed, rather than integrated as core system goals. Policy actions that simply tweak the minor parameters of this system (e.g. consumer information initiatives, industry-led responses, etc.) will do little to address these deeper political economy drivers.

Conclusion

A number of important changes in food actor configurations and power relations have occurred in recent decades, with important implications for healthy and sustainable food systems. Power has shifted in three directions. First, *upwards* as globalisation has given rise to more complex and globally integrated food systems governed increasingly by transnational food corporations and international organisations. To what extent are international forms of public and private regulation effective in addressing food systems sustainability challenges? In this new context, how can governments protect their domestic policy space to achieve food systems' sustainability? Second, power has shifted *downwards* as urbanisation and decentralisation of authority in many countries give cities and sub-national actors a more prominent role in food governance. What governance mechanisms are available (and needed) to achieve healthy and sustainable food systems at this level? What can be done to bolster the commitments and capacities of sub-national governments in devolved contexts? Third, power has shifted *outwards* with a greater role for market and civil society (i.e. private) actors, with an expansion in food industry power and increasing preferences for more market-orientated and decentralised forms of governance. The expansion in the geographical scale and complexity of food systems, in the power of food companies relative to nation states, and in the international rules governing national food economies has diminished the power of governments to influence food system activities, both within and beyond their territorial borders. What can be done to preserve and expand the power of national governments and non-corporate food system actors in this new context? The answers to these questions can, in part, be found in the following chapters in Part IV. In particular, the complexities outlined and the challenges identified in this chapter can begin to be acted on by focusing on:

- policy (Chapter 16)
- people's food-related practices (Chapter 17)
- practitioners' advocacy (Chapter 18).

References

Abbott, K. W., & Snidal, D. (2009). The governance triangle: Regulatory standards institutions and the shadow of the state . In *The politics of global regulation*. Princeton, NJ: Princeton University Press, pp. 44–88.

Baker, P., Hawkes, C., Wingrove, K., Demaio, A. R., Parkhurst, J., Thow, A. M., & Walls, H. (2018). What drives political commitment for nutrition? A review and framework synthesis to inform the United Nations Decade of Action on Nutrition. *BMJ Global Health*, 3(1), e000485.

Baker, P., Kay, A., & Walls, H. (2014). Trade and investment liberalization and Asia's noncommunicable disease epidemic: A synthesis of data and existing literature. *Globalization and Health*, 10(1), 66.

Brons, A., & Hospes, O. (2016). Food system governance: A systematic literature review. In A. Kennedy, & J. Liljeblad (eds), *Food systems governance*. New York: Routledge, pp. 13–42.

Challies, E. (2013). The limits to voluntary private social standards in global agri-food system governance. *International Journal of Sociology of Agriculture & Food*, 20(2), 175–195.

Clapp, J. (2014). Financialization, distance and global food politics. *Journal of Peasant Studies*, 41(5), 797–814.

Clapp, J., & Fuchs, D. A. (2009). *Corporate power in global agrifood governance*. Cambridge, MA: MIT Press.

Clapp, J., & Scrinis, G. (2017). Big Food, nutritionism, and corporate power. *Globalizations*, 14(4), 578–595.

Corduneanu-Huci, C., Hamilton, A., & Ferrer, I. M. (2012). *Understanding policy change: How to apply political economy concepts in practice*: Washington, DC: World Bank Publications.

Dauvergne, P. (2010). *The shadows of consumption: Consequences for the global environment*. Cambridge, MA: MIT Press.

Garnett, T. (2013). Food sustainability: Problems, perspectives and solutions. *Proceedings of the Nutrition Society*, 72(1), 29–39.

Gaventa, J. (2006). Finding the spaces for change: A power analysis. *IDS Bulletin*, 37(6), 23–33.

Havinga, T., van Waarden, F., & Casey, D. (2015). Conceptualizing regulatory arrangements: Complex networks and regulatory roles. In T. Havinga, F. van Waarden, & D. Casey (eds), *The changing landscape of food governance: Public and private encounters*. Cheltenham: Edward Elgar, pp. 19–36.

Hawkes, C. (2006). Uneven dietary development: Linking the policies and processes of globalization with the nutrition transition, obesity and diet-related chronic diseases. *Globalization and Health*, 2(1), 4.

Hawkes, C. (2015). *Enhancing coherence between trade policy and nutrition action*. Rome: United Nations Standing Committee on Nutrition.

Hawkes, C., & Halliday, J. (2017). *What makes urban food policy happen? Insights from five case studies*. London: International Panel of Experts on Sustainable Food Systems.

Henson, S., & Reardon, T. (2005). Private agri-food standards: Implications for food policy and the agri-food system. *Food Policy*, 30(3), 241–253.

HLPE (High Level Panel of Experts). (2014). Food losses and waste in the context of sustainable food systems: A report by the High Level Panel of Experts on Food Security and Nutrition of the Committee on World Food Security. Rome: Committee on World Food Security. Available at: www.fao.org/3/a-i3901e.pdf

HLPE. (2017). Nutrition and food systems: A report by the High Level Panel of Experts on Food Security and Nutrition of the Committee on World Food Security. Rome: Committee on World Food Security.

IFPRI (International Food Policy Research Institute). (2017). Global nutrition report 2017: Nourishing the SDGs. Washington, DC: International Food Policy Research Institute (IFPRI).

IPES-Food. (2015). The new science of sustainable food systems: Overcoming barriers to food systems reform. London: International Panel of Experts on Sustainable Food Systems.

IPES-Food. (2017). Too big to feed: Exploring the impacts of mega-mergers, consolidation and concentration of power in the agri-food sector. London: International Panel of Experts on Sustainable Food Systems.

Lang, T. (2005). Food control or food democracy? Re-engaging nutrition with society and the environment. *Public Health Nutrition*, 8(6), 730–737.

Lang, T. (2006). Food, the law and public health: Three models of the relationship. *Public Health*, 120, 30–40.

Marsden, T. (2013). From post-productionism to reflexive governance: Contested transitions in securing more sustainable food futures. *Journal of Rural Studies*, 29, 123–134.

Mason, P., & Lang, T. (2017). *Sustainable diets: How ecological nutrition can transform consumption and the food system*. London: Routledge.

McMichael, P. (2009). A food regime genealogy. *The Journal of Peasant Studies*, 36(1), 139–169.

Meija-Costa, A., & Fanzo, J. (2012). *Fighting maternal and child malnutrition: Analysing the political and institutional determinants of delivering a national multisectoral response in six countries*. Brighton: Institute of Development Studies.

Swinburn, B. A., Kraak, V. I., Allender, S., Atkins, V. J., Baker, P. I., Bogard, J. R., … Dietz, W. H. (2019). The global syndemic of obesity, undernutrition, and climate change: The Lancet Commission report. *The Lancet*. doi:10.1016/S0140–6736(18)32822–32828.

Willett, W., Rockström, J., Loken, B., Springmann, M., Lang, T., Vermeulen, S., … Wood, A. (2019). Food in the Anthropocene: The EAT-Lancet Commission on healthy diets from sustainable food systems. *The Lancet*, 393(10170), 447–492.

16

POLICY TO PROMOTE HEALTHY AND SUSTAINABLE FOOD SYSTEMS

Tim Lang

Introduction

It is widely accepted across diverse disciplines that the food system is in trouble. On the one hand, never has there been so much food. This has been the success of the post-Second World War "productionist" policy and its priority to produce more food. And yet, on the other hand, serious problems threaten its future if current practices and trends remain (Lang & Heasman, 2015) There is too much food, gross societal dietary inequalities, extensive systematic waste and damage to ecosystems on which food production relies. Whereas in the first half of the twentieth century, it was reasonable to argue there was a need for more food, by the end of that century, a toxic combination of malnutrition, undernutrition and overconsumption had emerged globally, hunger alongside obesity even within low-income societies. For those viewing food from a public health perspective, it meant having to consider a new feature: systemic environmental damage with regard to biodiversity, water use, soil health and climate change due in part to how food is produced. Methods of farming, processing, retailing and even cooking became part of the discourse linking public health to environmental and society. For policy-makers, this meant a new reality of multiple and systemic problems across the food system. New problems replaced the old pattern of the early twentieth century. Obesity alongside hunger. Climate change alongside soil erosion. Food waste at the farm alongside food waste by consumers. All this having different manifestations in different parts of the world. Facing the conflict between food evidence and food reality sits at the heart of the policy challenges charted in this book. This chapter explores whether we now have what we can call a "policy lock-in", in which the wrong policies exacerbate rather than resolve problems.

Evidence-policy reality gap

A short summary of the state of evidence to support policy for healthy and sustainable food systems might present a catalogue such as this:

- Agriculture and food systems are major sources of environmental damage threatening planetary health (UNEP et al., 2009). Food systems help undermine planetary dynamics (Rockström et al., 2009). Food systems are major drivers of biodiversity loss (WWF & Zoological Society of London, 2015), and water use (Rockström et al., 2014).
- Agriculture alone contributes 14 per cent to global greenhouse gas (GHG) emissions (Stern, 2006; HLPE, 2012). In rich societies, food accounts for a third of average consumer GHG emissions (Tukker et al., 2006; Tukker et al., 2011).
- Meanwhile, consumption patterns have changed and become more complex. Dietary factors are major factors in premature deaths from non-communicable diseases (NCDs) (WHO, 2015), surpassing hunger, which also remains stubbornly high (FAO, IFAD, UNICEF, WFP, & WHO, 2018).
- Agriculture and food sectors are the biggest employers on the planet yet are characterised by low (and sometimes no) wages and difficult working conditions (International Labour Organisation, 2018).
- An avalanche of new food products flows at consumers, intended to add economic rather than nutritional value and to compete in over-supplied markets; around 20,000 new food products a year come on to the US market (USDA ERS, 2017), and giant food transnationals increase market share, wielding unprecedented power. Advertising messages are shaped for sales not health (PLoS Medicine Editors, 2012).
- Globally, an estimated third of all food produced is wasted, with rich society consumers wasting post purchase, while in low-income countries food is wasted nearer production, often due to inadequate storage and infrastructure (FAO, 2011; Institute of Mechanical Engineers, 2013).

It was no longer possible for policy-makers to support "business-as-usual" while claiming that their policies were evidence-based. The evidence called for new policies. Table 16.1 lists some major reports on the global food system recommending system-wide change. The point is that there is no shortage of such policy advice to decision-makers. Their reluctance to accept that systemic change is needed has to be faced. It is not for lack of evidence.

The data now question not just the grossly unfair mal-allocation of food by supposedly efficient markets but how food is produced, processed and consumed. Policy attention surely thus needs to focus on what happens to food after it leaves the land and yet this has been hard to win, despite it being obvious that late twentieth-century capitalism has created highly complex and long supply chains with multiple actors having little to do with farming, yet using it. Thirty years ago, development analysts argued that this "food systems" critique came from analysts in rich societies, and that it was not applicable to developing countries that still suffered problems of under-production. By the 2000s, when obesity and its ill-effects such as diabetes type 2 had risen rapidly in developing countries, alongside other diet-related NCDs, a new realism began to be voiced, arguing that the twentieth-century policy package now needed to be reformed (Maxwell & Slater, 2003). Optimists thought this new thinking would triumph, and that its evidence would sweep across public policy. This was not so. When the oil and commodity price crisis took hold in 2007–2008, creating the Great Recession, it was notable how the world's leading economies reverted to the default productionist policy position. More food was needed, they cried (G8, 2009).

One thing certainly has to change. There is little point shouting doom messages ever louder at policy people who do not understand or speak the language. It does not unlock the

TABLE 16.1 Some major reports pointing to need for integrated food systems change

Date	Report title	Sponsoring bodies	Comment
2008	International Assessment of Agricultural Science and Technology Development Knowledge (World Bank, 2008)	World Bank and the FAO	Global and regional perspective
2009	"L'Aquila" Joint Statement on Global Food Security (G8, 2009)	G8	Political statement of concern by rich economies about global food system
2010	Australia and food security in the changing world	Australian government	Global analysis by Australian science body
2011	The Future of Food and Farming: Challenges and choices for global sustainability. Final Report (UK Government, 2011)	UK government	Global review by UK chief scientist Foresight panel
2012	Big Food (PLoS Medicine Editors, 2012)	PLOS Medicine	Collection of papers calling scientists to debate the politics of current food system's winners and losers
2014	Agrimonde: Scenarios and Challenges for Feeding the World in 2050 (Paillard, Treyer, & Dorin, 2014)	French government	Global scenarios prepared by French government science body
2016	The Global Food System: an analysis (Gladek et al., 2016)	WWF	Large conservation NGO recognises that its biodiversity interests are shaped by the food system dynamics
2018	Opportunities for future research and innovation on food and nutrition security and agriculture: The InterAcademy Partnership's global perspective (InterAcademy Partnership, 2018)	Coalition of 130 international scientific bodies	Science overview which provides sober analysis and calls for better research and integrated action
2018	Creating a Sustainable Food Future (Searchinger et al., 2018)	World Resources Institute	Final report in a three-year series from ecosystems perspective
2019	EAT-Lancet Commission on Healthy Diets from Sustainable Food Systems (Willett et al., 2019)	EAT Foundation and *The Lancet*	Models how a healthy diet can be delivered and the changes this requires

policy lock-in. That said, we must remember that the fable in which a boy falsely warned villagers of an approaching wolf actually concludes with the boy crying "wolf, wolf" being ignored on the occasion when the wolf really was at hand. From that perspective, it is important to maintain the production of good data and gently to issue warnings. And some argue that the gap between evidence and reality is so great that only a crisis will unlock the lock-in, hence the persistent interest in collapse theory (Diamond, 2005). This chapter explores how to ask questions that would make a difference: Can we pitch positive not just negative futures? What would unlock the lock-in? Is evidence the only change agent?

We need better understanding of how the food system works and why the known big problems seem resistant to change. For a start, we need to reject the notion that policy-makers need only to pull a few policy levers to engineer change. By definition, complex systems are a web of dynamics rather than simple dynamics, which is why there is emerging interest in looking at food as systems using multi-criteria approaches. Some recent reports thus propose multi-level, multi-actor, multi-sector, multi-method approaches to change. Interdisciplinary approaches are required. Indeed, scientists and evidence gatherers might do well to consider what kind of evidence would impress policy-makers. Three decades or so of studies providing economic costs of failure to change seem barely to have dented the shape of the food economy.

How did we get here? The role of facts in policy-making

To address the philosophical and practical questions raised above, we must see if we can agree on how the current food system state of affairs came about. A number of interpretations are possible. It could be a failure of policy, or the result of a loss of political interest in food (until there was a crisis, such as happened in 2007–2008) or the unintended consequences of what used to be a rational and good food policy at the time, but which has become inappropriate today.

Rule number one in any policy conundrum is to face reality. This is easily said, but only part of the situation. Facts are only part of food reality. And the facts are themselves frag-mented: health facts, environmental facts, economic facts, cultural facts, political facts all vie for attention. Part of the success of the twentieth-century productionist paradigm has been that it brought food prices down as incomes rose – if one was lucky enough to live in an expanding economy. In low-income economies, of course, this was and remains not the case. In low-income, less-developed economies, consumers can spend half to two thirds of their incomes on food, whereas rich consumers in highly developed economies might only spend less than a twentieth. Economic 'facts' – shaped by policies which judge food as good if it is relatively cheap – trump the health 'facts' that highly processed, cheap foods externalise their 'cost' onto the health budget rather than food's budget. To which 'facts' do the policy-makers listen? Part of much scientific anxiety about resistance to change comes from a mistaken view about the power of evidence.

Facts are not the only features that matter. Views, ideologies, positions, experience, bal-ance of interests and societal forces, those too are part of reality. In particular, how the pro-blem is conceived or "framed" matters considerably. If obesity is framed as the result of a failure of consumer willpower, less attention will be given to how the consumer is sur-rounded by endless messages to consume, consume, consume. Vice versa, if the consumer is framed as a passive victim, there is little that can be done until the messages are turned off.

That is why modern food policy analysis charts these more complex dynamics, in the course of which it is essential to bring out whatever assumptions have "framed" and shaped policy. The framing assumptions are those perspectives and known features which are brought to any analysis. Facts are not simply facts. There is no paternalist science supremo who can genially ordain food change based solely upon the facts. Change happens for lots of reasons, among which may be the facts; but also other considerations come into play: the economy, jobs, political commitments, ideology, assessments of who will be winners and losers if there is change. And sometimes change does not happen at all but simply the state of affairs drifts on or gets worse – despite the rising cacophony of facts (Lang & Rayner, 2007).

How did we get here? Analyses that the food system is in serious difficulty, even crisis, are not new, as we saw above. Indeed, modern food policy as a distinct focus of intellectual and political debate can be traced to the mid to late eighteenth century, certainly in Western thought. The might of Ancient Rome depended on a vast flow of grain through its port of Ostia to keep the city's one million citizens fed. When Ostia was pillaged and later silted up, that dependency became clear. This was an early lesson – not lost on classically trained civil servants centuries later – in the need to have "policies" on how to maintain food flows. Throughout history, every marauding army had a de facto "policy" on how it would feed itself, often simply by corralling or pillaging food supplies wherever it went. Part of that brutal approach was often to lay waste to the enemies' capacity to feed itself, hence burning crops, taking draught animals, destroying farms. The word "policy" is given in quotation marks because, while these were attempts to shape food supplies, they were clear and sharp rather than subtle and trying to balance multi-criteria interests.

Modern food policy, in the sense that it is discussed and studied today, however, starts more recently than classical Rome, Egypt, Greece or China. Most agree that this means beginning at the emergence of industrial capitalism from the mid to late eighteenth century with the transition to post-feudal societies. This is when there is a confluence of transitions which turn food into a flexible item on the public policy agenda; and it is when the choices and options about food become both more complex and more overt. Chemistry begins to show that appearances are not the truth and that food is not what it seems. Mass harnessing of condensed energy in the form of water or coal enables a scaling-up of food production. Engineering exceeded the capacities of the Romans or Arabs, allowing towns to grow everywhere across Northern Europe. Accumulation of capital from western colonialism unleashed a search for new opportunities and outlets. New canals, railways and modes of traction outpaced the horse and oxen in what could be hauled. The distances for food to travel and the scales of transport expanded. Money flowed into and from food on an unprecedented scale. Entire new industries emerged with new technologies. Tiny villages turned into large manufacturing towns, all creating demand for food, while undermining it by attracting labour off the land. This combination of factors and features, push and pull, was something altogether new.

Above all, food took on new meaning and dangers with this emergence of industrial capitalism. Rural-urban splits become a dominant feature of society. The grip of old social relations were weakened. Vast populations worked in towns which began to take on their own dynamics, severed from the land and forging a new urban-rural split, reshaping what the land is for. A new dependency on food supplies produced beyond the town generated an infrastructure which enabled factory labour, output and creativity to be unleashed.

Founding thinkers about political economy as diverse as Adam Smith, Thomas Malthus and Karl Marx agreed that the food trade enabled other economic activity to happen. Managing and shaping that food trade became a topic for political discourse. All the social goals, including the arguments about what direction policy charts, the assessment of impacts, follow from that primary urban-rural split. Malthus was among the first to consider this new dependency relationship. Not enough food could be produced to feed growing populations, he argued. On the one side, his analysis was claimed by imperialists (who said this is why Britain needed its colonies) and then by eugenicists (who claimed this was the reason to control who should be allowed to breed), and more recently by deep green ecologists, although treated with kid gloves because that eugenicism had slipped into Nazism and the

Final Solution. Malthus was and remains vilified as an apologist for authoritarianism; undoubtedly he offered what to us seem stark policy suggestions – to delay human breeding patterns or to import more food (on which he did a U-turn). Marx argued against Malthusian determinism, arguing that societal change would feed people. In fact, it was "scientific" agriculture which sidelined Malthus by showing that the land could be milked harder to produce more food. This "productionism" became the dominant approach to food policy in the twentieth century. Demographers have also showed Malthus' mechanistic analysis to be wrong: provide incomes, technical support, and healthcare, particularly for women, and then rates of childbirth drop. Towards the final quarter of the twentieth century, a policy mix which offered enough food and better quality of lives looked deliverable.

In fact, this was the calm before the storm. Already in the 1980s, evidence was emerging of the immense impact of diet-related NCDs: heart attacks, strokes, diabetes, etc. And simultaneously, burgeoning environmental sciences showed how the wonder technologies of the agricultural revolution were "fixing" problems of output but having unforeseen consequences elsewhere: pollution, run-off, wildlife loss, weakened soil structure. The juxtaposition of massively increased outputs alongside massive externalised problems was clear by the end of the twentieth century.

What to do about food thus re-emerged as one of the big challenges of the twenty-first century. The United Nation's Millennium Development Goals (MDGs), formulated in the late 1980s, continued to frame under-nutrition and hunger as the great evils to be tackled. The 2015 UN Sustainable Development Goals (SDGs), which superseded the MDGs only 15 years later, recognised a far more complex reality; allied to the 17 SDGs are 166 targets, of which 70 or so require action on food. Table 16.2 illustrates how the broad goals can be translated into food terms.

TABLE 16.2 Examples of how UN Sustainable Development Goals (SDGs) can be translated into food terms

SDG	Goal	Significance for diet and food
SDG 1	End poverty	Inequalities determine access to diet; c.80% of the world's poor are rural, many working on food
SDG 2	End hunger	c.800 million are hungry; c.2 billion overweight or obese
SDG 3	Health and well-being	Ensure healthy lives and promote well-being for all at all ages
SDG 6	Clean water	Crops and livestock account for 70% of all water withdrawals
SDG 7	Energy	Food systems use 30% of global energy resources
SDG 12	Sustainable consumption and production	An estimated 30% of food is wasted; changing dietary patterns increase food's footprint
SDG 13	Combat climate change	Diet is a major contributor to climate change, accelerating with the nutrition transition
SDG 14	Oceans, seas and marine resources	C.29% of commercially important assessed marine fish stocks are overfished; c.61% are fully fished
SDG 15	Life on land; biodiversity	A third of land is degraded; up to 75% of crop genetic diversity is lost

Source: Based on FAO (2016).

Defining food progress: from single to multi-criteria analysis

If the brilliance of productionism was that it distilled nineteenth- and twentieth-century food problems into matters of production and distribution, today's problems are more complex. Although for years the policy mantra remained "produce ever more food", by the 2000s, that was becoming thin within scientific discourse if reviewed across the terrain. If one remained in particular policy "boxes", it was business-as-usual. This new complexity stretched existing policy analysis (Lang & Heasman, 2004). Environmental and health analyses showed problems which required different solutions, some regarding land use but many more regarding processing, marketing, retail and the systematic moulding of consumer consciousness. Few nutrition policy-makers, for example, took biological diversity within food systems seriously. And farming and food manufacturing everywhere saw nutritional public health as a matter of consumer choice, not their problem. Tacitly, they adopted the "wrong consumer" theory. To parody this somewhat, the argument was that existing food production was and is fine; it's just that consumers will not act rationally! Public health campaigners saw it differently, arguing that industry messages distorted or undermined consumer knowledge.

Almost every issue in food has similar competing positions. Powerful corporations have different interests to small farmers or shop-keepers, but sectors are also divided. Policy-making is about understanding, exploiting and negotiating those divisions and interests, and about having or creating processes which enable decisions to be made, and events to change to maximise the public interest. But that too is contested, as was argued earlier. What is "progress"? What price health? What value to long-term ecosystems balance? Part of the challenge for policy-makers today is to work out whether, in fact, they do have the right institutions and policy levers. Is there an agency or scientific advisory body which can provide independent and evidence-based advice? Are there existing processes which can be canalised or copied? Is there sufficient support within the appropriate bodies to steer policies through to acceptance? Will new policies make a difference? Will consumers see short-term change as worth long-term gain? These are political questions with which policy-makers tussle.

An even bigger question is: what is food policy for? Not so far beneath the surface of any policy discourse is the issue of progress. The advantages of this or that policy are claimed as "for progress". The trouble is that they do not necessarily agree on what is meant by progress. If one is alert to the centrality of defining Progress (note the capital 'P' now), some clarity on what the arguments and blockages are to policy processes can be gained.

A conservation group, for instance, might see a plot of land as the terrain where biodiversity can be revitalised. An agricultural interest sees it as a chance to farm profitably. A nutritionist sees it as the source of food. An employer sees the type of land as raising the thorny matter of whether to invest in labour-saving equipment or to hire cheaper labour, whether to farm intensively in terms of labour use or capital use. A consumer might see it just as where her or his food comes from. A romantic sees landscape and beauty (or degradation). And so on. Their interpretation and aspirations for the same place have variations. Arguing over these different versions of reality and the future are ultimately matters for political processes.

Again, over the last two decades, the data have shown ever more clearly that the current food system is unsustainable and that policies are not steering it in a better direction. Academic papers and reports have continued to push sustainability up the food policy agenda. Climate change initially appeared to be the leading issue within dominant policy-making circles from twenty years ago. But other issues quickly crowded behind and alongside it: obesity, the range of NCDs, societal inequalities, biodiversity loss, soil quality, landscape preservation, labour processes, consumption patterns. Each of these policy zones had compelling data and arguments. Biodiversity, for example, had been recognised as a crisis area back in the 1980s and, by 1992, the relatively new UN Environment Programme (UNEP) had won international support for the Convention on Biological Diversity (UN, 1992). But these issues kept on being addressed in their separate policy boxes.

By the 2010s, it was clear that food sustainability is not just about embedded carbon (climate change) but also about embedded water, embedded labour, embedded social values, embedded health, and so on. This impinged on what was meant by a "good" diet. For nutrition science and public health policy, this meant that good diets had to be about more than just nutrients or affordability – the A's analysis of access, affordability, availability and absorption. A new approach to public health was approaching, seeing human health as back-to-back with eco-systems health – what this author and his colleagues call "ecological public health" (Rayner & Lang, 2012; Mason & Lang, 2017). For policy-makers, the ecological public health challenge is how to juggle food's multi-functionality and how to manage competing interests and versions of the way forward, i.e. defining what we mean by Food Progress.

Conventional policy-makers say, at this point, that some trade-offs are inevitable. It's one thing to accept the multi-functionality and multi-criteria nature of food and it is another to say that Progress means improvements on all fronts. Policy realists will argue that one criterion will win over others. You cannot have, they argue, a policy where everything wins; "win-win" scenarios are a fiction. This may be true in the cut-and-thrust of daily politics where timetables dictate what happens. Deadlines, party loyalties, skill in policy processes (such as knowing the procedures), marshalling of outside supporters at the appropriate time, these are all the variables which food activists and scientific advisers and participants in policy-making processes learn to use.

Anyone arguing for healthier and more sustainable food systems must appreciate how important the juggling of these competing factors and features is. But yet, surely we cannot ignore the compelling evidence that food systems need to change across the entire set of criteria by which they are judged. This is why the 2019 EAT-Lancet Commission report called for a Great Food Transformation to begin, a transformation of what is produced, how, when and where (Willett et al., 2019). The food system as a system must be steered in a different direction, not gain in one area traded off for loss or continued damage in another. The world, countries, regions, consumers, farmers, and food sectors, everyone needs new frameworks to help reorient the drivers of the food system, from production to food culture to consumption.

This is a tussle over where food fits into conceptions of Progress. Do we judge Progress solely or mainly as about quantity and sufficiency, as productionism did? Or can we combine the data, the thinking, and the solutions from across the sciences to create multi-criteria approaches and win cultural change? Different insights are needed to help policy-makers. Just shouting louder from one perspective will neither convey the complexity nor produce the kind of systemic change that the overview analyses have increasingly realised are necessary. Assessments need to be made in each country or region as to what is the best and fastest way to begin the Great Food Transformation. This is a new radical pragmatism where science and evidence do not claim to dictate what happens; rather they inform societal processes of engagement.

Policy reactions and options

In theory, the United Nations is where a new multi-criteria policy approach ought to be manifest. In fact, this has been slow to emerge. While both human and environmental health concerns are represented and debated by the UN, it is rare for them to be addressed simultaneously. Like all vast policy machines, the UN addresses issues within policy boxes. And the boxes come in different sizes. The Food and Agriculture Organization (FAO) has a huge budget compared to the World Health Organization (WHO_, and both dwarf UNEP's budget. The joint FAO-WHO second International Conference on Nutrition (ICN2) in 2014 side-stepped discussion of sustainable diets, sticking to the important but old priorities of under-nutrition and NCDs, mapped in 2011 (UN, 2011), and keeping away from integrating these with ecosystems health (Brinsden & Lang, 2015).

Happily, both the SDGs and the Climate Change Accord agreed in 2015 to change this. A new level of policy engagement, one that specifies goals, targets and commitments is now agreed, but the process of their translation, particularly with regard to consumer behaviour is proving harder to achieve. The EAT-Lancet Commission was clear that the full range of policy instruments must be available, from "soft" measures, such as information, labels and education to "hard" measures, such as taxes, rationing and bans. The Nuffield Council on BioEthics' Ladder of Policy Interventions is one useful schema for situating policy actions. Table 16.3 summarises this with the first rung on the ladder indicating the application of "soft" policy measures, while by the eighth rung at the top, "harder" measures are indicated (Nuffield Council on Bioethics, 2007).

Too often, policy-makers shy away from food change and remain on the lower rungs, putting responsibility on consumers, citing the language of the market, and resorting to the "wrong consumer" explanation if and when required change does not follow. If the policy reflex is to stay soft, those seeking Progress in the name of health, environment and social justice must therefore consider what alters the balance of competing forces. Political realities might be fighting over information and counter-information, fact and factoid, "fake news" accusations, but above all, what matters is public sentiment (Nestle, 2018). A certain cynicism and defeatism can easily be fanned. "They" are too powerful. "We" are too weak and underfunded. But any campaigner will tell us that this is always initially the case. If ecological

TABLE 16.3 The Nuffield Ladder of Policy Interventions

Rung	Policy Option	Measures implied
8.	Eliminate choice	Channel actions only to the desired end and isolate inappropriate actions
7.	Restrict choice	Remove inappropriate choice options
6.	Guide choices through disincentives	Apply taxes or charges
5.	Guide choices through incentives	Use regulations or financial incentives
4.	Guide choice by changing default policy	Provide "better" options
3.	Enable choice	Enable individuals to change behaviour
2.	Provide information	Inform or educate the public
1.	Do nothing	No action or only monitor situation

Source: Nuffield Council on Bioethics (2007).

public health is Food Progress, then long-term strategies need to be formulated around which many actors can unite, drawing on sound science and doing their policy research homework by mapping the policy terrain, not assuming rationality will triumph. There are always weak points in opponents. While funding might be scarce, there are always resources which have not yet been tapped, and strengths in the form of people, if not cash, which can be marshalled.

This author is an optimist about our capacity to forge better food policies. A multi-criteria approach to food opens up clear options for action. We do not need to accept lock-ins as permanent. Institutional failures and policy sclerosis can be analysed and overcome. Ideological opposition is inevitable. The twentieth century saw the emergence of powerful oppositions to Food Progress at the societal level. The policy default is a notion of democracy through the everyday "vote" of consumer choice at the checkout. But this assumes well-informed consumers.

The overwhelming power of the evidence that the food system must become sustainable means that policy-makers must be encouraged to change and to adopt more subtle and multi-level, multi-sector engagement. Some argue that the role of science is simply to produce evidence and to leave policy to the policy-makers. The Intergovernmental Panel on Climate Change (IPCC) provides another model. It does the science but models the policy options. Now, it says, is not the time for "studied distance"; only by engaging can we see what evidence is effective and can we help frame solutions which answer the policy-makers' problems. This chimes with the history of the public health movement. Public health has always required engagement. It is about changing the conditions in which humans live. Seeing food from an ecological public health perspective reinvigorates science for the public interest.

Conclusion

This chapter has proposed that food policy requires a multi-criteria approach. We are in a "multi" era of food: multi-level, multi-sector, multi-discipline, multi-actor, multi-institution. This transforms what we mean by Food Progress. New policy frameworks are beginning to emerge at the global level, but the Great Food Transformation which is now required is not yet happening. Movements in that direction are emerging but it remains to be seen whether these are strong enough to defeat opposition and to unlock the policy lock-in. We can feel confident that modern analysis of the complexities of the food system are useful and can help refine and inform policy processes. Ultimately, the prize is to feed people differently to how they were in the twentieth century. The stakes are high.

References

Brinsden, H., & Lang, T. (2015). Reflecting on ICN2: Was it a game changer? *Archives of Public Health*, 73(42), doi:10.1186/s13690–13015–0091-y.

Diamond, J. (2005). *Collapse: How societies choose to fail or survive*. London: Penguin Books.

FAO (Food and Agriculture Organization). (2011). *Global food losses and food waste: Extent, causes and prevention*. Rome: FAO.

FAO. (2016). *FAO and the 17 Sustainable Development Goals*. Rome: FAO. Available at: www.fao.org/3/a-i4997e.pdf

FAO, IFAD, UNICEF, WFP, & WHO. (2018). *State of food insecurity 2018: Building climate resilience for food security and nutrition*. Rome: Food and Agriculture Organisation, International Fund for Agricultural Development, UNICEF, World Food Programme and the World Health Organisation.

G8. (2009). "L'Aquila" Joint Statement on Global Food Security. L'Aquila Food Security Initiative (AFSI), 10 July 2009. Rome: G8 Leaders. Available at: www.g8italia2009.it/static/G8_Allegato/LAquila_Joint_Statement_on_Global_Food_Security%5B1%5D,0.pdf

Gladek, E., Fraser, M., Roemers, G., Sabag Muñoz, O., Kennedy, E., & Hirsch, P. (2016). The global food system: An analysis. Available at: wwf.panda.org/wwf_offices/netherlands

HLPE. (2012). *Food security and climate change: A report by the High Level Panel of Experts on Food Security and Nutrition of the Committee on World Food Security*. Rome: Food and Agriculture Organization.

Institute of Mechanical Engineers. (2013). *Global food: Waste not want not*. London: Institute of Mechanical Engineers.

InterAcademy Partnership. (2018). *Opportunities for future research and innovation on food and nutrition security and agriculture: The InterAcademy Partnership's global perspective*. Rome: IAP.

International Labour Organisation. (2018). *World employment and social outlook: Trends 2018*. Geneva: ILO.

Lang, T., & Heasman, M. (2004). *Food wars: The global battle for mouths, minds and markets*. London: Earthscan.

Lang, T., & Heasman, M. (2015). *Food wars: The global battle for mouths, minds and markets*. 2nd ed. Abingdon: Routledge.

Lang, T., & Rayner, G. (2007). Overcoming policy cacophony on obesity: An ecological public health framework for policymakers. *Obesity Reviews*, 8(S1), 165–181.

Mason, P., & Lang, T. (2017). *Sustainable diets: How ecological nutrition can transform consumption and the food system*. Abingdon: Routledge.

Maxwell, S., & Slater, R. (2003). Food policy old and new. *Development Policy Review*, 21(5–6), 531–553.

Nestle, M. (2018). *Unsavory truth: How food companies skew the science of what we eat*. New York: Basic Books.

Nuffield Council on Bioethics. (2007). *Public health: Ethical issues*. Cambridge: Cambridge Publishers/Nuffield Council on Bioethics. Available at: http://nuffieldbioethics.org/project/public-health/

Paillard, S., Treyer, S., & Dorin, B. (eds) (2014). *Agrimonde: Scenarios and challenges for feeding the world in 2050*. Berlin: Springer.

PLoS Medicine Editors. (2012). Big Food. *PLOS Medicine*, 9(6), e1001246. doi:10.1371/journal.pmed.100124.

Rayner, G., & Lang, T. (2012). *Ecological public health: Reshaping the conditions for good health*. London: Earthscan.

Rockström, J., Falkenmark, M., Allan, T., Folke, C., Gordon, L., Jägerskog, A., ... Varis, O. (2014). The unfolding water drama in the Anthropocene: Towards a resilience-based perspective on water for global sustainability. *Ecohydrology*, 7(5), 1249–1261. doi:10.1002/eco.1562.

Rockström, J., Steffen, W., Noone, K., Persson, Å., Chapin, F. S., Lambin, E., ... Foley, J. (2009). Planetary boundaries: Exploring the safe operating space for humanity. *Ecology and Society*, 14(2), 32. Available at: www.ecologyandsociety.org/vol14/iss32/art32/

Searchinger, T., Waite, R., Hanson, C., Ranganathan, J., Dumas, P., & Matthews, E. (2018). *Creating a sustainable food future: A menu of solutions to feed nearly 10 billion people by 2050*. Washington, DC: World Resources Institute.

Stern, N. (2006). *The Stern Review of the economics of climate change: Final report*. London: HM Treasury.

Tukker, A., Goldbohm, R. A., De Koning, A., Verheijden, M., Kleijn, R., Wolf, O. ... Rueda-Cantuche, J. M. (2011). Environmental impacts of changes to healthier diets in Europe. *Ecological Economics*, 70(10), 1776–1788.

Tukker, A., Huppes, G., Guinée, J., Heijungs, R., de Koning, A., van Oers, L. ... Nielsen, P. (2006). *Environmental Impact of Products (EIPRO): Analysis of the life cycle environmental impacts related to the final consumption of the EU-25. EUR 22284 EN*. Brussels: European Commission Joint Research Centre.

UK Government. (2011). *The future of food and farming: Challenges and choices for global sustainability. Final report, Foresight project*. London: Government Office for Science.

UN (United Nations). (1992). Convention on Biological Diversity. Available at: www.cbd.int

UN. (2011). *UN General Assembly 66th Session, prevention and control of non-communicable diseases: Report from the Secretary General, May 16, 2011, A/66/83*. New York: United Nations. Available at: www. un.org/ga/search/view_doc.asp?symbol=A/66/83&Lang=E

UNEP, Nellemann, C., MacDevette, M., Manders, T., Eickhout, B., Svihus, B., ... Kaltenborn, B. P. (2009). The environmental food crisis: The environment's role in averting future food crises. A UNEP rapid response assessment. Arendal, Norway: United Nations Environment Programme/ GRID-Arendal.

USDA ERS. (2017). New products. Washington, DC: US Department of Agriculture Economic Research Services.

WHO (World Health Organization). (2015). *WHO estimates of the global burden of foodborne diseases*: Geneva: World Health Organisation, Foodborne Diseases Burden Epidemiology Reference Group, 2007–2015.

Willett, W., Rockström, J., Loken, B., Springmann, M., Lang, T., Vermeulen, S., ... Murray, C. J. L. (2019). Food in the Anthropocene: The EAT-Lancet Commission on healthy diets from sustainable food systems. *The Lancet.* doi:10.1016/S0140-6736(18)31788–31784.

World Bank. (2008). *International Assessment of Agricultural Science and Technology Development Knowledge*. Washington, DC: World Bank.

WWF, & Zoological Society of London. (2015). *Living Blue Planet report 2015: Species, habitats and human well-being*. Gland, Switzerland: WWF and ZSL.

17

PEOPLE'S FOOD-RELATED PRACTICES TO PROMOTE HEALTHY AND SUSTAINABLE FOOD SYSTEMS

Lada Timotijevic

Introduction

Food choice reflects one's cultural background and personal factors, such as motivation, preferences and habits, but is largely dependent on food provision (production, distribution and waste management) (Kearney, 2010). Food has deep cultural meanings, and is inextricably linked to the practices of different social groups. Food-related social practices are social phenomena, such as shopping, cooking and eating, in which their performance involves the reproduction of cultural meanings, values and infrastructures (Shove, Pantzar, & Watson, 2012). The factors driving food practices relate not only to beliefs and values about health but also to broader sets of beliefs transcending the immediate individual benefits, including animal rights, the future of the planet and social justice (Kearney, 2010). The range of values that underpin food practices is demonstrated by dramatic shifts in eating habits in the UK and the EU over the past fifty years in quantity, range and quality of diets (Foster & Lunn, 2007). For instance, increasing numbers of people are adopting vegetarian and vegan diets due to ethical, health and environmental concerns (The Vegan Society, 2018). Raw food diets and a trend towards reduced processing are evident with the growth of fruit and vegetable markets and fresh cut produce (Santermo et al., 2018), as well as the steady decrease in meat consumption in developed countries (Kearney, 2010). At the same time there is a trend towards localism and organic food consumption as people seek to reduce their food miles (Blake, Mellor & Crane, 2010; Kearney, 2010).

Policy actions directed towards people's food-related practices are any actions intended to promote healthier and more sustainable food systems by modifying the beliefs, values and social practices of individuals and groups. Due to the complexity of the modern global food system, achieving this aim will need careful balancing of the values underpinning policy decisions. Reviews of existing policy actions suggest that policy acceptability will depend on the extent to which policies are perceived to promulgate these values (Steg & Vlek, 2009), including equity, liberty, security and efficiency. Weighing them up ultimately requires considerations of where the responsibility for action rest – within an individual or a collective; and what kind of change is hoped for. Bearing in mind these two core questions, this chapter presents a review of policy actions for healthy and sustainable food systems aimed at people's food-related practices, and which are classified as:

- policy action based on the rational choice model (utilitarianism, libertarianism);
- policy action based on the predictable irrationality model (paternal libertarianism – nudge);
- policy action based on the social learning models (communitarianism).

Policy action based on the rational choice models

Consumer science has long been dominated by reductionist models that attempt to explain social practices through rational individual choice. Interventions based on rational choice models are rooted in Bentham's (1948 [1789]) argument that humans are motivated primarily by a utilitarian desire to maximise gain and pleasure while minimising loss and pain. This philosophy shaped one of the earliest theories of decision-making – the maximising expected utility (MEU) theory (Lindley, 1985), which attempts to explain choices based on the expected utility of outcome. This approach has influenced food policy in modern neoliberal societies, which hinge on a strong belief in a free market economy and define humans as autonomous decision-makers. The cost-benefit principle assumes that any social value can be monetised, which, through a simple cost-benefit calculation, can predict the preferred behavioural option.

In the context of food-related social practices, this would translate into achieving optimal benefit (e.g. health) at a minimal cost (time, resources). According to this rationale, intervening in the food system to promote healthy and sustainable diets for all is not considered necessary except in cases of information asymmetries and market failures. Rather, pursuit of liberty (freedom of choice) and efficiency (cost-effectiveness) are the driving values of food policy. Thus, the focus has long been on food product innovation and market-based interventions to maximise convenience (e.g. processed food, convenience meals), to extrapolate maximal value from less-than optimal food (e.g. food reformulation, such as fortification, fat and salt reduction) and to increase the quantity of foods available for a smaller price (e.g. price promotion and portion management policies). Consumers are simultaneously expected to respond to ever-expanding nutritional education, information provision and marketing efforts that put the onus on their ability to identify the optimal course of action based on the increasingly complex and often contradictory information presented to them. Nutrition labelling is a prototype rational choice behavioural paradigm for a policy that aims to provide information about nutrients without interfering with consumer choices.

Evaluation of policy action based on the individual rational choice models

Evidence is mounting at both the conceptual and empirical levels concerning the merit of basing policy actions on MEU theory. Kahneman and Tversky (1979; 2013) have demonstrated that, because humans are subject to many cognitive distortions ("biases and heuristics"), merely providing accurate information, for example, about risks, is not enough to facilitate a utility-maximising decision. Norms and values have also been repeatedly shown to influence the decisions of consumers who, for example, may sacrifice self-interest to invest in fairness norms. The unfettered individualism posited by the MEU theory appears particularly weak in explaining altruistic and biospheric value-based behaviour observed in pro-environmental domains (Dietz & Stern, 1995).

Reviews of the literature on the ability of financial incentives to influence dietary choice have reported mixed results. Such incentives appear to be effective only over a short period of time, with some studies suggesting they may even be counter-productive over longer periods (Paul-Ebhohimhen & Avenell, 2008; Purnell, Gernes, Stein, Sherraden, & Knoblock-Hahn, 2014). In fact, financial motivation may actually undermine long-term health and environmental goals (Kane, Johnson, Town, & Butler, 2004; Moller, McFadden, Hedeker, & Spring, 2014), arguably because they avert attention away from the common good and diminish long-term commitment to the social practices that are necessary to achieve these goals.

Evidence of the effectiveness of nutritional labelling upon healthy eating is also inconclusive. A recent Cochrane Review (Crockett et al., 2018) has shown that provision of nutrition labelling in out-of-home setting can indeed lead to the decrease in the overall calorie intake. However, the researchers sound a note of caution and suggest that nutrition labelling on its own is insufficient to substantially change established food and diet-related practices. The general agreement is that information provision only influences simple behavioural domains (e.g. reduction of salt) and that its effectiveness diminishes upon encountering behavioural barriers (Stern, 1999). Environmental impacts of current dietary practices, treated as externalities, are not directly addressed by these policy options except through food product innovation and information provision to incentivise consumers towards sustainable diets and better waste management, which on their own, have had a limited impact.

Policy action based on harnessing cognitive heuristics and biases: predictable irrationality models

Daniel Kahneman and Amos Tversky (Kahneman & Tversky, 1979; 2013) have refuted the dominant understanding of humans as rational maximisers. Through a series of cleverly crafted studies which manipulated the context of decision-making, including the wording, the reference value and level of certainty of probability information, they have shown that people's judgements are often made without due concern for benefit maximisation. Instead, people demonstrate the following tendencies:

- *reference-dependence* – rather than focusing on absolute payoffs, people instead make decisions with reference to arbitrary information that is typically irrelevant to the problem at hand;
- *loss aversion* – people are more sensitive to losses relative to reference points than to equally sized gains;
- *bounded rationality* – people evaluate utility and risks using cognitive heuristics as a way of coping with limitations in cognitive ability, time available and problem-specific constraints.

This has revolutionised thinking, not only about human nature and cognitive capacity, but also about policy approaches to achieving behavioural and social change. Thaler and Sunstein (2008: 6) synthesised the disparate evidence from economics and psychology into the umbrella concept of "nudge" theory:

A nudge, as we will use the term, is any aspect of the choice architecture that alters people's behaviour in a predictable way without forbidding any options or significantly changing their economic incentives. To count as a mere nudge, the intervention must be easy and cheap to avoid. Nudges are not mandates. Putting fruit at eye level counts as a nudge. Banning junk food does not.

The idea purports that, rather than assuming a capacity for making rational choice based on utility-maximising preferences, policy-makers should capitalise on the reliable irrationality of humans, using "choice architecture" – the subtle changes in the context of human behaviour – to gently nudge individuals towards a desirable outcome. This has led to a series of policies being introduced based on the premise that changing food practices may not, after all, require individuals to engage in deep information processing.

Various typologies of nudging have now been developed in the field of sustainable food practices (e.g. Blumenthal-Barby & Burroughs, 2012; Hollands et al., 2013; Lehner, Mont, & Heiskanen, 2016), including symbol nudges, priming, accessibility, functional design nudges, ambience and social nudging. For instance, symbol nudging, as shown in Figure 17.1, includes presentation of an image or a symbol which can trigger heuristics or shortcuts to signal the "right" behaviour.

While experimental research suggests that on-the-product symbols, such as traffic lights labelling and health logos, can facilitate identification of healthier alternatives (Grunert, Wills, & Fernández-Celemín, 2010) and are likely to increase purchase intentions of more healthful foods (Wilson, Buckley, Buckley, & Bogomolova, 2016), the extent to which this is translated into optimal food choice in the real world remains unclear (Hodgkins et al., 2015).

Evidence on the ability of eco-labelling on grocery and food products to nudge consumers towards more sustainable products (e.g. environmental sustainability certification labels, carbon footprint labels) is scant. While consumers appear to be willing to pay higher premiums for "green" products (Young, Hwang, McDonald, & Oates, 2010), this has yet to be confirmed in real-world contexts. When Vanclay et al. (2011) examined the purchase of

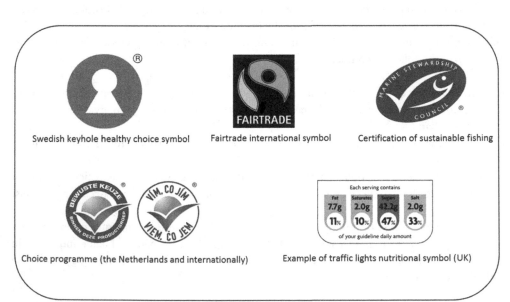

FIGURE 17.1 Examples of symbol nudges

groceries with the CO_2 emissions symbol nudge in a grocery store, they observed a shift towards purchasing green-labelled products of 4 per cent over a two-months period, the shift which, though substantive, was non-significant. The significant shift towards sustainable products was only observed when the green-labelled products were also the cheapest.

Social nudges in the food domain have included prompts to think about normative food-related behaviours, such as the amount of food people eat in social contexts (Robinson, Thomas, Aveyard, & Higgs, 2014; Vartanian, Spanos, Herman, & Polivy, 2015), or by indicating normative waste-management behaviour (Kallbekken & Sælen, 2013). It is hypothesised that people would follow socially normative behaviour as it can provide clues about what constitutes "correct" behaviour, and can enhance a sense of belonging because of conformity pressures. Robinson et al. (2014b) carried out a narrative review of the literature testing the influence of social norms on both the quantity and the quality (e.g. calorie density) of food consumed, and concluded that there was consistent evidence of moderate effect of norms upon food choice. Focusing more specifically upon the type of norm that influences food choice, Robinson et al. (2014a) looked at the role of descriptive norm (normative behaviour, i.e. what the majority of people do) and injunctive norm (expected behaviour, i.e. what people think you should do) and found that the effect existed for descriptive norm only and was limited to those consumers who report initial low fruit and vegetable consumption.

Evaluation of policy action based on predictable irrationality models

The majority of nudge-related food consumption studies did not measure the long-term effect of normative messages. Nudging has been criticised for its short-term effect and proximal context-dependency, meaning they are shown to mainly be effective when presented where the behaviour takes place (e.g. on a product or on an advert banner). Current evidence seems to suggest that its effectiveness varies depending on

- the behavioural goal (e.g. it is less effective in moving people away from unhealthy food but more effective in moving people towards healthy food) (Hollands et al., 2015);
- the social context (less effective in a less controlling environment) (Lehner, Mont, & Heiskanen, 2016);
- people's initial values and attitudes (less effective when they are not in line with the required behavioural shift) (Thomas et al., 2017).

Furthermore, nudging has been applied to food domains mainly as a way of dealing with the obesity epidemic, rather than with the view to promote environmental causes in food consumption, for example, reducing meat consumption and food waste (Lehner et al., 2016). We therefore have limited understanding of the effectiveness of nudges in promoting sustainable diets. Evidence from nudge studies shows that more complex behaviours are more difficult to influence. Sustainable food practices are indeed highly complex, incorporating many dimensions that must be considered; some of these are future-oriented (e.g. long-term effects of current meat consumption on climate), and some are others-oriented issues of social justice (e.g. animal welfare, food insecurity, poverty). The ethical underpinnings of the nudge approach have also been called into question. Issues of what constitutes the "common good" and who holds the power to decide the direction of change are a source of continuous dispute in the food domain (e.g. Rich, Monaghan, & Aphramor, 2011). The debate about the ethical acceptability of the nudge approach on issues characterised by heterogeneous, sometimes intractable values, calls for an alternative vision of human nature and new possibilities for change that strive to overcome bounded rationality.

Policy action based on harnessing human reflexivity through social learning

Food connects people to their social, religious, or moral communities, and, increasingly, due to the global and inter-connected nature of the food system, to their political community. Food consumption therefore is not merely a matter for the private sphere, and critical questions are being posed about human potential for reflexivity, learning, collective responsibility and collective action vis à vis food and food systems (De Tavernier 2012; Renting, Schermer, & Rossi, 2012).

A new concept of food citizenship is emerging, one which emphasises the complex relationship between an individual and the food system (Lozano-Cabedo & Gómez-Benito, 2017) and calls for consideration of the rights and responsibilities incumbent upon us as part of that system. Food citizenship is defined as "the practice of engaging in food-related behaviours that support, rather than threaten, the development of a democratic, socially and economically just, and environmentally sustainable food system" (Wilkins, 2005: 271).

Policy interventions that focus on individuals as self-interested or non-reflexive consumers have failed to combat problems of obesity, food insecurity and climate change. It is increasingly argued that what is needed is a reconceptualisation of people as members of communities and moral agents (and not simply as consumers), in other words, as citizens (Etzioni, 2004; Wilkins, 2005). By asking questions about how commodification of food affects our society and the environment, the food citizenship movement calls upon communities to engage in discussion about the areas of our food system that should not be subjected to market norms. It allows the deliberation about which aspects of our food-related practices should follow the logic of market economy, and which should be based on moral judgements (Sandel, 2013). Collective action is ultimately about social learning and exercise of human agency, through which people not only expand their semantic knowledge of the problem but also develop new skills and cognitive capacities with which to tackle it (Bandura, 2001), while also furthering the principles of food democracy (Lang, 1998).

Food acts to maintain and propel human agency, which is essential in ensuring transitions towards sustainable food systems (Lockie, 2009). Participatory and deliberative approaches to developing sustainable food policy are increasingly advocated because they can facilitate the process of co-production of solutions that will prove not only broadly acceptable but also desirable for increasingly pluralistic societies (Etzioni, 2004).

Evaluation of policy action based on social learning models

Interventions based on participatory and community action are a minor policy orientation often propelled by grassroots food networks and oppositional and constructive advocacy groups, such as the food justice movement and food cooperatives (e.g. parents associations, association of small farmers) (Gottlieb, 2010). Despite the growing incidence and power of such movements, they do not represent the mainstream food governance approach and there is paucity of systematic research to understand their prevalence, effectiveness, impact and potential to generate a step change in current food practices. Given the mounting crisis in the current food system, there exists an urgent need to develop systematic studies to identify best practices in participatory approaches to changing food practices.

Conclusion

The current review of policy actions at the level of people's food-related practices has brought to light a number of lessons. First, in trying to understand the impact of actions, we must contend with the ontological origin of the policy action, in particular, the way in which human nature is conceptualised within, and in relation to, dominant social and political systems. This chapter has noted that currently the predominant rationale for policy action to achieve sustainable food practices supports the neoliberal agenda of unfettered consumerism and the sanctity of market forces, targeting change at the level of individual rational or unconscious (irrational) decision-making.

Second, evidence suggests that neither of these approaches is achieving the change required to address the "wicked" (complex, multifaceted) problems facing the global food systems. New, emerging rationales for policy action recognise the embedded and interconnected nature of food production and consumption and simultaneously call for greater reflexivity – pragmatic as well as ethical – on the origins of the problem and possible solutions to the dysfunctional food system. What research does exist provides hope that through community-level engagement and deliberation to decide which versions of the future we, as society, would like to pursue, citizens can enact system change.

Finally, the process of policy development is deeply contested, a feature of our increasingly pluralistic and global society. Transparency about the values that drive our choices of policies and the trade-offs that are necessary to achieve a socially and ecologically desirable future is crucial in transforming current food governance system and practices.

Thus, in order to enable policy actions that are fit for the future challenges of food systems, several recommendations can be made:

- Policy solutions should be framed openly and transparently, through reflexive deliberation about the values that drive our actions and the versions of the future we would like to pursue.
- We should devise policy options that address a range of human capacities : for economic decision-making as well as moral judgement; for heuristic judgement as well as deliberative engagement for the common good.
- Public acceptance of policy can be harnessed by fostering greater ownership of the solutions, but to achieve this, public engagement is necessary. Community-level deliberation about policies can help link the particularities of individuals' food-related practices with the universal need to make food production and distribution both sustainable and just.
- Evaluation of a policy action is inseparable from its planning – evaluating impact should open up the debate about the criteria, the values and paradigms, through which we will judge the social desirability of the future the policy is helping to bring into being.

References

Bandura, A. (2001). Social cognitive theory: An agentic perspective . *Annual Review of Psychology*, 52(1), 1–26.

Bentham, J. (1948 [1789]). *An introduction to the principles of morals and legislation*. New York: Hafner Publishing Co.

Blake, M. K., Mellor, J., & Crane, L. (2010). Buying local food: Shopping practices, place, and consumption networks in defining food as "local". *Annals of the Association of American Geographers*, 100 (2), 409–426.

Blumenthal-Barby, J. S., & Burroughs, H. (2012). Seeking better health care outcomes: The ethics of using the "nudge". *The American Journal of Bioethics*, 12(2), 1–10.

Crockett, R. A., King, S. E., Marteau, T. M., Prevost, A. T., Bignardi, G., Roberts, N. W., ... Jebb, S. A. (2018). Nutritional labelling for healthier food or non-alcoholic drink purchasing and consumption. *The Cochrane Library*. CD009315.

De Tavernier, J. (2012). Food citizenship: Is there a duty for responsible consumption? *Journal of Agricultural and Environmental Ethics*, 25(6),895–907.

Dietz, T., & Stern, P. C. (1995). Toward a theory of choice: Socially embedded preference construction. *The Journal of Socio-Economics*, 24(2), 261–279.

Etzioni, A. (2004). *The common good*. Cambridge: Polity Press.

Foster, R., & Lunn, J. (2007). 40th Anniversary Briefing Paper: Food availability and our changing diet. *Nutrition Bulletin*, 32(3), 187–249.

Gottlieb, R., & Joshi, A. (2010). *Food justice*. Cambridge, MA: MIT Press.

Grunert, K.G., Wills, J.M., & Fernández-Celemín, L. (2010). Nutrition knowledge, and use and understanding of nutrition information on food labels among consumers in the UK. *Appetite*, 55(2), 177–189.

Hodgkins, C. E., Raats, M. M., Fife-Schaw, C., Peacock, M., Gröppel-Klein, A., Koenigstorfer, J., ... Gibbs, M. (2015). Guiding healthier food choice: Systematic comparison of four front-of-pack labelling systems and their effect on judgements of product healthiness. *British Journal of Nutrition*, 113 (10), 1652–1663.

Hollands, G. J., Shemilt, I., Marteau, T. M., Jebb, S. A., Kelly, M. P., Nakamura, R., ... Ogilvie, D. (2013). *Altering choice architecture to change population health behaviour: A large-scale conceptual and empirical scoping review of interventions within micro-environments*. Cambridge: Cambridge University Press.

Hollands, G. J., Shemilt, I., Marteau, T. M., Jebb, S. A., Lewis, H. B., Wei, Y., ... Ogilvie, D. (2015). Portion, package or tableware size for changing selection and consumption of food, alcohol and tobacco. *The Cochrane Database of Systematic Reviews*, (9). CD011045. doi:10.1002/14651858. CD011045.pub2.

Kahneman, D., & Tversky, A. (1979). Prospect theory: An analysis of decision under risk. *Econometrica, Journal of Econometric Society*, 47, 263–291.

Kahneman, D., & Tversky, A. (2013). Choices, values, and frames. In L. C. MacLean & W. T. Ziemba (eds), *Handbook of the fundamentals of financial decision making: Part I*. Singapore: World Scientific Publishing Co., pp. 269–278.

Kallbekken, S., & Sælen, H. (2013). Nudging hotel guests to reduce food waste as a win–win environmental measure. *Economics Letters*, 119(3), 325–327.

Kane, R. L., Johnson, P. E., Town, R. J., & Butler, M. (2004). A structured review of the effect of economic incentives on consumers' preventive behavior. *American Journal of Preventive Medicine*, 27(4), 327–352.

Kearney, J. (2010). Food consumption trends and drivers. *Philosophical Transactions of the Royal Society B: Biological Sciences*, 365(1554), 2793–2807.

Lang, T. (1998). Towards a food democracy. In S. Griffiths & J. Wallace (eds), *Consuming passions: Cooking and eating in the age of anxiety*. Manchester: Manchester University Press, pp. 13–24.

Lehner, M., Mont, O., & Heiskanen, E. (2016). Nudging: A promising tool for sustainable consumption behaviour? *Journal of Cleaner Production*, 134, 166–177. Lindley, D. V. (1985). *Making decisions*, 2nd edn. Chichester: John Wiley and Sons, Ltd.

Lockie, S. (2009). Responsibility and agency within alternative food networks: Assembling the "citizen consumer". *Agriculture and Human Values*, 26(3), .193–201.

Lozano-Cabedo, C., & Gómez-Benito, C. (2017). A theoretical model of food citizenship for the analysis of social praxis. *Journal of Agricultural and Environmental Ethics*, 30(1), 1–22.

Moller, A. C., McFadden, H., Hedeker, D., & Spring, B. (2014). Financial motivation undermines maintenance in an intensive diet and activity intervention. *Journal of Behavioral Medicine*, 37(5), 819–827.

Paul-Ebhohimhen, V., & Avenell, A. (2008). Systematic review of the use of financial incentives in treatments for obesity and overweight. *Obesity Reviews*, 9(4), 355–367.

Purnell, J. Q., Gernes, R., Stein, R., Sherraden, M. S., & Knoblock-Hahn, A. (2014). A systematic review of financial incentives for dietary behavior change. *Journal of the Academy of Nutrition and Dietetics*, 114(7),1023–1035.

Renting, H., Schermer, M., & Rossi, A. (2012). Building food democracy: Exploring civic food networks and newly emerging forms of food citizenship. *International Journal of Sociology of Agriculture and Food*, 19(3), 289–307.

Rich, E., Monaghan, L. F., & Aphramor, L. (eds) (2011). *Debating obesity*. London: Palgrave Macmillan.

Robinson, E., Fleming, A., & Higgs, S. (2014a). Prompting healthier eating: Testing the use of health and social norm based messages. *Health Psychology*, 33(9), 1057.

Robinson, E., Thomas, J., Aveyard, P., & Higgs, S. (2014b). What everyone else is eating: A systematic review and meta-analysis of the effect of informational eating norms on eating behavior. *Journal of the Academy of Nutrition and Dietetics*, 114(3), 414–429.

Sandel, M. J. (2013). Market reasoning as moral reasoning: Why economists should re-engage with political philosophy. *Journal of Economic Perspectives*, 27(4), 121–140.

Santermo, G., Carlucci, D., De Devitiis, B., Seccia, A., Stasi, A., Viscecchia, R. & Ardone, G. (2018). Emerging trends in European food, diets and food industry. *Food Research International*, 104, 39–47.

Shove, E., Pantzar, M., & Watson, M. (2012). *The dynamics of social practice: Everyday life and how it changes*. London: Sage.

Steg, L., & Vlek, C. (2009). Encouraging pro-environmental behaviour: An integrative review and research agenda. *Journal of Environmental Psychology*, 29(3), .309–317.

Stern, P. C. (1999). Information, incentives, and proenvironmental consumer behavior. *Journal of Consumer Policy*, 22(4), 461–478.

The Vegan Society. (2018). Available at: www.vegansociety.com/news/media/statistics (accessed 13t December 2018).

Thaler, R. H., & Sunstein, C. R. (2008). *Nudge: Improving decisions about health, wealth, and happiness*. New Haven, CT: Yale University Press.

Thomas, J. M., Ursell, A., Robinson, E. L., Aveyard, P., Jebb, S. A., … Higgs, S. (2017). Using a descriptive social norm to increase vegetable selection in workplace restaurant settings. *Health Psychology*, 36(11), 1026.

Vanclay, J. K., Shortiss, J., Aulsebrook, S., Gillespie, A. M., Howell, B. C., Johanni, R., … Yates, J. (2011). Customer response to carbon labelling of groceries. *Journal of Consumer Policy*, 34(1), 153–160.

Vartanian, L. R., Spanos, S., Herman, C. P., & Polivy, J., (2015). Modeling of food intake: A meta-analytic review. *Social Influence*, 10(3), 119–136.

Wilkins, J. L. (2005). Eating right here: Moving from consumer to food citizen. *Agriculture and Human Values*, 22(3), 269–273.

Wilson, A. L., Buckley, E., Buckley, J. D., & Bogomolova, S. (2016). Nudging healthier food and beverage choices through salience and priming. Evidence from a systematic review. *Food Quality and Preference*, 51,.47–64.

Young, W., Hwang, K., McDonald, S., & Oates, C. J. (2010). Sustainable consumption: Green consumer behaviour when purchasing products. *Sustainable Development*, 18(1), 20–31.

18

PRACTITIONER ADVOCACY TO PROMOTE HEALTHY AND SUSTAINABLE FOOD SYSTEMS

Christina Pollard, Andrea Begley and Claire Pulker

Introduction

The solutions to the "wicked" problem of achieving healthy and sustainable food systems are as complex, unclear and contested as the description of the problem (Lawrence, Friel, Wingrove, James, & Candy, 2015). A paradigm shift is required to transform our current food system to one that has health, environmental sustainability and prosperity as both policy drivers and outcomes. Restraining the drivers of food production and consumption using integrative, cross-sectoral and population-wide policies addressing agriculture and food supply, availability and access to food, physical activity, welfare and social benefits, fiscal policies, and information and marketing is sensible (Reisch, Eberle, & Lorek, 2013). Advocacy is essential to initiate and maintain shifts across the system.

Calls to transform food systems often are met with interest from citizens and organisations, but face political apathy and resistance from powerful commercial interests. The actions to address the problem are difficult to define due in part to the lack of an agreed understanding of the problem plus the contested political context. As Lang and Rayner (2012: 2) assert, for public health to alter the circumstances to enable health and sustainability, advocacy "requires a political savvy not reflected in the mantras of evidence-based policy" and "needs to be understood in terms of visions and movements".

Public health advocacy is simply "organised influence" to address public health issues and achieve policy goals by activating action. Advocacy is a combination of individual and social actions designed to gain political commitment, policy support, social acceptance and systems support for a particular health goal or programme (WHO, 1992). For public health practitioners, it is an accepted yet underutilised core professional competency (Barry, Allegrante, Lamarre, Auld, & Taub, 2009; Frenk et al., 2010).

The ever-changing nature and the uncertainty of the food system mean that constant and complex advocacy is necessary (Lang, 1999). There are many leverage points across the food system to effect change and many stakeholders are responsible for doing so. Theoretical models have been developed to simplify and help in understanding of issues, relationships, mechanisms, interactions, influencers and leverage points for action across the food system (Lang & Rayner, 2012; Lawrence et al., 2015). This understanding is important for effective advocacy.

Advocacy actions to promote healthy and sustainable food system can, and need to, be undertaken by a range of individuals, groups and organisations and this chapter will focus particularly on advocacy for practitioners more directly engaged with the food system. The remainder of this chapter describes why advocacy is important, the advocacy process, and finishes with two "advocacy for healthy and sustainable food systems" case studies.

Why is advocacy important?

Healthy and sustainable food systems require a constant balancing of complex considerations and their contribution to healthy dietary patterns and food security (Lang, 2017). It is challenging to consider the environmental footprint of population dietary intake along with other components of healthy and sustainable food systems, such as: supporting humane treatment of animals; paying agricultural and food processing workers a fair wage; avoiding land clearance; and minimising food and packaging waste (Broom, 2010; Lang & Barling, 2012). Advocacy strategies need to raise awareness of the complexity of the challenge and require investment in building local expertise and evidence. Healthy and sustainable food systems are geographically unique so international data and local solutions are not necessarily transferable. For example, the factors influencing a healthy and sustainable food supply will be different in a food-producing country compared to a country with net food imports, between large and small countries, or those with differing climactic conditions.

The opposition to healthy and sustainable food systems action occurs at numerous points, and joined-up responses are required as many of the necessary changes are not under the direct influence of the government departments or agencies with health and/or environmental responsibilities. Advocacy is needed to mobilise resources (different distribution of funds to what is currently in place); change opinions (change a decision-maker's perception or understanding of a problem or issue); catalyse change (influence choices that will be considered in formulating decisions); and ultimately cause action.

The advocacy process

Although the advocacy process does not always occur in a linear fashion, it can be planned by considering the four steps outlined in Figure 18.1 (Shilton, 2006; Brownell & Warner, 2009; Lobstein et al., 2013; Public Health Advocacy Institute of Western Australia, 2013; Chapman, 2015) and reviewing them along the way.

Why? Define the issue and why it matters, the context in which it is occurring

Evidence is used to identify the problem, its seriousness and magnitude; to assess alternative intervention options; to appraise the likely consequences of each policy action; and to evaluate the outcomes of the process (Lobstein et al., 2013).

It is not uncommon for policy-makers and/or opponents of the proposed policy to demand evidence to support a politically feasible option over the status quo, or to assist in building the case for withstanding calls for unfeasible interventions. The relationship between evidence, knowledge, policy-making and power is important. Vital evidence to understand the operation

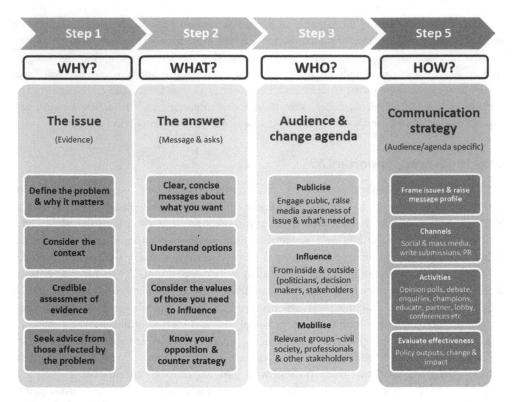

FIGURE 18.1 The four-step advocacy process
Source: Adapted from Shilton (2006); Brownell & Warner (2009); Lobstein et al. (2013); Public Health Advocacy Institute of Western Australia (2013); Chapman (2015).

of food and beverage markets and private sector is held by commercial organisations and is not available or too expensive for advocacy organisations to obtain (Lobstein et al., 2013).

Advocates rely on research to make their case, and often, even when evidence is available, it may not be suitable. Evidence must be appropriately framed to be useful. The lack of objectivity in advocacy messages, the personal demands of the process, information overload, and the mismatch of randomised thinking with non-random problems can lead to policy inaction (Brownson, Royer, Ewing, & McBride, 2006).

What? The message and agenda

Clear messages and agreed advocacy asks are paramount. The challenge is to bring together food systems thinking across food, nutrition and environmental sustainability (Burlingame, 2014). Although there have been decades of concern and understanding of the health and environmental impact of food systems (Gussow & Clancy, 1986; Gussow, 1999; McMichael, Powles, Butler, & Uauy, 2007; Wegener, 2018), often there is a lack of agreed agenda or clear messages across sectors.

Experts can assist in deciding the relative importance of advocacy priorities. The EAT-Lancet Commission on Food, Planet, Health brought together 20 scientists across the globe to develop a consensus statement on what constitutes a healthy diet from a sustainable food system and identify actions to speed up and support food system transformation (Willett et al., 2019). The results can help frame advocacy messages and provide evidence for advocacy asks.

The ways governments decide policy priority are not always transparent, but are usually based on political ideology and timing. As an example, although in Australia a "comprehensive cross-sector strategy and implementation plan to ensure a sustainable food supply for health" was considered important by public health experts, it did not rank as an advocacy priority due to perceptions of low political feasibility (Pollard, Pulker, & Devenish, 2015), see Table 18.1.

Environmental advocacy groups have not had as much success in generating relevant news stories due to the partisan and ideologically polarised nature of many of the issues (Swenson & Olsen, 2017). Articulating the issue to draw the links between policy, science, pressure groups, and public actions that resonate widely is the aim in framing advocacy messages (Swenson & Olsen, 2017). Environment and health issues need to be framed as bipartisan, particularly in the current neoliberal political environment. When considering which actions to advocate for, whether it is at a global or local level, remember that "for change to occur ... the power of vested interests needs to be challenged and the policy problem, solution and political climate all need to align" (Cullerton, Donnet, Lee, & Gallegos, 2016).

TABLE 18.1 Australian expert opinion ranked order of food and nutrition advocacy priorities, from 1 highest advocacy priority to 16 the lowest advocacy priority

Rank	Advocacy task
1	National food & nutrition policy, implementation strategies, monitoring & evaluation
2	Benchmark & monitor the healthiness of the Australian food system
3	Improve the quality of the food supply, e.g. reformulation, portion sizes, proportion of nutritious foods available
4	Implement incentives and disincentives to impact affordability of foods consistent with the Australian Dietary Guidelines
5	Comprehensive nutrition education campaigns to increase population knowledge, skills and abilities to comply with the Australian Dietary Guidelines
6	Address marketing and promotion of unhealthy food
7	Nutrition label standards and regulations on the use of claims and implied claims on foods
8	Set incentives and rules to create a healthy retail environment
9	Offer healthy foods and set standards for food provided in public institutions and other specific settings
10	Comprehensive cross-sector strategy and implementation plan to ensure a sustainable food supply for health is for effective food and nutrition advocacy
11	Strengthen nutrition workforce capacity
12	Challenge vested interests and undue influence
13	Assess and communicate the impacts of trade and investment agreements on the healthiness of the Australian food supply
14	Ensure social policies guarantee food equality
15	Challenge miscommunication to increase credible, reliable nutrition information through the media
16	Nutrition advice and counselling in health care settings

Source: Pollard et al. (2015).

Invariably practitioner advocacy activities for healthy and sustainable food systems encounter opposition, particularly from those with commercial interests to protect. These messages need to be countered using well-designed advocacy strategies (Brownell & Warner, 2009). Unhealthy commodity industries have strong, well-resourced advocacy strategies to prevent interventions that reduce their economic prosperity. Table 18.2 highlights industry strategies used against the environment movement and moves to reduce consumption of tobacco, unhealthy food, alcohol and pharmacological products (Beder & Boston, 1999; Dixon & Banwell, 2004; Dixon, Sindall, & Banwell, 2004; Kraak et al., 2012; Moodie et al., 2013). Many of these strategies, and more, will be used to counter advocacy for healthy and sustainable food systems.

Who? Targets for advocacy including government, practitioners and citizens

The United Nations (UN) identifies and promotes government actions for sustainable development and is uniquely positioned to take action on the issues confronting humanity, including climate change, sustainable development, human rights, humanitarian and health emergencies, governance and food production. The UN's Food and Agriculture Organiza-tion (FAO) and the World Health Organization (WHO) set goals requiring cooperation from governments, the private sector, and citizens (UN, 2015). The Decadal Nutrition Plan of Action 2016–2025 (United Nations) and the Global Compact Blueprint for Business Leadership (UN, 2017) advocate for action to achieve the Sustainable Development Goals (SDGs) (UN, 2015). They provide online advocacy resources, especially suitable for public health practitioners, explaining the need for healthy and sustainable food systems, the current problems and possible solutions.

Political will, whether or not decision-makers are supportive of policy change, is under-pinned by public will, the mood and policy preferences of voters (Cullerton et al., 2016). Consumers are both the targets of advocacy efforts and advocates for change. Consumers need to be motivated and able to make healthy and sustainable food choices. Although consumers understand deforestation, the environmental impact of human use on land and water, and recyclable packaging, their understanding and motivation to adopt healthy, sus-tainable and plant-based diets are limited (Van Loo, Hoefkens, & Verbeke, 2017). Food citizens are developed by pursuing social values, engaging interest groups and encouraging debate across society (Lang & Rayner, 2012). Building food systems literacy, and empower-ing citizens as consumers to develop a more complex understanding of the food system, are another advocacy priority (Widener & Karides, 2014).

How? The approach

The news media has traditionally been used to frame messages to build support for initiatives, influence those with the power to change or maintain laws, enact policies and fund inter-ventions (Chapman, 2004). Those deciding which issues are given media attention and how they are framed ultimately have the power to generate audience engagement and normalise the acceptability of actions (Swenson & Olsen, 2017). The proliferation of social and other media channels reaching a variety of audiences is both an asset and a barrier to enlisting public support for healthy and sustainable food systems.

TABLE 18.2 Some corporate strategies to resist policy actions for public good

Purpose	Strategies
1. Communications and media	*Influence and frame the communication agenda*
Expand communication scope, brand values, address controversial topics	Partner with media organisations or become media producers and creating own platforms for stories (Swenson & Olsen, 2017)
Influence the media agenda	Hire public relations firms and use paid media to frame agenda
Refute the science, frame public debate and maximise perceptions of legitimacy	Co-opt professionals who are media experts to speak for industry Professional capture
	Establishment of front groups and think tanks
	Use reputable bodies to advance the science supportive of industry products
	Engage high-profile spokespersons from food companies, trade associations and their political allies
Repair reputations and re-establish credibility by distracting, confusing, posturing	'Greenwashing' or 'bluewashing' dis-information from organisations (Laufer, 2003)
Stall, delay or influence regulatory, policy or other relevant decisions	Hire professional lobbyists/lobby government and decision-makers
	Participate in private public partnerships Encourage voluntary options, industry self-regulation
	Identify COI among members of key scientific committees
	Encourage debate within science, divide and conquer
Limit public participation, delay action	Use of lawsuits
2. Research	*Undermine science and add credibility to bad science*
Produce research or stimulate controversy	Establish networks of sympathetic consultants
Promote corporate citizenship through corporate research, counter science	Industry-funded research
	Develop programmes to generate support for 'junk science'
	Third party endorsements
Influence research process	Sit on committees overseeing the research
Discredit research and confuse	Question the research methodology being used by bodies considered to be hostile to the industry
Interpretation of findings	Develop a contingency plan, should the preliminary results be leaked
Dissemination of findings	Develop communications in advance of the study results
Discredit individuals, professional organisations	Research opposition to the industry
3. Influence future generations	*Undermine science and add credibility to bad science*
	Finance pro-industry education programmes for schools

Source: Adapted from Beder & Boston (1999); Dixon & Banwell (2004); Dixon et al. (2004); Kraak et al. (2012); Moodie et al. (2013).

Social platforms offer a far-reaching and timely approach to advocacy while at the same time, they can make it harder to distinguish message sources. New partnerships with media organisations allow corporations to expand the scope of their sustainability communication, amplify their brand values, address controversial topics, and closely analyse audience engagement with messages (Swenson & Olsen, 2017).

Case studies of effective advocacy activities

CASE STUDY 18.1 GARNERING POLITICAL SUPPORT FOR ENVIRONMENTALLY SUSTAINABLE DIETARY GUIDELINES

As long as science continues to support advice to reduce consumption of targeted foods, the guidelines will continue to elicit political controversy.

(Nestle, 2018: 148)

As the government-endorsed, credible and reliable source of nutrition advice, national dietary guidelines (DGs) form the basis for promotion, programmes and policies to support dietary changes that ultimately affect the food system. Attempts to integrate the principles of environmental sustainability, as well as health outcomes, into DGs have met with commercial and political resistance in some countries. For instance, following the release of the 2015 US DG scientific committee recommendations that dietary patterns should be lower in red and processed meat, the beef industry mobilised 30 US Senators to complain to the U.S. Department of Agriculture and the U.S. Department of Health and Human Services that those DGs were anti-meat (Nestle, 2018). The scientific committee was directed to focus on nutrient recommendations with the DG being decried as an inappropriate vehicle for policy conversation about sustainability. There was no mention of the word sustainability or the recommendation to reduce red meat, despite strong evidence of the health benefits (Nestle, 2018). Nevertheless, in recent times more and more countries are integrating sustainability considerations into their national DGs. Here we showcase the advocacy activities associated with the development of the Brazilian DGs, one of the first countries to integrate sustainability considerations into national DGs.

Why?

Brazil introduced a number of nutrition policies in the 1990s to address undernutrition, including the Zero Hunger Project, the driver of legal instruments introduced to guarantee and protect the human right to adequate food. Brazil's DGs are also rooted in a human rights approach to an adequate and healthy diet. The right to adequate food is written into the Brazilian Constitution, which requires the government to implement policies and actions to protect population food and nutrition security. Despite an ongoing decline in childhood malnutrition, which is still prevalent in some sub-population groups, Brazil also faces increasing overweight and obesity. To address this, DGs were first published in 2006. The Brazilian Ministry of Health revised the guidelines for the food, meals and eating practices to promote the health and well-being of the population due to the social changes that were affecting Brazil.

What?

The importance of food sovereignty is also recognised by Brazilian law, whereby people have the right to define policies that affect sustainable production and consumption of food. The "nutrition transition", which has occurred in many countries, including Brazil, describes the rapid change in dietary patterns that coincide with economic development. Natural and minimally processed local foods have been increasingly replaced by ultra-processed foods that are typically ready-to-eat. Along with addressing changes in dietary patterns, the guidelines aimed to highlight the importance of enjoying eating with family and friends, and the need for social and environmental sustainability in the food system.

Who?

Development of the DGs involved a coordinated consultation process that commenced in 2011. There were two national meetings of researchers, health professionals, educators, and representatives of civil society organisations. Regional meetings were held in the 26 Brazilian States and the Federal District with civil society groups. The draft guidelines underwent public consultation, receiving 3,125 responses, followed by extensive revision. Five principles guided development of the DGs, and special attention was given to prevention of under-nutrition.

How?

The guidelines address the general population directly, as well as health professionals. The document is illustrated and available online in English, Spanish and Portuguese. Copies of the DGs were distributed throughout the country to health centres, schools, hospitals, and health professionals. They were designed to enable the general population to make better choices for themselves, contribute to ensuring food and nutrition security for all, and demand the human right to adequate food. For example, the fifth chapter recognises that there are likely to be obstacles to following the DGs, and suggests ways to overcome them. The DGs have also been designed to support policies, programmes, and actions that encourage and promote public health and food and nutrition security of the Brazilian population.

Conclusion

The Brazilian Constitutional recognition of the human right to adequate food was a powerful context for advocacy action for developing DGs to address the "nutrition transition". Mobilisation of citizens on a nationwide scale during earlier development phases generated an enormous public response to the consultation phase.

Sources: (Jaime, 2014; Ministry of Health of Brazil, 2014; Monteiro et al., 2015).

CASE STUDY 18.2 MOBILISING ACTION: THE EATING BETTER ALLIANCE

Why?

The Eating Better alliance is a fair, green, healthy future alliance that aims to help the UK population eat less meat and dairy foods, and more foods that are healthy and sustainable, in order to create more sustainable food systems. The alliance, comprising 52 supporting organisations, partner networks, and local and community organisations, came together to address the challenges of feeding a growing and more affluent global population healthily, fairly, and sustainably. Their vision is "a world in which everyone values and has access to healthy, humane, sustainable diets".

What?

The focus is on meeting the challenges of eating better, and less, meat. They do this by: (1) raising awareness of the need to have a conversation about the issue; (2) building support to demonstrate to those with the position or power to make a difference that the time is right to address the issue; (3) stimulating long-term shifts in the cultural values attached to the issue, so that the message is compelling and inclusive. Advocacy addresses government policies, business practices and policies, and public awareness and behaviour change.

Who?

The alliance aims to strengthen their leadership by encouraging more organisations to collaborate with them to achieve the goal of less and better meat consumption, and more plant-based eating. They also aim to make change happen in government and business policy-making, by generating advocacy support and providing practical solutions. The core focus of their work aims to raise awareness of the need to eat less and better meat among the UK population, as well as policy-makers and businesses.

How?

They have summarised scientific evidence from academic researchers and specialist reports to determine guidelines for healthy, sustainable diets; and they compile reports and commission research to provide leadership on issues relevant to eating less and better meat. Communication channels include a website, blogs, monthly e-newsletters, social media, conference presentations, and media commentary. They convene organisations within the alliance to work collaboratively to develop shared positions or responses to submissions. In 2016, Eating Better was selected to provide a challenge to an advertising industry initiative that donates expertise to good causes resulting in the "Are you veg-curious?" mass media campaign to target young men. "The future of eating is flexitarian: Companies leading the way" report for businesses features case studies of twenty food retailers and manufacturers and shows practical ways for companies to help the population eat less and better meat, and more plant-based foods (Eating Better, 2017). It also provided examples of civil society organisations working in partnership with businesses to achieve these goals. The alliance has used the mass surveys from YouGov to provide population-level statistics to demonstrate cultural shifts towards acceptance of eating less and better meat.

Conclusion

The Eating Better advocacy campaign has successfully mobilised diverse organisations to raise one specific issue on the political agenda. The campaign reached multiple audiences, with targeted messages, over a sustained period of time to generate a conversation about the role of meat in the diet and challenge cultural norms.

Conclusion

For practitioners, the key advocacy message for a healthy and sustainable food system is that the current food system is broken and contributes to poor health, and we need to act now for the health of the planet and future generations. Creativity is needed to find ways to simply describe the system so that its complexity is clear and opportunities for intervention are obvious. Compelling evidence and knowledge that inspire action are needed. We must be mindful and understand the context in which we operate and measure both the effectiveness and unintended consequences of our actions. Collective action across sectors (e.g. from trade, agriculture, to technology and retail) and at all levels (e.g. globally and locally, and from citizens to organisations to governments) is required. Successful public health advocates recommend choosing a small number of key tasks. Although we subscribe to this point of view, it is also important to acknowledge the complexity of the challenge, the role of differing sectors, and the need for "fit-for-purpose" approaches to achieve a healthy and sustainable food system. The complexity of the healthy and sustainable food system calls for advocacy at all levels and so building coalitions for change is essential. Be prepared to compromise, but not too much; take small wins while keeping your eye on the big picture. Finally, advocates need to enjoy themselves, finding like-minded people helps and, of course, never give up!

References

Barry, M. M., Allegrante, J. P., Lamarre, M. C., Auld, M. E., & Taub, A. (2009). The Galway Consensus Conference: International collaboration on the development of core competencies for health promotion and health education. *Global Health Promotion, 16*(2), 5–11. doi:10.1177/1757975909104097.

Beder, S., & Boston, T. (1999). Global spin: The corporate assault on environmentalism. *Alternatives Journal, 25*(4), 42.

Broom, D. M. (2010). Animal welfare: An aspect of care, sustainability, and food quality required by the public. *Journal of Veterinary Medical Education, 37*(1), 83–88. doi:10.3138/jvme.37.1.83.

Brownell, K., & Warner, K. (2009). The perils of ignoring history: Big Tobacco played dirty and millions died. How similar is Big Food? *The Milbank Quarterly,* 87(1), 259–294.

Brownson, R. C., Royer, C., Ewing, R., & McBride, T. D. (2006). Researchers and policymakers: Travelers in parallel universes. *American Journal of Preventative Medicine,* 30(2), 164–172. doi:10.1016/j.amepre.2005.10.004.

Burlingame, B. (2014). Grand challenges in nutrition and environmental sustainability. *Frontiers in Nutrition*, 1(3), 3. doi:10.3389/fnut.2014.00003.

Chapman, S. (2004). Advocacy for public health: A primer. *Journal of Epidemiology and Community Health*, 58(5), 361–365.

Chapman, S. (2015). Reflections on a 38-year career in public health advocacy: 10 pieces of advice to early career researchers and advocates. *Public Health Research and Practice*, 25(2), e2521514. doi:10.17061/phrp2521514.

Cullerton, K., Donnet, T., Lee, A., & Gallegos, D. (2016). Playing the policy game: A review of the barriers to and enablers of nutrition policy change. *Public Health Nutrition*, 19(14), 2643–2653. doi:10.1017/S1368980016000677.

Dixon, J., & Banwell, C. (2004). Re-embedding trust: Unravelling the construction of modern diets. *Critical Public Health*, 14(2), 117–131.

Dixon, J., Sindall, C., & Banwell, C. (2004). Exploring the intersectoral partnerships guiding Australia's dietary advice. *Health Promotion International*, 19(1), 5–13.

Eating Better. (2017). The future of eating is flexitarian: Companies leading the way. Available at: www.eating-better.org/uploads/Documents/2017/Eating%20Better_The%20future%20of%20eating%20is%20flexitarian.pdf

Frenk, J., Chen, L., Bhutta, Z. A., Cohen, J., Crisp, N., Evans, T., … Zurayk, H. (2010). Health professionals for a new century: Transforming education to strengthen health systems in an interdependent world. *The Lancet, 376*(9756), 1923–1958. doi:10.1016/S0140–6736(10)61854–61855.

Gussow, J. (1999). Dietary guidelines for sustainability: Twelve years later. *Journal of Nutrition Education*, 31(4), 194–200. doi:10.1016/S0022-3182(99)70441–70443.

Gussow, J., & Clancy, K. (1986). Dietary guidelines for sustainability. *Journal of Nutrition Education*, 18(1): 1–5.

Jaime, P. (2014). The 2014 Brazilian dietary guidelines: The guide based on food and meals for everybody now and in future. *World Nutrition*, 5(12), 1085–1096.

Kraak, V. I., Harrigan, P. B., Lawrence, M., Harrison, P. J., Jackson, M. A., & Swinburn, B. (2012). Balancing the benefits and risks of public–private partnerships to address the global double burden of malnutrition. *Public Health Nutrition*, 15(3), 503–517.

Lang, T. (1999). Food policy for the 21st century: Can it be both radical and reasonable? In M. Koc, R. MacRae, L. Mougeot, & J. Welsh(eds), *For hunger-proof cities: Sustainable urban food systems*. Ottawa: International Development Research Centre, pp. 216–224.

Lang, T. (2017). Re-fashioning food systems with sustainable diet guidelines: Towards a SDG 2 strategy. Paper presented at Food Climate Research Network, Oxford, April.

Lang, T., & Barling, D. (2012). Food security and food sustainability: Reformulating the debate. *The Geographical Journal*, 178(4), 313–326.

Lang, T., & Rayner, G. (2012). Ecological public health: The 21st century's big idea? *BMJ*, 345, e5466. doi:10.1136/bmj.e5466.

Laufer, W. S. (2003). Social accountability and corporate greenwashing. *Journal of Business Ethics*, 43(3), 253–261.

Lawrence, M. A., Friel, S., Wingrove, K., James, S. W., & Candy, S. (2015). Formulating policy activities to promote healthy and sustainable diets. *Public Health Nutrition*, 18(13), 2333–2340. doi:10.1017/S1368980015002529.

Lobstein, T., Brinsden, H., Landon, J., Kraak, V., Musicus, A., & Macmullan, J. (2013). INFORMAS and advocacy for public health nutrition and obesity prevention. *Obesity Review*, 14(Suppl. 1), 150–156. doi:10.1111/obr.12083.

McMichael, A. J., Powles, J. W., Butler, C. D., & Uauy, R. (2007). Food, livestock production, energy, climate change, and health. *The Lancet, 370*(9594), 1253–1263. doi:10.1016/S0140–6736(07) 61256–61252.

Ministry of Health of Brazil. (2014). Dietary guidelines for the Brazilian population. 2nd edn. Translated by C. A. Monteiro. Available at: http://189.28.128.100/dab/docs/portaldab/publicacoes/guia_alimentar_populacao_ingles.pdf

Monteiro, C. A., Cannon, G., Moubarac, J. C., Martins, A. P., Martins, C. A., Garzillo, J., … Jaime, P. C. (2015). Dietary guidelines to nourish humanity and the planet in the twenty-first century: A blueprint from Brazil. *Public Health Nutrition,* *18*(13), 2311–2322. doi:0.1017/s1368980015002165.

Moodie, R., Stuckler, D., Monteiro, C., Sheron, N., Neal, B., Thamarangsi, T., … Lancet, N. C. D. A. G. (2013). Profits and pandemics: Prevention of harmful effects of tobacco, alcohol, and ultra-processed food and drink industries. *The Lancet,* *381*(9867), 670–679. doi:10.1016/S0140-6736(12) 62089–62083.

Nestle, M. (2018). Perspective: Challenges and controversial issues in the dietary guidelines for Americans, 1980–2015. *Advances in Nutrition*, 9(2), 148–150.

Pollard, C., Pulker, C., & Devenish, G. (2015). Food and Nutrition Advocacy Priorities. Discussion guide, Round 1, Delphi results. Perth, Western Australia: Curtin University.

Public Health Advocacy Institute of Western Australia. (2013). Public health advocacy toolkit, 3rd edn. Perth, Western Australia: Curtin University.

Reisch, L., Eberle, U., & Lorek, S. (2013). Sustainable food consumption: An overview of contemporary issues and policies. *Sustainability: Science, Practice and Policy*, 9(2), 7–25.

Shilton, T. (2006). Advocacy for physical activity-from to influence. *Promotion & Education*, 13(2), 118–126.

Swenson, R., & Olsen, N. (2017). Food for thought: Audience engagement with sustainability messages in branded content. *Environmental Communication*, 1–16. doi:10.1080/17524032.2017.1279202.

UN (United Nations). (2015). Sustainable Development Goals. Available at: https://sustainabledeve lopment.un.org/?menu=1300

UN. (2017). Global Compact Blueprint for Business Leadership. Available at: http://blueprint.ungloba lcompact.org/

Van Loo, E. J., Hoefkens, C., & Verbeke, W. (2017). Healthy, sustainable and plant-based eating: Perceived (mis)match and involvement-based consumer segments as targets for future policy . *Food Policy*, 69, 46–57. doi:10.1016/j.foodpol.2017.03.001.

Wegener, J. (2018). Equipping future generations of registered dietitian nutritionists and public health nutritionists: A commentary on education and training needs to promote sustainable food systems and practices in the 21st century. *Journal of the Academy of Nutrition and Dietetics*, 118(3), 393–398. doi:10.1016/j.jand.2017.10.024/

Widener, P., & Karides, M. (2014). Food system literacy: Empowering citizens and consumers beyond farm-to-fork pathways. *Food, Culture & Society*, 17(4), 665–687.

Willett, W., Rockström, J., Loken, B., Springmann, M., Lang, T., Vermeulen, S., … Murray, C. J. L. (2019). Food in the Anthropocene: The EAT-Lancet Commission on healthy diets from sustainable food systems. *The Lancet*. doi:10.1016/S0140-6736(18)31788–31784.

WHO (World Health Organization). (1992). *Advocacy strategies for health and development: Development communication in action*. Geneva: WHO Division of Health Education.

CONCLUSION

Transitioning towards healthy and sustainable food systems

Mark Lawrence and Sharon Friel

Through 18 chapters of interdisciplinary insights, we have shone a light on the nature and scope of the health, environmental and equity problems arising from modern industrialised food systems, which themselves are being impacted by environmental changes. Rather than simply pathologising the problems, the book has examined food systems from the perspective of their functioning as coherent wholes consisting of many parts – the supply chain, the food environment and the various actors involved in the system – and importantly discussed what kind of transformation is needed to ensure a sustainable resilient food system that provides healthy diets for all now and into the future.

The book provides a systematic, comprehensive and up-to-date coverage of the intersectoral issues pertinent to achieving healthy and sustainable food systems. More than 30 international experts across a diversity of disciplinary and sectoral fields have provided valuable insights into and critical analyses of the problems emerging from modern industrialised food systems, the causes of those problems and practical suggestions for moving forward towards healthier and more sustainable food systems.

A systems perspective has been a fundamental focus of this book. This recognition of multiple, dynamic and interconnected parts offers hope for the future. Systems thinking tells us that the food system is not static, it is changing and adapting constantly. The opportunity and imperative therefore are to influence the changes in ways that ensure healthy and sustainable food systems emerge as a consequence.

Although the book has recognised that the food system is interconnected to a vast number of other systems and that actions in those systems have profound implications for healthy and sustainable food systems, we have by necessity had to contain our focus to the already highly complex food system. We believe this provides valuable insight into the many entry points for policy and action to take place.

The main themes and lessons from the book

A number of common themes emerged across the chapters despite the individual chapters focusing on specific aspects of healthy and sustainable food systems. The first main theme is the scale and urgency of the problem. A key lesson is that poor nutritional health, unprecedented environmental degradation and major social inequities are pervasive, each tightly connected to the other via food.

A second main theme that the chapters reveal is the workings of a complex dynamic system – a food system that is interconnected with other systems including economics, social, political and of course the Earth's system – and that changes and actions in one system affect the others, which can result in trade-offs and negative unintended consequences. Two key lessons from this systems insight are that: (1) whole system change is needed, not just individual-level dietary change or just change in specific components of the food system; and (2) attention must be paid to potential negative externalities that can arise from actions taken in sectors and systems beyond the food system.

Across the chapters there was general consensus that modern industrialised food systems are broken and will continue to exacerbate health, sustainability and equity problems unless meaningful and decisive changes are made. Five core characteristics of these changes can be synthesised from the chapters:

1. *Aspirational*: With the overwhelming power of the current neoliberal ideology's dominance of the food system and the degradation of many environmental resources, the question arises, 'Is it realistic to aim for radical system change or is it more pragmatic to work within the current settings to look for solutions that might be more achievable immediately?' Although pragmatism will be a key consideration in achieving change, if this means compromising on achieving outcomes that are immutable, such as protecting the Earth's ecological foundations, it will fail to secure necessary change. Pragmatism can be a slippery slope when it is used to construct an alternative narrative to the existence of ecological realities. It risks being used as an excuse to avoid challenging assumptions about the global economic growth agenda characterised by greater economic integration, trade and investment liberalisation and increased agriculture production. If we are not guided by aspirations of the type set out in the UN's Sustainable Development Goals (SDGs) but instead accept compromise from the start, on what basis do we inform decisions and set objectives?

2. *Transformative*: If the aspirations of the SDGs are to be achieved, then there is a need for collective action to drive transformative change in the food system. Transformative change requires policies and actions to work in a coordinated way across government sectors and across civil society, NGOs and corporate sectors. Just as the nature and scope of the food system challenge are unprecedented, so must be the approach taken for its solution. The action cannot be simply tweaks, nudges or adjustments to the structure and operation of individual components of the system, such as framing it as a food production or food reformulation agenda. Action must be about refocusing the structure and operations of all parts of the food system and done in such a way that it is based on principles of health, environmental sustainability and equity.

3. *Holistic*: The dietary patterns and types of food and beverage choices made by people play an important role in ensuring good health and environmental sustainability. There

is ample evidence to articulate the general characteristics of healthy and sustainable dietary patterns, thereby providing guidance to consumers and policy-makers concerned about public health, nutrition and environmental sustainability. Such dietary patterns would be based on four overarching principles: (a) any food or beverage that is consumed above a person's energy requirement represents an avoidable environmental burden in the form of greenhouse gas emissions, use of natural resources and pressure on biodiversity; (b) reducing the consumption of foods and beverages that are not necessary for health, i.e. those that are energy-dense and ultra-processed and packaged, reduces both the risk of dietary imbalances and the excessive use of environmental resources; (c) a global diet comprising less animal and more plant-derived foods; and (d) reducing food waste at each stage of the food supply and consumption chain. Formulating appropriate national and international policies on animal source foods that recognise both the benefits of reductions in high consuming countries and the need for more equitable distribution remains an important global challenge that will require intersectoral actions and good global governance. These principles and policies are informed by a holistic worldview of the causes of and solution to nutrition problems, i.e. a focus on changing the consumption of dietary patterns and foods and beverages. Yet, recently there has been a relatively large amount of policy activity in a number of countries informed by a reductionist worldview of the causes of and solutions to nutrition problems, e.g. excessive use of nutrient profiling algorithms to inform policy activities. Focusing on changing nutrient consumption out of context of the foods and diets within which those nutrients exist is inconsistent with nutrition science principles and risks exacerbating dietary imbalances and being irrelevant for sustainability considerations.

4. *Participatory and inclusive governance*: Essential to the repurposing of food systems is dealing with matters of national priorities; trade and investment arrangements; market deregulation; fiscal policy, and climate change mitigation and adaptation policy. Fundamentally, repurposing food systems is about rebalancing the concentration of power in global food chains, which requires attention to governance and the degree to which policies and processes are inclusionary of different sectors, disciplines and involve democratic decision-making. Addressing these structural factors will empower states, other key public sector institutions and citizens. For example, inclusive and participatory governance and regulatory frameworks can create a national policy space that enables government to introduce policies that tackle corporate pressures such as irresponsible food marketing. And all the time operating to governance models that are transparent and free of conflict of interest.

5. *Urgent*: Food-related health and sustainability problems are happening now and escalating and so we need to act urgently. Lack of knowledge is not an excuse, we already have much knowledge about the problems and potential solutions. Part of the reason for such limited action is the inherently political nature of food. With the food system interwoven with social, economic, and political concerns, any transformation is by nature not only going to be substantial but that level of change will impact like a tsunami through many other systems. It will be met with resistance from those actors who benefit from maintaining the status quo. Addressing such resistance involves fostering a process of "political empowerment", whereby people, organisations, and nations gain control over the decisions that affect them and their vision for healthy and sustainable food systems.

Encouragingly, coalition building has started among food and nutrition NGOs and some governments in relation to restrictions on marketing of food to children, nutrition labelling, and fiscal and pricing policy. In Mexico, for example, an active civil society network worked together with a receptive government and policy advocate in the health minister to generate wide support for the successful introduction of a national level soda tax (a tax on sugar-sweetened beverages). While the soda tax success may seem like a drop in the ocean in relation to the transformation of food systems, and addresses only one part of the necessary system-wide response, it is a start. Similarly, the actions being taken by some countries to include sustainability in their dietary guidelines or to promote collaboration around the Code of Marketing Breastmilk Substitutes. The global nutrition and health community can build on these social actions and learn salient lessons from other cases of policy changes that have resulted in the effective and safe tackling of other public health challenges such as access to medicines and tobacco control.

Understanding how to foster that political empowerment will require ongoing engagement between sectors, disciplines and literatures including political science. Doing so may give hope that, despite long odds, recalibrating the power inequities in the industrial food system may be possible through a variety of approaches, including coalition building, social mobilisation, and institutional strategies. Essential to success is the creation of cohesive networks of nutrition-related actors, identifying potential partners and new foot soldiers in the quest for healthy and sustainable food systems (e.g. the linking of nutrition, food systems and climate issues to broaden the coalitional base), compelling issue framing, and, importantly, high profile and powerful policy advocates who can use their discursive powers effectively.

Next steps, opportunities and challenges for the future

The messages may be grim at times and the challenges substantial, but there are also many positive activities from committed experts doing great things. We hope that the book highlights that there are indeed many opportunities with which to create the type and scale of transformation that is needed within the current food system. In terms of evidence, we know much more today than ever before about the extent of the food-related health, social and environmental problems. As Part II of the book illustrates, significant progress has also been made over the past few decades in understanding the relationships between the different parts of the food system and these negative outcomes, and accordingly the types of policies and actions that are needed to rectify the health and environmental harms. In addition, it is encouraging that there is increasing attention among the research community not only to the pathologies and the technical aspects of these relationships but also to the political, policy and social processes that enable or hinder progressive action in the food system. This literature points towards a much greater appreciation of the political economy of food and the power of social movements, highlighting the many advocacy groups that are motivated to engage and bring about food system transformation for the well-being of our own and future generations.

INDEX

Note: bold page numbers indicate tables; italic page numbers indicate figures; page numbers containing n indicate chapter endnotes.

Printed in the United States
by Baker & Taylor Publisher Services